DEATH OF THE BEAUTY PHARM

Kevin Horak

DEATH OF THE BEAUTY PHARM

First published in the United Kingdom in 2025 by Wolf House Publishing Ltd.

FIRST EDITION

A catalogue record for this book is available from the British Library.

ISBN: 978-1-9192638-0-9

MIX
Paper | Supporting responsible forestry
FSC www.fsc.org FSC® C007785

WOLF HOUSE

Wolf House Publishing Ltd
8 Shoplatch, Shrewsbury, Shropshire,
SY1 1HF
United Kingdom

Further information is available at
kevinhorak.com, wolfhousepublishing.com, or
deathofbeauty.com

Jacket artwork by Kevin Barlett, who has granted an exclusive license for perpetuity to Kevin Horak or nominated assignees. Author photograph by Leanne Pugh.
This is a work of fiction; any references to historical events, places and incidents are used fictitiously, and any resemblance to actual persons living or dead is entirely coincidental.

Printed in Great Britain by Bell and Bain Ltd, Glasgow

Contents

In a leading scientific report in 2022, the global non-invasive aesthetic market was valued at $61.2 billion. The same report suggests that by 2030, it will be valued at $190 billion.

Leading countries for the use of non-invasive treatments include the United States, Japan, China, South Korea and India.

In the United Kingdom, a variety of reports suggest that 11% - 13% of the population have had some form of aesthetic treatment.

Patient knowledge reports vary, but it is acknowledged that a very high percentage have little understanding of what is being injected into their skin.

KnightArk
PHARMACEUTICAL

A MESSAGE FROM OUR CEO

Since 1973, Knightark Pharmaceutical has been at the forefront of cosmetic science. We are committed to quality and innovation, never taking shortcuts, and pioneering the development of revolutionary new treatments for you.

We will continue to invest in development and lead the industry.

Just over two years ago, our board supported my vision, which has now become a reality with the opening of our new laboratory in South America. Here, we have developed cutting-edge techniques that utilise the region's most natural resources. Through rigorous testing, we ensure the highest quality of our products. Our new line of cosmetic fillers is exceptional, and I'm especially proud of the innovations with our Hydra-Fillixir range – they really are the first of a kind, and I guarantee you'll experience the benefits immediately. You won't be able to wait for your next cosmetic procedure, because making you feel good is our mission. Achieving beauty and well-being will help you evolve to your best self. I'm confident that you will choose us time and again. Here's to the future!

Always remember, you are in safe hands with Knightark Pharmaceutical.

Yours most sincerely,

Darius Neith, CEO
Knightark Pharmaceutical

"Depend on Ingenuity"
Knightark.com

Chapter One

MAIDA VALE, LONDON, UNITED KINGDOM

"Good morning!" Alison said as she entered the kitchen, though her two children barely acknowledged her, offering only the briefest of grunts.

"Come on, you two, don't act like that," she said, pulling Joshua, her seven-year-old, toward her and kissing him on the cheek.

"Mum, get off!" he complained, trying to push her away.

"Please don't talk with your mouth full," she reminded him.

Joshua swallowed his toast but seemed more interested in the game he was playing on his phone.

"Morning, Alison!" Joanne called out from across the kitchen.

"Hi, Joanne," Alison replied, her face lighting up as she accepted a cup of coffee from the children's nanny. She leaned down to kiss her eldest child on the head. "Are you prepared for your French test later?"

Jody, almost eleven years old, gave a little shrug.

"Come on, sweetheart! You want to do well, don't you?" Alison gently took the phone from Jody and placed it face down on the counter.

"Mum, seriously!" Jody said, her voice filled with frustration.

"You'll see your friends soon enough at school. Now, finish your breakfast."

Alison nodded at Joanne, signalling that she wanted to speak privately. They moved to a corner of the kitchen. "Joanne, I know you're trying, but please do your best to keep the kids off their phones at the breakfast table."

"I do try, Alison. They know they're not supposed to use them."

"Well, please keep trying. Do you have everything you need for today?"

"Yes, I'll go shopping right after I drop them off at school."

"Thank you. Do you have enough money on the debit card?"

"Yes, it should be fine; today's newspaper is on the side if you want a look."

"Good morning, my lovely!"

Mike wrapped his arms around Alison's shoulders and kissed her on the neck.

"Morning, darling. Do you have time for a coffee?"

"No, I need to get into the office."

Alison glanced at Mike, her husband of twelve years. "Oh, okay. We're still on for this evening, right? You haven't forgotten?"

Mike leaned over the kitchen island, took a piece of toast from Joshua's plate, and nodded. "Yes, it's all good. I know we need to be there by seven-thirty."

Alison nodded. "You will be on time, won't you? It's important. I need their support for my campaign. I've invited Helen Lord as well; she's up to speed on what's going on, and we've been working on a massive story. I need to discuss that with you because it could lead to complications; the story could change everything."

Mike smiled and kissed Alison on the forehead. "Yes, I promise. But I wish you wouldn't spend so much time with that member of parliament. None of them can be trusted."

"With what's coming up, I'll need her help. Besides, I trust her."

"More fool you. Anyway, what complications, what's going on?"

"Not now, not in front of the kids. I'll talk to you about it later," she whispered.

Mike nodded with some uncertainty. "If you're sure."

Alison smiled and affectionately placed her right hand on Mike's face. "It'll be fine, I promise you."

Mike swallowed his toast and waved at Joshua and Jody. "Catch you later. Bye, you two. Have a good day at school."

"Bye, Dad."

Alison watched as both children acknowledged their father's departure. She raised her eyebrows, knowing he was their favourite. Aside from these brief moments in the morning, she had barely seen her children lately. Since starting her job at Channel 8 television, her life had become consumed by its demands, forcing her to work late into the night.

The nanny, ensuring she was out of earshot of the children, walked back over to Alison. "Are you nervous about this evening?"

Alison sipped her coffee. "I wouldn't exactly call it 'nervous,' but my name is constantly in the media—especially now with Helen's support. I'm facing a lot of negativity and hate online. I need the right people standing by me; this issue is not going away." She pulled the nanny aside and added, "Look, I haven't shared all the details, but Helen and I have been collaborating on a project for the past few weeks, and what we've uncovered has made us both uneasy. There's something significant happening right now—something that has the potential to escalate to almost epidemic proportions. I'm anxious about that, to be honest. Having more support can only help."

"Really? What is it?"

Alison sipped her coffee and said, "It's probably best if I don't say anything for now. I haven't even discussed it with Mike yet, but I plan to later."

Joanne nodded and lowered her voice even more. "I've seen some of the online comments, and I genuinely worry about you."

Alison shook her head, finished her coffee, and set her cup down. "Please don't worry. It comes with the territory. If there's ever a reason for alarm, I will let you know. I promise." She glanced at her watch.

"Okay, if you're sure," Joanne replied, then directed her attention to the children. "Come on, you two. It's time for school. I'll clean up when I get back. Joshua, please put on your shoes."

The children checked to make sure they had their phones before leaving the table and heading to the hallway to retrieve their shoes and school bags. "Please let me know if anything is bothering you. I know it's not easy," Joanne added.

Alison walked to the side and picked up the newspaper. "Thank you," she said, scanning the front page. "You know, Helen has been receiving hate mail at home. Her address was leaked online through one of the many pro-surgery forums. She's had to take security advice from the Serjeant at Arms department at Westminster."

"Are they helping?" Joanne asked.

Alison shrugged as she opened the newspaper. "She's a backbench MP, which means she isn't entitled to any physical security unless she pays for it herself. There would be a public uproar if taxpayers were to cover the cost of her safety. I think the police are assisting where they can, and..."

"Oh, good, you're ready then." Their conversation was interrupted as Jody returned to the kitchen. Joanne grabbed the car keys from the side. "If you need anything today, Alison, please let me know."

"Thank you, I will."

"Joshua, put on your shoes, please. We need to go," Joanne instructed.

Alison motioned to Jody. "Come on, give Mum a squeeze."

Jody sighed, "All right."

They shared a quick hug before Alison went into the hallway and kissed Joshua on the head. "Hopefully, I'll see you both later. I have a meeting tonight, but I'll be home in between."

"Again," Jody muttered under her breath.

"Yes, all right. It's just a busy time at the moment."

"Right, come on," Joanne said as she opened the front door, ushering Joshua and Jody outside. "I'll message you in a bit, Alison."

"Thank you, have a great day. Good luck with the test, Jody," Alison called out.

Jody didn't respond as the front door closed. Alison rechecked her watch. Finding little of interest in the newspaper, she tossed it aside and grabbed her coat from the row of hooks next to the front door. She rushed back into the kitchen for her keys, hurriedly slipped on her coat and shoes, and snatched a piece of leftover toast. With her laptop bag over her shoulder and her purse in her jacket pocket, she headed out of the front door.

It was a bright summer day. As she stood outside, she took a deep breath, contemplating the long day ahead of her. In this upscale area of London, the street was lined with approximately forty identical three-story Georgian houses. The neighbourhood was generally quiet, making these homes highly sought after. With their white walls and columns atop a short flight of stairs, it was a rare place in London where residents could park directly outside their homes, though finding a parking space was a daily challenge. Her small black Mercedes was parked in front of the house two doors down. It was practical and easy to manoeuvre through the city. Like many of her neighbours, she had found that the necessity of owning a car had diminished over time. Mike had relied on train and tube travel for the past couple of years. Still, she had resisted this change, detesting the thought of taking the underground, especially during summer when the heat below ground was oppressive, particularly during rush hour.

After descending the short flight of stairs, she spotted her neighbour across the street, standing at his front window. She raised her right hand, smiled, and waved as she stood next to her car, fiddling with her keys. Holding the vehicle remote forward, she felt the warmth of the morning sun and looked up at the sky, which promised good weather for the day. Deciding she didn't need her jacket, she headed back up the stairs, opened the front door, and hung her coat back on the hook. Noticing her neighbour wave back, she smiled again and, from the top of the stairs, pressed the unlock button on her car remote. However, nothing happened; the side mirrors didn't fold out as they usually did when she unlocked the car. She turned to lock the front door and pressed the remote again from the top of the stairs. Alison frowned as she noticed the rear lights flashing more quickly than usual. As she began to walk down the stairs, a massive ball of fire suddenly erupted from the front of the car. The explosion propelled Alison into the air, sending her crashing backwards against the railings. As her car's rear windscreen shattered, windows of nearby houses were torn from their frames, and several other vehicles ignited. Alison fell at the base of the rails, her right arm pinned through the railings as shrapnel ripped through her in several places, tearing clothing from her body in an instant. A steady stream of blood ran from her lips, nose, and right eye as her head bobbed back and forth, and fluid ran from her right ear.

Multiple car and house alarms rang loudly as she lost consciousness.

++++

"We are now bringing you some breaking news of a reported explosion in central London. Our reporter, Gareth Araya, is on the scene. Gareth, what can you tell us?"

The TV reporter nodded and lifted the microphone. "Anna, the police have cordoned off the road at both ends. This is as close as I can get. If the camera can zoom over my shoulder, you will see behind me that several houses are missing windows, and building debris is strewn across the street. There are charred remains of several cars. I was told there was a small fire that was rapidly contained. However, this is remarkable in this exclusive and usually quiet part of London."

"Have the police given any details of injuries or what is suspected to have happened? Reports are of an explosion."

"Nothing has been said as yet in an official capacity, although I've been told there will be a statement from the Metropolitan Police in the next few hours. However, until that time, there is intense speculation online. You can see the white tent on the left behind me, further down the road. The owner of that particular house is drawing this story, and a lot of speculation surrounds it. I've already seen that there are an incredible forty thousand comments across all social media platforms, as that house is known to be Alison Harwood's family home. A lady whose views have monopolised certain themes in social media."

"Well, there is no bigger theme today than beauty. I'm presuming this is the same Alison Harwood who is the head of policy at Channel 8 television?"

"Yes, quite. That very same lady was appointed to the channel following a major lawsuit brought against it by a reality TV contestant. You may recall that the case gained worldwide notoriety following what was proven to be botched surgery. It was the first, and to date, the only time a full body surgery makeover was offered as a prize in a television show."

"I'm sure our viewers will recall it very well. That lawsuit was the tipping point against reality TV, prompting people to seek damages from production companies and media channels. It was a floodgate moment."

"Well, it did. Although the exact particulars of that settlement were conducted privately, it is still widely believed that more than fifty million pounds in compensation was paid to the former reality TV star, Megan Launders. A non-disclosure agreement, or gagging order if you will, prevents her from detailing the exact nature of the settlement and the full extent of her surgery complications."

"Can you remind us exactly what happened and what the lawsuit alleged?"

"Well, Megan Launders, the winning contestant of the now-cancelled reality show called The Beauty Beach, won the series and elected to receive a full body makeover involving extensive surgeries. Although she was initially physiologically and psychologically assessed before the show, it was alleged that there was very little aftercare. That was allegation number one. After the show, her name dominated the tabloid press and social media for a short period, but that soon took its toll on her mental health, as a percentage of social media users turned against her, citing that she was fake. Her TV appearances slid, and she was the victim of a considerable amount of online bullying that led to multiple arrests; some of those cases are still going through the courts. That was allegation number two: she was not ready for her life in the public eye and the attention that came with it. This was effectively someone who came into the public eye from nowhere, and, as her later admission showed, she couldn't cope. But it was a ruptured breast implant some months after her makeover that allegedly led to a raft of other medically related issues. That was the main allegation and the basis of the lawsuit's main complaint. The surgeon concerned closed his practice in London and relocated to the Far East, where he has since established a thriving new practice. Nevertheless, it was the production company that engaged the surgeon and, as Channel 8, commissioned the series; they were deemed culpable."

"And it was this case that opened the floodgates?"

"Well, yes. Other contestants from the same show came forward to discuss how the show had negatively affected their lives, which proved to be the catalyst for a landmark case. Megan Launders' legal success paved the way for multiple lawsuits against major networks worldwide. For that very reason, we rarely see those types of reality TV programmes. Alison Harwood was brought into Channel 8 to try to revolutionise how we see television programmes. Her view that television presenters and others in the public eye should be free of surgery and make-up propelled her campaign to embrace natural beauty. Nothing has been off the table; she's challenged the pharmaceutical trade and cosmetic companies, even led a campaign about abolishing energy drinks and smoking, and she has been very vocal about the drug problems that the UK faces right now. The main drive of her campaign is that cosmetic surgery is still in its infancy. In her opinion, many people are unaware of what is being put into their bodies and the potential lasting effects. She is a pioneer of a global movement championing natural beauty. Her critics and supporters of cosmetic procedures label her as trying to crush freedom of choice, and it is from her campaign that the term, the so-called death of beauty, has emerged."

"Gareth, is there any suspicion that Alison Harwood was targeted specifically in this attack?"

"As you know, there is no official comment as yet, but residents have told me her car exploded and that she was badly injured in this attack. So..."

The television was turned off, and the remote was placed gently on the old oak desk. Darius pressed the internal call button on his phone, and his assistant answered immediately.

"Yes, Mr Neith."

"The board need to meet; start making calls, will you?"

"Yes, Sir, do you have a timescale in mind?"

"The location, time and date will be confirmed in due course, but it will be as soon as possible."

"Yes, Mr Neith, I'll begin arrangements immediately."

Darius Neith, the Chief Executive Officer of Knightark Pharmaceutical, took an unregistered phone from his blazer pocket and connected the battery and SIM card from his desk drawer. After gaining power, he scrolled through the recent call list. He selected the number he needed, and his call was answered within a few rings.

"I take it you've seen the news. If the reports are to be believed, you failed to complete your task." He listened intently as the other voice responded. "This situation is about to escalate. Certain board members will be very dissatisfied; a significant amount of time and money has gone into this endeavour." Darius's voice remained calm, his words carefully controlled. He nodded as he absorbed the information. "We'll need to meet in the usual place. I'll be in touch once I've spoken with my senior colleagues."

As he hung up, Darius removed the battery and SIM card from his phone and placed them in the pocket of his blazer. With a steady hand, he began to rap his fingernails against the green leather on his desk. The gravity of the situation settled heavily on his shoulders; Alison Harwood was not meant to survive. There would always be repercussions, but if she pulled through, the problem would become more complicated. With what she knew, she might become even more determined. They needed to proceed with phase two sooner than anticipated.

Chapter Two

Dr John Farmer, a shareholder and junior board member of Knightark Pharmaceutical, had contributed his insights to the board for eight years. Inspired by his father, a former shareholder and esteemed senior board member, John's journey into the company was deeply rooted in family legacy. Following his father's passing, John inherited not only a legacy but also a coveted position on the board as the sole heir to his father's vision. Despite his father's unquestionable reputation and years of service, the board was required to vote on his appointment. This vast, profit-driven company was not merely a corporate entity; it was a pioneer in the cosmetic pharmaceutical industry, dedicated to discovering and developing innovative products, holding numerous patents, and ensuring its position at the forefront of medical innovation. Admission to the board was a rigorous process. Financial stability was a minor consideration, as it was generally assumed; however, your investments were closely scrutinised to prevent any potential conflicts of interest. Key factors included education in the private sector, family heritage, and political acumen. Each prospective board member underwent a lengthy screening process without their knowledge or consent. Evaluations considered associations, trustworthiness with sensitive information, sexual preferences, and, importantly, how you engaged with others in these aspects. The need for secrecy stemmed primarily from the company's innovation development division, particularly its advancements in cosmetic surgery. The pharmaceutical industry was fiercely competitive, especially when substantial financial rewards were involved; trust was essential, with no room for mistakes or interference.

It was no surprise that a board meeting had been called. Such meetings had become commonplace, due to the ongoing concerns about declining profits over the past year and a half. Although the company remained profitable, its earnings were significantly lower than projected. This discrepancy led to numerous protests from board members and stakeholders alike, emphasising the urgent need for change and a new strategic direction. The turning point was triggered by a lawsuit against a television channel, which initiated widespread change. The country was flooded with lawsuits and demands for a return to "naturals," meaning individuals without cosmetic enhancements. Alison Harwood led a movement to exclude anyone with even minor cosmetic procedures from appearing on Channel 8 programs. She effectively used social media to advance her agenda. While this initiative sparked outrage and raised concerns about human rights, her mission was clear. She believed that only essential medical procedures should be allowed, and anyone who had undergone non-essential surgeries would not be permitted to appear on the channel in any role. Many supported her initiative, prompting others to adopt similar practices. All front-of-camera staff signed agreements to this effect. Violating the agreement would lead to termination of their employment with the channel and could also result in legal action for breach of contract. If an individual chose not to sign, their position was offered to someone else, with no regard for their views or rights.

John had received a call from the secretary of Mr Darius Neith, the company's most senior board member and CEO. Neith was a significant shareholder and held the most voting rights. The location, date, and time of the upcoming board meeting had not yet been disclosed. Recently, details about board meetings have been kept confidential from anyone outside the board. Usually, John would receive an email via their secure servers, but this time, that did not happen. Something felt different; he suspected that the senior decision-maker wanted to avoid leaving a trail of evidence, making the forthcoming meeting even more confidential than usual. Despite his years of service on the board and his late father's good standing within the company, he was still considered a junior member. Others had been involved longer and had access to private meetings. Their inner circle was nearly impenetrable. While board meetings were a matter of business process, he understood that the four members of the inner circle were the ones who truly made the decisions.

He sighed deeply, dropped his newspaper onto the table, and rose to his feet as the bell rang from the gate at the end of the driveway. Security within the company was taken seriously. For years, concerns had been raised about the company's substantial profits, with investigative journalists probing and alleging misconduct in its accounting practices. The disappearance of a British journalist named Charles D'Anno in Brazil just over a year ago had drawn unwanted attention to all senior members of the company. He has never been found, but the media reported that he was investigating the company at the time of his disappearance. Allegations in the press suggested he may have gotten "too close" to the truth, and the story eventually faded away.

Leaving his sitting room, John walked across the white marble tiled kitchen floor toward the heavy oak front door. He understood the security protocol: no one could enter the house without a prior appointment, and he had none today. He pressed the control screen on the wall to the right of the door, activating the CCTV camera. The screen displayed a man standing at the front gate. His heavy looking walking boots and tactical jacket suggested he was a former military person.

"Yes, who is it?" John called out.

"Is this Dr Farmer?" came the direct and blunt response.

John studied the man at the front gate, who was holding a small envelope.

"Who is asking, please?" John replied.

The man unzipped his jacket and removed an identity card from his pocket. He held the card up to the camera. "My name is Stephen, and I'm from SETI Special Projects. I have an urgent delivery for Dr Farmer."

John studied the ID card and recognised it; the man was from the specialist security company that Darius occasionally engaged. "I'm Dr Farmer. If you look to your left, you'll see a post box where you can leave it," he suggested.

"I'm sorry, sir, but I cannot do that. I have instructions to deliver this to you in person. It's important, as I understand. I must either present it to you by hand or not at all," the security man insisted, his body language firm and stern.

"We've never met before. How do you know I'm Dr Farmer?" John asked.

The security man leaned closer to the camera. "Trust me, sir, I know exactly what you look like."

John smiled with amusement; he was definitely one of Darius's men. "Okay, fair enough," he replied, pressing the button to open the gates. After unclipping the security bolts on the front door and turning two locks, John opened the door and stepped out onto his driveway to greet his unexpected guest.

"Dr Farmer, thank you for receiving me," the man said, marching briskly down the driveway. "I have this urgent letter for you. It must be delivered by hand. Before I give it to you, could you please hold out your right hand? I need to scan your index finger."

"You can't be serious! I thought you said you would recognise me," John retorted.

"I do, sir. But on this occasion, there is a matter of procedure; other board members need to conform as well," the security man explained.

"Very well," John said, shaking his head as he held out his right hand. "I'm sure an email would have sufficed."

The security officer took a scanner from his pocket and replied, "I'm unaware of the contents of the letter, sir."

The security officer took John's hand and said, "Please place your index finger on the scanner, sir."

John complied while the intimidating man observed the device. "Thank you, sir," he said, putting the scanner back in his pocket and handing over an envelope. "I'll be off now. Take care."

John nodded, though it was never reassuring when security personnel reminded him to take care. He turned the envelope over; it was blank, with no name printed on either side. Once he was certain the security officer was out of sight, he walked back into the house and closed the door behind him. Watching the monitor, he pressed the button to ensure the gates closed before opening the envelope. Inside, only a few words were printed on the unsigned letter: "Emergency Meeting" was the title. It included an address, a date, and a time, but no agenda was specified.

The timing was intriguing; he had seen the news about the recent attempt on Alison Harwood's life. Her anti-surgery campaign made her very well-known to the board, and she was considered the number one problem. Her constant accusations and worldwide lawsuits plagued their entire industry. He ran his fingers through his hair; he didn't trust the senior board. He hoped to God this had nothing to do with them.

++++

EVENTS SURROUNDING MEGAN LAUNDERS AND THE LEGAL CASE

Twenty-six months previously.

Dubbed the most radical beauty televisual fest, The Beauty Beach became Channel 8's flagship programme. With significant investment and international distribution, it attracted over twelve million viewers in the UK alone. The series was syndicated worldwide and reportedly had over fifty million regular viewers. Despite running for only one season and being abruptly cancelled midway through its second, the programme sparked both outrage and delight. Many social media commentators supported it, influencers capitalised on the viewership, and the "cult of cosmetic surgery" began to emerge. The series emphasised the importance of looking younger and actively promoted this notion, sparking worldwide debates and mainstream media coverage. Parents and political opponents questioned why young people needed surgery, which added to the show's polarising effect, drawing in viewers and lucrative sponsorship deals. The winning prize, awarded to Megan Launders, was a complete body makeover with a top surgeon from London's Harley Street. The tabloid press actively supported the programme, while broadsheet publications dismissed it. At just twenty-four years old, Megan Launders became a focal point for critics who labelled the series "the death of beauty." Every contestant was screened and psychologically tested, not only to assess their ability to handle the physically and mentally demanding nature of the series but also to determine their suitability for a full body enhancement. This comprehensive surgical makeover could involve significant changes. To participate, each contestant signed a non-disclosure agreement and underwent a thorough physical assessment, including scans of their internal organs and evaluations of their fitness to withstand the stresses of surgery. The qualification process was simple and open to all genders, but contestants needed to believe they had a specific flaw in their appearance. Scars or skin conditions were not the focus or purpose of the programme. Instead, it aimed to address radical changes, such as an uplift and/or liposuction, where a contestant may have lost weight quickly, resulting in sagging skin, or they might feel their breasts are too small, too large, or their backside is too large or not large enough. A couple of male contestants were opting for implants to enhance their physiques and appear more muscular, without having any interest in going to the gym. The list of procedures was extensive: lip surgery, facial implants, scarification, and even a request from one contestant for subdermal horn implants, which would create the appearance of having devil's horns on their skull. The list felt endless, and the possibilities seemed limitless. Contestants and applicants were required to share their stories and explain how these experiences impacted their lives. Their highly intimate stories were broadcast, giving viewers insight into their perceived flaws and their desires to feel more confident and "perfect." The show focused exclusively on cosmetic procedures aimed at achieving an ideal appearance, rather than addressing any procedures related to health conditions. By the end of the first season, contestants had become temporary household names. Some earned quick incomes and, despite not winning the competition, were able to afford their surgeries. Others secured sponsorships for their procedures, with two contestants receiving free surgery from unknown doctors.

However, despite the initial excitement and television exposure, these contestants quickly faded from public view. They returned to their previous careers, often finding themselves relegated to the Z-list of fame. For Channel 8 and the production company they engaged, the show was highly profitable, and the flaws, along with the promoted messages, were largely overlooked. That was until the crash, when the lawsuit changed everything and nearly bankrupted the channel.

The winner of the series, Megan Launders, underwent extensive surgery, which included a tummy tuck, breast augmentation, breast uplift, fat removal from her backside, calf implants, facial tightening and a nose reduction. The cosmetic process was completed in just three weeks, leading to much consternation in the press about the physical demands placed upon the winner in such a short period. The recovery process took an additional six weeks, and Channel 8 was eager to promote the newly transformed winner. Competing channels labelled the Launders parade as almost "a look at what you could win." Surgery costs were never publicly disclosed, and arrangements between the production company and the surgeon were kept private. Social media buzz suggested that, because the surgeon and his practice were heavily promoted, any costs associated with his work would likely have been only a fraction of what others would pay. However, one broadsheet newspaper estimated that the surgery costs alone could exceed one hundred thousand pounds, not including the subsequent recovery process. Megan Launders was quickly thrust into the spotlight and became a regular feature in many weekly magazines. She posed nude in various publications as part of her contractual agreement. Often, she found herself on beaches where paparazzi were already waiting, having been tipped off in a premeditated move by her then-agent. Her private life, specifically, who she had and was currently dating, became the subject of worldwide news stories. One major gossip and lifestyle magazine even reported that she wanted children, sparking speculation about a potential new series in which men would compete for her hand.

But it never happened. A ruptured breast implant and a reaction to her calf implants changed everything. She collapsed in a nightclub in New York City after complaining of feeling unwell, all in full view of the press. Hospital assessments revealed that she had blood poisoning. The calf implants were removed, leaving her with extensive scarring, and she spent weeks in rehabilitation afterwards. Her silicone breast implants were removed as well, only to be replaced later. The pressure from the various surgical procedures she underwent caused her to age prematurely. The medical bills in the United States surpassed three-quarters of a million dollars. Her insurance company refused to cover the costs, arguing that she had not disclosed the procedures she underwent when she took out the policy, and it was these very procedures that led to her multiple health issues.

Aware of the upcoming lawsuits, the production company behind The Beauty Beach show suddenly declared bankruptcy. As a result, Megan Launders' lawyers filed a lawsuit directly against Channel 8. After two years of litigation and sensing an imminent defeat, Channel 8 chose to settle out of court for an undisclosed amount. However, this was just the beginning of a series of lawsuits within the industry. Globally, the cosmetic surgery business and its practitioners became immediate targets, with many eager to capitalise on alleged wrongdoing. Thousands of lawsuits were filed against television and film production companies, their agents, and film studios. Insurance companies began refusing coverage for anyone who had undergone non-essential surgeries, creating controversy around what constituted "non-essential" treatment.

Ageing became a focal point of discussion, with Megan Launders herself appearing on chat shows worldwide to advocate against cosmetic surgery. Major pharmaceutical companies suffered significant financial losses, and many beauty practitioners who once thrived on the high street went out of business. The repercussions were vast: the responsibility for health and well-being shifted onto individuals, regardless of age, sexual identity, or lifestyle. The insurance industry underwent a dramatic transformation, requiring anyone seeking private medical care to undergo a comprehensive assessment. Additionally, the British National Health Service, following changes in law due to government reforms, began charging for corrective surgeries. The Beauty Beach was the tipping point that ignited a modern legal revolution. Channel 8 narrowly survived, but its programme commissioners faced a new mandate regarding the content they could broadcast. Freedoms were restricted, leading to safer programming. The emerging claims culture influenced what was presented and discussed on air, with lawyers meticulously reviewing every word broadcast. The potential for individual offence became increasingly costly. Channel 8 learned a valuable lesson: the practice of making quick, easy money by exploiting others had to change. Alison Harwood was appointed as the new head of policy with a clear mandate: eliminate lawsuits and issues, focus on creating profitable programming, and promote the idea of natural beauty.

Chapter Three

EMERGENCY BOARD MEETING – CHANNEL 8 TELEVISION. LONDON

"Turn the television off; I can't bear to hear the news any longer." Ben Tasker dropped a stack of paperwork onto the boardroom table and took his seat. He was the last to enter the room. As the channel's Chief Operations Officer, he was chairing the emergency meeting.

As the TV was switched off, he locked eyes one by one with the other eleven senior executives sitting around the table. He received looks of concern and fear, noticing some had tears in their eyes.

"What's the latest? Does anyone know?" he asked.

"I've been informed that Alison's condition is serious but stable. However, she is in the high-dependency unit at the hospital, and I'm sorry to say she will have life-changing injuries... that's what I've been told." Julie Bateman glanced around at her colleagues. As the channel's Chief Commissioner, her involvement in the lawsuit surrounding The Beauty Beach put her in a difficult position when everything went wrong. Holding on to her position by the skin of her teeth, she had played a key role in appointing Alison to the board. Julie was desperate to distance herself from the legal case; this attempt on Alison's life had the potential to drag her back in.

"I've tried calling her husband, but, not surprisingly, he isn't answering his phone," Ben said as he leaned back in his seat, shaking his head. "This is what I think it is. It has to be."

A few people nodded, but most avoided making eye contact.

"We have little further information beyond what's being reported by our competitors." They turned to look at Jennie Upland, a relatively new appointment brought in after the scandal to add social value to their programming. She shrugged her shoulders and looked around the room. "But let's face it, the police are being tight-lipped. Even with the persuasive skills of our crew on the ground, it seems glaringly obvious," she continued, leaning forward on the desk to ensure she had everyone's attention. "That car didn't explode just by accident. Seriously, who does something like that? Who has the capability to carry out actions like this?"

"It's a professional hit; someone tried to take her out."

"Jesus, Brian, don't use such crass language when discussing this? We're talking about a friend of ours!" Jennie replied.

As a senior producer, Brian Clement was known for speaking his mind. He didn't subscribe to politically correct culture and disliked the channel's direction. To him, ethics and social value were simply buzzwords for people trying to justify their existence. "Well, how else would you like me to put it?" he replied.

"Alison was forthright with her views, but let's be honest: they are perspectives that most of you have supported to save this channel," Ben said as he glanced at Brian, who shook his head and looked away in disagreement.

"We've seen a global shift in the media since The Beauty Beach; everyone is now looking at us, and we are respected and revered in equal measure. In effect, this channel is becoming the standard. We are judged more in the press than anyone else. Millions, if not billions, have been paid out in compensation cases worldwide."

"And that's why they've tried to silence her, Ben. There are many people out there who are pissed. I've heard the term 'the death of beauty' being used," he gestured with despair, "more like the death of choice and the death of freedom!"

"Brian, your views are well known to all of us. But tell me, who could be responsible for something like this? Who is malevolent enough to target Alison? What vendetta could they possibly have against her? Does anyone have any ideas?"

Debbie Rachels leaned back in her seat and crossed her arms. As the head of public relations, she had a qualified opinion. "Her social media presence does face backlash; we all know that. But for every negative comment, there are two positive ones. Overall, there is general respect and support for her."

"All of our socials face backlash; being associated with this channel guarantees that."

"While that may be true, Sharron, as our senior news anchor, I hate to say it, but some of this comes with the territory. That's the age we live in, like it or not."

"You receive abuse, Sharron, due to your aggressive interview techniques; that's why people bitch and whine about you."

Sharron's mouth dropped open in shock, reflecting her disgust at Brian's persistent lack of tact. She glared at him while he remained unfazed.

"That's enough, Brian," Ben interjected, raising his hands to calm the group. "We need answers! I've checked, and our in-house security has provided little new information; they are as in the dark as we are. There were no known threats to Alison, except for those posted on her social media accounts. Most of those comments were not reported because they were deemed nothing more than clickbait intended to provoke others. Debbie and I have repeatedly advised you all to be cautious about what you post and to avoid engaging with negativity. Either ignore such comments or delete them. If any of you have concerns regarding social commentary or personal security, you must discuss them with Debbie; that is part of her role. If security needs to be arranged, I will look into it, and if police involvement is necessary, I will support it."

Ben closed his eyes and rubbed his temples. "I'm going to the hospital shortly to see how she is and to try to gather more information." He glanced at the ceiling as he collected his thoughts. "Debbie, we need to issue a press statement. For now, let's communicate that she has been in an accident and that the police are investigating. We have no further comments at this time, other than wishing her a speedy recovery and expressing our thoughts for her family. I'd advise against revealing anything else, but we are still in the dark. Not one of you should mention a possible assassination attempt." Ben pointed around the desk, "I mean it. Your jobs depend on it. We will not engage with speculation; the media is already doing enough of that. We will remain resolute and dignified. No loose talk in this building or anywhere else, am I clear?"

The silence in the room suggested that he had been heard.

Brian removed his glasses and placed them on the table as he rubbed his eyes. "You know, something severe is being glossed over here. Is this not a subject any of you want to discuss? An assassination attempt has been made!" He slammed his fist on the table. "Are we next? Who has she angered, or have we upset someone? Was she investigating something outside of our knowledge? Does anyone know? Has her PA said anything to anyone? Because I know shit all and frankly, I'm worried about it. I have family, you know!"

Everyone present noticed that Brian's hands were shaking.

"Does anyone have anything to add to that?" Ben added.

Not a word was spoken; only a few heads shook in response.

"Brian, look, don't think we aren't concerned. As head of this network, I feel that more than most," Ben said softly. "I know you're looking to me for answers, and I'm sorry to say that I don't have any. Alison never confided in me about anything that could have led to this escalation. The very thought that someone wanted to take her life…"

"You're missing the point, Ben," Brian quickly interrupted. "This isn't just about someone wanting to kill her. This was not a home invasion or a burglary gone wrong; this was a professional hit, and she was specifically targeted. Who could have that kind of knowledge and, in this country, have access to explosives or whatever is needed? Come on, everyone!"

"As I say, and with respect, Brian, we only know what everyone else knows at this point. Julie, given your connections with production companies and journalists, surely one of your contacts has a reliable police connection. Can't we find out anything more?"

Julie nodded. "I can try."

"Well, do so quietly, leave no noise that anyone else can pick up on."

"Whoever is behind this has serious connections, can't you see. I can't just go to the supermarket and buy bits needed to make a car bomb, that and get away with it." Brian threw his arms in the air in frustration.

"You say that, Barry, but I watched a programme once where..."

"Oh, fuck off, Debbie, get serious, will you?" Brian folded his arms and continued, "We haven't done anything to provoke a terrorist group or radicals from the far reaches of some ass end place; this is something else entirely. This has everything to do with what she is saying and what she is trying to accomplish. Who are the real losers in all of this... hmm?"

Ben frowned and shrugged his shoulders. "Well, we changed the front-of-camera presenters. Alison banned anyone who had undergone unnecessary cosmetic surgery from holding a broadcasting position. Other channels have followed suit, and..."

"Oh, get real! You don't seriously think a disgruntled TV presenter is behind this! This is all about the money; that's what this is about. Consider the claims culture that emerged after The Beauty Beach. Who did it really cost? Ask yourself that."

Debbie looked incredulous and practically laughed as she spoke. "You think there's some sort of beauty salon collective behind this?"

Brian nearly spat out his response in annoyance. "You need to think bigger! Who would have the resources to do this? Who would be motivated? Who did it ultimately cost?"

Ben shook his head. "You think it's the plastic surgeons? Although they were affected, much of their work is not cosmetic."

Brian shook his head in disgust. "No, you need to go further up the chain to see who it truly impacted. I believe the pharmaceutical industry is behind this, big pharma. They are trying to make a statement, and, whether we intended it or not, I think they have just declared war on us."

++++

HOUSES OF PARLIAMENT, WESTMINSTER - LONDON

Helen Lord, a government backbench MP, had developed an interest in cosmetic surgery after the collapse of the production company behind The Beauty Beach. This interest evolved into more than just a campaign; some of her peers and media outlets labelled her a maverick. Taking a bold step, she publicly supported Alison Harwood and sought to change the law regarding cosmetic surgery. Specifically, she advocated for an outright ban on unnecessary procedures.

As the chair of the All-Party Parliamentary Group on Cosmetic Beauty Management for the past fourteen months, she regularly urged select committee members to consider her views. She pressed hard for greater transparency and ethics from big pharmaceutical companies. However, their response was always the same: they claimed their "research and development arm was commercially confidential" and they were not obliged to answer her questions. Some members of her government reminded her that she was just a backbench MP and suggested she remove her focus from matters that did not concern her. On one occasion, she was confronted just outside the House of Lords by two members of the upper house who attempted to intimidate her into silence. Since then, she had avoided the Lords, weary of being the target of stares, aggressive gossip, and ridicule.

Until regulators in the field provided tangible scientific evidence and long-term health benefits, she called for a complete cessation of the so-called "beauty business." For her, it was nothing more than a pursuit of financial gain, often at the expense of others. While there was abundant scientific speculation about the use of cosmetic products, proven long-term side effects remained a matter of conjecture; nevertheless, reactions to surgeries and instances of malpractice occurred. Medical professionals who aligned with her viewpoints were often labelled as cranks and conspiracy theorists. She believed she had independent experts supporting her on two occasions, but she soon realised this was a misconception. Her parliamentary researchers did not have to dig deeply to uncover the connections between these experts and pharmaceutical companies, with Knightark Pharmaceutical being mentioned most frequently. She knew these companies employed underhanded tactics to gain access to parliament, and they were not even discreet about it. Their representatives often mingled in the Commons and the Lords, hosting social gatherings to impress potential clients and investors. It was particularly easy for Knightark Pharmaceutical, which had two members of the House of Lords on its payroll as "consultants." This arrangement was legally declared, and the payments the Lords received were documented in the register of members' interests. To her, this indicated that Knightark Pharmaceutical was essentially buying access to parliament and the associated advantages.

Her opinion was clear: the cosmetic industry suffered from lacklustre regulations and provided little proven evidence of long term physical and mental aftereffects. Across the board, the cosmetic business viewed her as troublesome, a meddler, and an irritant.

Despite her efforts, members of both Houses of Parliament offered her little support, and she rarely found a platform to voice her concerns. On her behalf, the secretariat of the All-Party Parliamentary Group frequently attempted to communicate with major pharmaceutical companies but often found themselves brushed off with scientific jargon, whilst these companies usually donated to associated charities. Pressing for a change in the law, she lobbied medical experts and made a habit of studying white papers daily. What began as simple research quickly became an obsession; she absorbed information like a sponge. Her knowledge grew to the point where she could discuss the topic for hours, and for those willing to listen, her opinions seemed almost 'qualified.'

Sitting in Portcullis House, the building adjacent to Parliament, she nervously sipped her tea. She hadn't eaten all morning, and her throat felt parched with worry. Upon arriving at work, one of her research assistants had expressed concern for her health, noting her pale complexion. She spent the morning watching news reports to learn more about what had happened to Alison, which was the leading story. After about thirty minutes of coverage, she felt compelled to go to Parliament, seeking refuge within its walls. She had gleaned little information about Alison's condition beyond what was publicly disclosed. Despite her position as an MP, the hospital would not share any details. She had attempted to contact Alison's husband, but his phone was off. All she had confirmed was that Alison was in the high dependency unit and that it was under police guard. Sipping her tea, she scanned her surroundings; Wednesday mornings were always the busiest time in Parliament. Typically, she used this time for people-watching. If a seat was available, she preferred to sit opposite the escalator that connected Portcullis House to the older part of Parliament, where Westminster Hall and the main chambers are located. Here, a spectacle unfolds that changes from week to week. One member of parliament rises the escalator while another descends, often finding that the one coming up has been vilified in the media by the one going down that morning. The mutual glares of disgust between the two parties never failed to amuse her; it was just a game of handbags in this adult playground. However, even the thick skin required to be a politician could be tested on the Portcullis escalator.

Having held her seat for over nine years with a healthy majority, she represented the constituency of Shrewsbury in Shropshire, located in central England. National polling suggested that her support had increased, but it was beginning to wane locally. Her constituents were vocal in challenging her for the time she spent fighting an unwinnable cause, often accusing her of neglecting local issues.

Glancing at her watch, she finished her tea; she only had a few minutes left to get to the chamber. As parliamentary etiquette dictated, she had submitted her request to the Speaker of the House the previous week. She had tabled a question she wanted to ask the Prime Minister during Prime Minister's Questions; on this occasion, it concerned a local issue in her constituency.

The current Speaker of the House has held the position across two parliamentary terms, although it was intended to be filled by a member who should not take a partisan stance. She found him unsupportive of her campaign, and any questions she directed towards the Prime Minister about the cosmetics and beauty industry were consistently ignored. However, this morning's events changed everything; what she had initially planned to ask was no longer the key question. Although it was not in the spirit of parliamentary etiquette, it was a risk she was willing to take. Now, she would pose a question about what had happened to Alison. As a sitting member of Parliament, she was entitled to parliamentary privilege, which meant that her question to the Prime Minister in the chamber would be legally protected from reprisals. Regardless, it would undoubtedly attract media attention.

She gathered her research papers from the table and looked across to the far end of Portcullis House, where a commotion was taking place. The Prime Minister was arriving, flanked by advisors and a couple of police officers providing close protection. The Prime Minister had various ways of entering the parliamentary estate. Today, he must have left Downing Street and entered Portcullis House through the back entrance, passing by the mailroom. She rechecked her watch; it was just a few minutes before noon, and the Prime Minister was going to the chamber for the weekly session of Prime Minister's Questions.

Rising, she placed her research papers into her bag and headed toward the escalator. The Prime Minister glanced in her direction but did not acknowledge her; his disdain for her campaign was apparent. The Government had shown no interest in her campaign, and it was not open to discussion. She had been summoned once to the Chief Whip's office, where her comments had been deemed too fractious, especially considering that a particular British pharmaceutical company was a significant donor to the party. The company in question again was called Knightark Pharmaceutical.

As Helen grasped the escalator railing and began descending, her thoughts turned to Alison. Alison had confided that she suspected she was being followed and had lost faith in her phone and email systems, fearing they might be monitored. The police had investigated numerous online threats made against both Alison and herself. Still, there had only been a few arrests, mostly of low-level offenders, while the more serious threats to their lives remained unresolved or were working their way through the legal system. Alison had noted that the police believed those responsible for the higher-level threats were well-versed in using the dark web, enabling them to cover their tracks easily. This indicated a higher level of sophistication and a determined threat.

Upon reaching the bottom of the escalator, Helen hurried down the corridor toward Westminster Hall. The Prime Minister was ahead of her, so she took a shortcut to reach her seat in the Commons chamber. She walked briskly through one of the cloakrooms and entered the central lobby. As was customary every Wednesday, cameras and journalists were positioned throughout the area. One reporter recognised and rushed toward her, asking, "Helen, will you give an interview after PMQs regarding what happened to Alison Harwood this morning? We know how close you are."

She raised her hand without comment and made her way down the corridor toward the main entrance of the chamber. Briefly stopping at the imposing statue of Winston Churchill, who stood proudly just outside the entrance, she gave Winston's foot a quick rub for luck and nodded at the ushers, who opened the doors for her. The chamber was packed as she shuffled past a few newer members who were standing. The chamber had been designed when there were fewer members of Parliament, so it wasn't big enough to provide a seat for everyone. Since she was in her third term, she had a seat on the backbenches. She nodded in respect toward the

Speaker's chair and headed to the dispatch box, taking the steps on the left-hand side. Other members shuffled along the bench to make room for her. One of the security ministers was speaking, but it seemed few were paying attention. There was the usual hubbub as members prepared for the weekly spectacle of Prime Minister's Questions. As she sat down, she glanced briefly at the Speaker of the House, catching his eye. She was second on the list and hoped he would permit her to ask her question. Feeling the heat in the chamber, she removed her jacket and took a deep breath.

The Prime Minister entered the chamber from behind the Speaker's chair as those seated on the cramped front bench shuffled to make room for him.

Alix Gregory was in his second term as Prime Minister. Much was made of his having attended an elite college, but he was reasonably popular. He spoke frankly, and the public appreciated his candour for a while. When he formed his government, the party's ratings were high. His administration decisively overwhelmed the opposition in a convincing victory, capturing 403 seats in the House, surpassing the 326 needed for a majority. They managed to win several long-held opposition seats in surprising contests, and the opposition's loss meant some members were now in the House of Lords.

The Securities Minister collected his paperwork after seeing the Prime Minister enter the chamber. Alix placed his prepared notes on the dispatch box and then sat. The Chancellor of the Exchequer sat on his left, and they exchanged a few words.

Helen did her best to catch the Speaker's eye again. She knew the Prime Minister would need to address the events from that morning, particularly the various media speculations about a potential terrorist attack. However, her question was pertinent. The chamber was the only place where her inquiry could be directed at the government and heard by millions.

The Speaker nodded at the Securities Minister to conclude, saying, "Order. Questions to the Prime Minister. Shelly Forsyeth"

The MP for Crewe and Nantwich in Cheshire stood up and said, "Question 1, Mr Speaker," before promptly sitting back down.

"Prime Minister," the Speaker beckoned.

Alix rose to his feet and addressed the Speaker, "Mr Speaker, I would like to express my shock regarding the incident this morning in our very capital. While the police are still investigating, I can report to the House that it is a fact that Alison Harwood, the Head of Policy for Channel 8 television, was seriously injured in what we understand to be an explosion. No one from the government, including me, will comment until the police have concluded their investigation. Our security services have assured me, along with the Right Honourable Home Secretary, that this appears to be an isolated incident. At this time, there is no indication of further incidents. I ask the media to refrain from speculating on these events and to report the facts as they become available. I would also like to express my regards and best wishes to her family for a quick recovery."

Supportive murmurs echoed from both sides of the House.

"Mr Speaker, this morning I had meetings with ministerial colleagues and others, in addition to my duties in this House. I shall have further meetings later today."

"Shelly Forsyeth," the Speaker called as the MP from the Cheshire region of the UK stood up again from the opposite side of the chamber.

"Thank you, Mr Speaker. Will the Prime Minister provide his perspective on my constituency within the beautiful Crewe and Nantwich and the constant broken promises regarding support for our care homes..." Cheers erupted from the opposition benches. "The care industry is one of our most critical services; it is understaffed, and care workers must work longer than twelve-hour days..." The noise grew louder. "New developments and new homes have not materialised; what has the Prime Minister done about it?" Shelly Forsyeth pointed at Alix, and the noise in the chamber intensified.

The Speaker rose again. "Order! We will have order here. I think we have the gist of the honourable member for Crewe and Nantwich's question. Prime Minister." The Speaker then sat back down as Alix rose to his feet.

Alix took a sip of water. "To answer the honourable member's question, since this government took over from the mess they left behind…" He pointed at the opposition front bench. "We have invested over three hundred and twenty million pounds in developing new care homes nationwide." There were appreciative cheers from the government side of the house. "We have raised the national living wage and are investing in further training for all care staff…"

"They don't need training; they need to be paid more," the MP who had asked the question heckled.

Alix raised his voice. "And I'll take no lessons from them about the state of the care profession; you all neglected it for years!"

Cheers erupted from the government side of the house as Alix grabbed the folder holding his prepared notes and sat down.

"Helen Lord," the speaker announced.

Muted supportive cheers emerged as Helen swallowed and stood up. "I appreciate the Prime Minister's words regarding my friend Alison Harwood, although they are just that, words." Alix crossed his arms, and no one from the government front bench turned to look at her.

"Will he be visiting her in the hospital? Will he be investigating who carried out this attack? For far too long, many members in this house and the upper house have had their pockets lined by major pharmaceutical companies." Cheers and jeers filled the chamber, with one member sounding like he was making animal noises in an out-of-control zoo. Helen noticed the speaker frown as he stood up. She immediately sat down.

"Order! Order here, on both sides of the House. I would ask the honourable lady to stick to the original question she had tabled," the Speaker said, sitting back down and gesturing for Helen to stand.

"Thank you, Mr Speaker. As I was saying, what will the Prime Minister and this government do to investigate this shocking attack on the streets of London? This was not just an incident; it was an assassination attempt on someone who speaks out, and he knows it!"

Uproar erupted in the chamber when a member from her side threw a schedule of business at her. Furious at such a breach of parliamentary decorum, the Speaker shot to his feet. "Enough! The honourable member was warned. Serjeant-at-Arms, remove the member from Shrewsbury from the Chamber."

As Helen made her way down the short flight of steps, the jeers and raucous barracking enveloped her as the Serjeant-at-Arms extended an arm to assist her, but she waved him off, saying, "I'll walk myself out, thank you," she declared, her voice firm against the chaos around her.

The spectacle of a parliamentarian being escorted from the Commons would make national headlines, and Alix knew it. With the opposition and cameras watching his every move, he remained resolute, his face a mask of calm as he focused on the dispatch box. The noise only intensified with MP's waving papers until Helen was finally ushered out of the chamber.

Once more, the Speaker rose, asserting his authority against the noise of disruption. "The Prime Minister does not need to address what the honourable member for Shrewsbury said," he declared, casting a disinterested glance at his paperwork before calling for the next MP to speak, and sat back down.

Alix felt the pressure knowing the opposition leader would soon take the initiative and ask him difficult questions. Helen's unruliness was a liability; party donors would be very unhappy. Her defiance was becoming costly, and action needed to be taken against her.

++++

After watching Prime Minister's Questions, Darius leaned back in his seat and placed his hands behind his head. That bloody politician was entirely out of control. It was quite unprecedented for a member of parliament to behave in such a manner. PMQs had concluded, and the debate show on the BBC was focused solely on Helen Lord being escorted out of the chamber. There was little discussion about the Prime Minister's performance, aside from his failure to address the points she raised. The Speaker's intervention, asking for the questions to be dismissed, was seen as a sign of weakness on Alix Gregory's part, according to a couple of the panellists. Lord would likely face disciplinary action from the Party Whip; no political party can afford an unruly backbencher, and his company could do without it as well.

However, that was just one concern. The main topic on television was cosmetic surgery, which was the focus of Helen's campaign. It would soon be all over social media, with influencers rallying around the rogue MP. Influencers who had shifted their agendas—those who hadn't had cosmetic procedures, that is. These new influencers focused on promoting a positive lifestyle, self-help, yoga, health retreats, meditation and ageing naturally, rather than showcasing images of beach holidays, luxury hotels, cars, and jewellery as the entitled few had done in the past. Followers of that more superficial lifestyle were more beneficial to the company, and he had sponsored enough of them in the past. Superficial lifestyles were great for business, but it was on the wane. Economic poverty was a worldwide issue, and people were tired of seeing others flaunt their so-called 'incredible' lives and ostentatious wealth. No one wanted to emulate these figures anymore; hero worship had declined, and the social revolt was more significant for those born into privilege.

Despite this bleak environment, Helen Lord faced an uphill battle getting her proposed bill through Parliament. Support for changing the law or even introducing amendments was limited. Meanwhile, the constant stream of medical horror stories shared on social media by her and her accomplice, Alison Harwood, became an ongoing nuisance and a financial burden. Together, they kept the debate alive by posting statistics on compensation payouts worldwide since the successful lawsuit regarding The Beauty Beach.

Darius rubbed his eyes in frustration. His company was not

involved in breast augmentation or the supply of implants; those issues belonged elsewhere. However, the winning contestant, Megan Launders, had used their fillers, and they were tainted by association. Following a significant investigation by a prominent newspaper that published a story on the matter, other media outlets quickly followed suit, collectively targeting major pharmaceutical companies with any stories they could find. They also attempted to dismantle media empires, such as Channel 8, and nearly succeeded.

As the major shareholder and senior board member, he had an obligation to report to the board, and profits were consistently declining. Phase two involved the discreet introduction of a new filler—something users couldn't live without. Three other senior board members were aware of this new product, which had been in development in their lab in Brazil at considerable expense. The product had only recently completed trials with remarkable success. Helen Lord's outburst would complicate matters further, but they had little choice but to press on; too much had been invested. The failed assassination attempt on Harwood would bolster Lord's campaign, and he was certain it was only a matter of time before they were photographed together in the press. Ironically, Harwood might now need cosmetic surgery. Darius smirked, imagining sending her a gift basket of cosmetic fillers from his company and a 'get well soon' card. He connected the battery and SIM card to his unregistered phone and dialled. He nodded as it was answered. "It's me. I mentioned earlier that I want to meet at the usual place. I need to see you within the hour; your failure requires a change in direction." Darius nodded as the voice on the other end agreed. "Okay, see you soon." He ended the call, disassembled the phone, and pressed a button on his office phone.

"Yes, Mr Neith?"

"Please have my car brought around to the front."

"Yes, Mr Neith, I'll call the concierge immediately."

Darius switched off the speaker, straightened his tie, and put on his suit jacket. He was familiar with the basics of surveillance and needed to ensure he wasn't being followed. He was meeting David Needam, a former member of the French Foreign Legion with a strong understanding of security matters, who had worked in the private sector for the past seven years. David brought a wealth of knowledge to the company and was usually an excellent problem solver and asset. Although he had failed with Harwood, Darius believed he would likely get a second chance. They also needed to decide how to handle the meddling member of parliament. If they were going to get the company back on track, they needed to consider a different approach before the rollout of the new product.

Chapter Four

Ben Tasker locked his car and walked toward the accident and emergency department. Before leaving Channel 8 to head to the hospital, he had spoken with the owner of the security company responsible for protecting the channel's headquarters. They had agreed to implement enhanced security measures, including more rigorous checks on building access and increased security patrols around the car park. Additionally, he planned to contact security consultants to assess and fortify their protocols.

Ben's primary safety concern wasn't being at work; it was the fact that his car would be left unattended, parked on the street in a residential area overnight. He would be lying if he said he wasn't nervous about starting his vehicle before heading to the hospital. At home, anyone could walk right up to his front door. While there was a six-foot-high wall at the end of his back garden, with a little effort, climbing over it wouldn't be difficult. After all, a professional had carried out the assassination attempt on Alison. Until now, he had never considered his own safety or that of his family. That was about to change, and he realised he needed to sit down and talk with his wife that evening. She had seen the news and called him immediately. He didn't lie to her; he told her what he knew, which was very little, and asked her not to worry, though his reassurance was quickly brushed aside.

He still hadn't been able to contact Mike, Alison's husband, but he would be surprised if Mike weren't here. So far, all he had gathered was that Alison was under police protection and was in the high-dependency unit (HDU).

As he entered the accident and emergency department, he immediately spotted various blue signs mounted on the walls, indicating the locations of different departments within the building.

The HDU, along with several other departments, was to the left. The A&E waiting area was busy; some people had fallen asleep, while others were holding their aching limbs. Following the signs, he walked through another set of automatic doors and down a corridor to the left. Almost immediately, he noticed two police officers standing next to a doorway. A sign above indicated that he had arrived at the high-dependency unit. Further down the corridor, he spotted Mike staring blankly at the wall in front of him.

"Excuse me," Ben approached a nurse at a desk to the side. "Can I please get an update on Alison Harwood?"

The nurse glanced at him dismissively. "Are you another journalist?"

"Oh..." Ben smiled, trying to clarify. "No, well, not anymore. I'm Alison's boss, and we are extremely concerned about her."

"I can't provide any information other than that she is in the HDU. That's all I can say at this time. Respectfully, I do not know who you are," the nurse explained.

Ben nodded. "That's understandable. However, may I speak to her husband? I see he is sitting over there."

The nurse nodded but added, "Someone else came in earlier claiming to know him. If you're not who you say you are, the police are armed, and I won't be rushing to help you." Ben glanced at her name badge; it read 'Shelly.' She offered a brief smile after finishing her statement. He returned her smile and said, "I understand."

The police officers observed him closely. One of them approached as he began walking down the corridor.

"I'm a friend of Alison's. I know I can't go in, but I would like to speak to Mike," he said, pointing down the corridor. "Her husband."

"And you are?" the officer asked.

"Ben Tasker. I work with Alison."

At that moment, Mike noticed someone approaching and waved him over. "He's okay, officer," he said.

The policeman allowed Ben to pass and turned to confer with his fellow officer.

Ben extended his right hand, and Mike took it. They shook hands and exchanged a brief hug. "Please, sit with me," Mike said, indicating the seats behind him. Judging by the number of empty coffee cups, it was clear he had been waiting for some time.

Ben took a seat. "I'm sorry. I got here as quickly as I could." As he settled in, he glanced to his left; both officers were watching him intently. "No one is saying anything, Mike. Seriously, what the hell has happened?"

Mike shook his head, his eyes bloodshot and his hands trembling from worry and an overdose of caffeine. He spoke barely above a whisper, "I had already left for work, literally only minutes before. I was outside the tube station when I heard the explosion." He shook his head again, tears welling in his eyes. "I still got on the damn tube; I was in such a rush to get to work. I couldn't tell where the noise came from." His eyes streamed with tears. "My Alison, my Alison," he pounded his chest in frustration at himself. "I feel sick, disgusted with myself."

As Mike's tears continued to flow, Ben had to look away. Over the past year, they had come to know each other reasonably well. "There's nothing you could have done. Don't let that weigh on your mind. Where are the kids?"

Mike glanced at his watch. "They'll be leaving school soon. They don't know anything yet. The nanny is collecting them as usual. I've told her to take them somewhere else, somewhere away from our road, somewhere away from the press. She has coordinated with the headteacher to ensure nothing is said until I see them. With so much press around, I must keep my distance for now. The nanny is using taxis; her car will be left on the school grounds overnight." Mike placed his hands on his thighs, his knuckles turning white as he gripped his knees in frustration, feeling helpless, knowing there wasn't a thing he could do. "I guess we'll need a hotel later."

Ben shook his head. "Not at all; you can all stay at my place."

Mike chewed on his lower lip. "Thank you. I'm not sure what to do at the moment. I can't figure out what the hell to do with myself." He rubbed his brow. "Tell me, what are the press saying? I can't bring myself to watch TV now; I've turned my phone off."

Ben took a deep breath. "Okay, are you sure you're ready to hear this?"

Mike's eyes, red and glistening with tears, held Ben's solemn look. "Go on."

"It's suspected this was a targeted attack. The police have not released any official statement."

Mike nodded, letting out a forced laugh. "I figured that out for myself, Ben. Cars don't just explode by themselves. She had been receiving threats, and she shielded a lot of it from me because she didn't want the kids or me to worry. The threats I was aware of were generalised, offensive, yes, but from accounts not necessarily linked to a living person. They were typically associated with recently created profiles featuring fake pictures and content. So please don't talk down to me or try to sugarcoat it. Tell me, was this a terrorist attack?"

"I don't know. Nothing is being said."

"Then what do you know? The police over there aren't telling me anything."

"I suspect they don't know anything to share. All I know is that your road is closed off; no one is allowed in or out, and everyone has been evacuated. One of our journalists said that the Royal Logistics Corps are there, searching every vehicle and every nook and cranny, but I can't wholly verify that. I saw in earlier news reports that barriers have been put up, so you can't see in or out. The only views being shared now are from drones and helicopters." Ben leaned closer. "Look, if this is suspected to be a planned attack, and I have to say, it looks like it, counter-terrorism will likely be on the ground, along with our security services. They will investigate thoroughly. But whether we will be given the facts is another matter."

"Who could do this, Ben? Seriously?"

Ben shook his head. "There has to be military involvement, probably special forces."

"Our people targeting us..."

"No, no, that's not what I mean. I'm talking about someone freelance, someone from the private sector."

Mike rubbed his eyes and sat back in his chair. "It's too much to comprehend."

Ben nodded. "It is. It's a shock to everyone. Tell me, how is she? What is her condition?"

"I'm still not fully sure. I know they are holding back from me. Severe facial lacerations, internal bleeding, organ disruption from the blast wave, God knows what else."

"Christ, it's difficult to know what to say to you, Mike. I'm sorry to ask, but is there something more going on? Has she mentioned anything to you that could be, well, off-topic? Something that might have enraged someone enough to lead to this?"

Mike shook his head. "I can't think of anything. She did mention the threats she received on social media, but they always followed the same pattern. The only person I can think of is Helen Lord. She spoke with her regularly and is the only figure of controversy that comes to mind. Helen's facing the same level of threats and abuse as Alison. Alison would often visit her in Parliament."

"Mmm. Well, she had a meltdown in the chamber today."

"What do you mean?"

"I saw it on my phone earlier. During PMQs, she went completely off the rails about Alison, challenging the Prime Minister in the process. The Speaker kicked her out of the chamber."

Mike turned in shock; his laughter was more a response of concern than humour.

"If you ask me, she's in the shit. The PM's face and body language were expressionless, but he wasn't fooling anyone; he was angry."

They paused briefly. Ben glanced down the corridor where the police officers were talking among themselves. "I don't suppose you've tried going home yet? Are they searching your house? You know they will."

Mike shrugged. "I have no idea. They have a key to get in. I guess they are. I'll leave here soon to see the kids, but will return afterwards. They may let me into the High Dependency Unit later, but she's sedated for now. I haven't even been able to see her." His words broke as tears streamed down his face. He sniffed loudly, rubbing the back of his hand over his nose. The noise immediately caused the officers to turn and face them. "Helen Lord. She's the only one I can think of. They used to talk all the time."

"Look, do you need anything right now?"

Mike shook his head.

"I'll come back to see you later, and the offer is open if you all want to stay at my place. Please be careful when you leave; the press is at the front of the hospital."

"Thank you, Ben. I appreciate it, and I know Alison would as well."

"You are family. I mean it. Anything you need, ask." Ben stood up. "I'll leave you in peace for now. Everyone from the office sends their love; a few wanted to come, but I told them no. I'll drop by later."

Mike remained seated, watching as Ben nodded to the officers and turned down the right corridor.

Ben glanced back to make sure he wasn't being followed. Satisfied that he was alone, he paused and placed a hand against the wall to collect his thoughts.

Alison had been in regular communication with Helen Lord MP. He knew they spoke to each other, but not how often. Every visit to Westminster left a trace; it was likely that the security services were monitoring her movements. He was intelligent enough to piece the situation together; this was likely an assassination attempt. Such actions required the resources of only the most serious individuals, and even fewer could carry out such a plan undetected.

He needed to return to the office. The only connection that made sense was between Alison and the politician. Unless Alison was hiding something, which he doubted, they might have been onto something significant together. He thought about Mike, but reminded himself that he had his own interests to protect; after all, he was her employer. He needed to understand what was happening and uncover the truth as quickly as possible.

++++

Darius parked his car and looked across the road at the mobile café. David was sitting outside next to the caravan, holding a mug in one hand and the front page of a tabloid newspaper in the other. He appeared to be scanning the headlines while seated in a worn, faded plastic garden chair on this remote and largely deserted industrial estate.

David noticed Darius but took his time getting up from his seat as the car drove away and parked further down the estate. This area of London was highly deprived, lacking CCTV surveillance, and with very few visitors. It resembled a wasteland, filled with abandoned warehouses and remnants of businesses that had long since closed.

After collecting his car from outside the reception of Knightark Pharmaceutical UK headquarters, Darius decided to dismiss his chauffeur for the day, wanting some private time with his professional problem-solver. In the rearview mirror, he saw David folding his newspaper and tucking it under his arm as he approached. Darius pressed the unlock button on the car, and David casually opened the passenger door and got in. The doors automatically locked as soon as he sat down. Impatient for answers, Darius calmly asked, "So, what went wrong?"

David glanced away. "I did as we planned, the way we discussed."

"Well, that's not entirely true. The problem remains, and I understand she is now under police guard."

David shook his head in frustration. "My work isn't a science; there are always extenuating factors. The IED detonated perfectly, and from what I've seen on TV, it destroyed surrounding cars and caused structural damage to a couple of nearby properties. The blast radius and the amount of explosives were correct. I can only assume she remotely unlocked the car door. If she had been right next to the car door when she unlocked it, her chances of survival upon detonation would likely be less than one percent. Let me be clear, Darius: this will never be accepted as a terrorist attack; it was too direct, too personal, and targeted. You knew the consequences. Nevertheless, MI5 will be on the ground along with other specialist units from the MET. I've covered my tracks as best as I can."

Darius tapped his fingers on the steering wheel, considering David's words.

"This was your plan," David asserted. "Even though a colleague of mine has been making constant threats to her through various social media accounts, many questions are being raised right now about who would want to do this and who has the capability. There were always going to be risks involved."

"I'm fully aware of the situation. A great deal of thought was invested in this by myself and the senior board. Nevertheless, you are our problem solver, and the problem remains unsolved. In fact, it may have just worsened; she needed to be silenced, permanently!" Darius paused to catch his breath. "If she pulls through, it will only galvanise her. That woman will be viewed as a martyr for her cause. Do you realise the consequences? This just became a whole lot worse."

"Don't take me for granted! You pay me well, but money is just money; I have what I need. I specialise in this field. Never underestimate those who take life," David replied sharply.

"I never would, but the facts are what they are!"

"I fully understand the dynamics of a master-servant relationship; however, I will never tolerate abuse from you."

Darius released the steering wheel and took a deep breath. "We need to change direction. We have a new streamlined product set to enhance one of our existing cosmetic fillers. We cannot continue down this path. The board is concerned, and our business is declining, just as our competitors' is. We have decided to take a stand to save this business on a global scale."

“What do you have in mind? Trying to go after her while she is in a city centre hospital is suicidal. Data trails will be left behind, and police ANPR cameras are practically everywhere. More factors mean greater chances of a compromise. If I get caught and my background is revealed, no one in their right mind will believe I acted alone. It will be obvious that I have an employer.”

“I know, and that’s why I don’t want you to go back on her, for now anyway. What’s done is done. If she doesn’t pull through, that would be for the best. However, I’m going to give you a new target.”

David frowned. “Who else could bring about the change you are looking for? If you’re considering going after the politician she collaborates with, that will lead to significant problems.”

“No, not her. Although I’ve given that some thought. Are you aware of Ben Tasker?”

“Of course. He’s the head of Channel 8. He figured prominently in my workups. Taking him out would cause chaos at that network; they’d all end up surrounded by bodyguards.”

“No, no, no. You misunderstand. I want him to work for us.” Darius turned to David with a malevolent grin on his face.

David let out a small laugh. “Okay, that would be interesting. But I don’t think he’ll be tempted by money, even with your coffers.” David threw the newspaper on the floor and crossed his arms. “Plus, even the threat of death will be tricky. There’s a good chance the police will start monitoring his communications now.”

Darius shook his head. “No, those methods won’t work. This is an assassination of a different kind; you could call it a corporate assassination.”

David nodded. “Go on.”

“I want you to surveil him, track where he goes and what he does. If possible, bug him directly. Identify his weaknesses, and once you do, build a friendship with him.”

“From my earlier research, I discovered that he is happily married with children.”

“Did you find out how long he’s been married?”

"From what I could gather, he's been married for over twelve years and was with his wife for a few years before they tied the knot."

Darius nodded. "Okay. I want him to do something for me. Have you heard of the American actor Gracy Ann Taylor?"

"I know who you mean. I think she's an Academy Award winner, very active on social media, and known for being pro-surgery."

"That's right, and she has had enough of our product in her face; she's the perfect role model for what we need."

David sat silently, still unaware of the connection.

"As you can probably imagine, celebrity surgery is beneficial for our business. We assist them with higher-level procedures that most people cannot afford. In return, they promoted our products, creating a successful business arrangement that lasted for years until The Beauty Beach disaster occurred, triggering a surge in lawsuits. What many don't know about our media darling, Gracy, is that she fell into some rather questionable circles. She briefly picked up the crystal habit, but it didn't last long because it affected her appearance too quickly, and some faces are simply beyond saving. She was weaned off it, and cocaine is now her choice of poison, which is much easier to manage."

"Darius, I'm still not following."

"Of course, her drug problem isn't common knowledge. Her last performance was somewhat lacklustre, so the signs are there, but I'm confident we can keep her under control."

David shook his head in confusion. "I don't understand. How are you keeping her under control?"

Darius laughed. "Because we got her hooked on crystal in the first place." He continued to laugh. "It was a backup plan; it took time to arrange. But we have people in the right places. Her cocaine supplier is a personal contact, and he keeps her dependent, along with a couple of other famous faces we've started working on."

David looked at Darius in shock.

"Well, do you think it's only you we work with?" Darius continued.

"We have connections everywhere. So, for all your talk about being a professional, never lose sight of the fact that you are expendable to this company. This is much bigger than just you or me."

David turned to look out the car window. "That still doesn't explain the connection to Tasker."

"I'm confident we can get this drug-addicted actor onto Channel 8. Of course, we need to be a bit subtle about it; she's too high profile to present a TV series or anything like that. Maybe we can feature her in advertisements for perfume, lingerie, or even haemorrhoid cream, who cares? However, in any case, we need to get her on the very channel that started banning cosmetics, and Tasker is the key; he can make it happen as long as we can find something to use against him. If the actor doesn't comply, we'll cut off her cocaine supply. It won't be long before the LAPD picks her up on a street corner somewhere. No more red carpets for her." Darius laughed. "She'll certainly be reminded of that if she refuses."

David nodded. "You've thought this through. You have been busy."

Darius began tapping on the steering wheel again. "This is business, David, and I'll do whatever it takes. If we can get her on the channel, it has the potential to change everything, returning to how things used to be, the days when everyone was happy. Once that's underway, we'll launch our new product. She will promote it, although she doesn't realise that yet." He paused, carefully considering his following words. "The so-called death of beauty will become a thing of the past." Darius looked at David, wanting to ensure he understood the importance of his point. "A lot of work has gone into this, money, time, and leveraging favours. Now we're handing the responsibility for the next phase over to you. We need to know if you can complete this."

"I've never let you down before. I can complete."

"Good. The senior board will be pleased. However, before we proceed, I need to convene a board meeting. We must discuss our new product in a private setting. Our discussions must remain confidential. Do you understand? Not a word should escape that room."

David nodded, "Yes, I think so. However, this is not my area of expertise; it requires a different type of specialist, someone who specialises in room sterilisation."

"Why? The more who know, the more problems we'll have. This is a tight circle! What do you mean? Do you have someone in mind?"

David nodded but avoided eye contact. "You know what you know, and I know what I know, but the scope of the specialist field is too broad. No one is an expert in everything. This situation requires a specialist with complementary skills who is trustworthy. He's an old colleague: English, a former Legionnaire. However, we went in different directions after our service."

"Okay. Tell me more about him."

"We both worked in freelance markets, but he was less principled than I was. For him, it was never about a cause; it was always about the money. Eventually, though, it became something entirely different." David took a deep breath as he gathered his thoughts. "He fell from grace and began taking jobs in places I wanted no part of. A lot of people died who didn't need to, and over time, he became progressively worse. After turning on his own men in a fit of rage, he kept moving, living in paranoia. His temperament deteriorated as he drifted from one country to another. He ended up in Nepal, where Buddhist monks took him into their monastery. He spent over two years there and emerged almost reborn. By all accounts, he became something of a holy man. I haven't worked with him for some time, but this is his area, and he continues to work."

"This does not sound like a trustworthy man to me. So, he has a high body count. What's the big deal? That's part of your profession; it's what you do. An unstable operator is someone we could do without. Why are you even considering him?"

"After returning from Nepal, he transitioned into the private sector and quickly demonstrated his resourcefulness. He took on various bodyguard jobs but struggled to adapt to civilian life. Eventually, he quit and decided to work independently. His expertise is in TSCM."

Darius shook his head. "What does that stand for?"

"Tactical Surveillance Counter Measures. He can conceal a camera anywhere, record anything, and bug people without their knowledge. If he's on your case, he'll know more about your daily activities than you do. If you are under surveillance, he can track those who are watching you without them realising it. As I mentioned, in this business, you cannot be a specialist in every field. I have a basic understanding of TSCM; he has a deeper knowledge of it. He's the one to bring in. He can search for and eliminate listening devices wherever you want to hold this board meeting. While I may know the basics, if you want to be certain, we should bring him in."

Darius nodded. "It sounds like he has the right skills, but can he be trusted? Do you think he'll take the job?"

"Yes, he can be trusted. As I mentioned, I haven't worked with him in a while, but he's well-known in my network and remains active. The good news is that he's very motivated by money again."

"Good. Money we have, which should give him the focus he needs."

"He sends all his earnings back to the temple in Nepal and leads a very frugal life, or so I've been told. He comes with my recommendation, but I need to discuss this with him first."

"I don't want to meet him, and I don't want him to know he's working for us. There will be no paperwork or trails; he works for you, and we will pay you."

David nodded. "I understand."

"Good. Look into it, will you? I'm selecting a location outside of London for the board meeting. It's only a three-star hotel because we do not want to attract attention. I've booked the entire fifth floor for a few days. Our usual security team will be in place to monitor who comes and goes. This time, we'll need to take it up a notch. I don't trust our headquarters for such a meeting."

“Do you have concerns about the board members as well?”

Darius nodded. “Just a feeling; I can’t quite put my finger on it yet. I’ll keep you updated.”

David leaned forward and picked up his newspaper. “Will there be anything else?”

“No. The payment will be made to you in the usual manner. Contact your colleague and let me know if you can fulfil our request. In light of recent events and the fact that the woman is still alive, we need to proceed immediately.”

David nodded and checked the side mirror to ensure no one was behind him. He pulled the car handle, heard the lock click open, and then swung the door open and stepped outside. “I’ll be in touch,” he said as he closed the car door.

Darius acknowledged his words and drove away.

Chapter Five

A lot had changed in the last hour as Helen Lord ascended the escalator back up to the main floor of Portcullis House. Defiant and resolute, she locked eyes with those who stared at her from the opposite side of the escalator with an expressionless stare until they descended. Among the thousands who work in Parliament every day, a significant number would have seen her removal from the chamber on television. While it wasn't unprecedented, it was certainly irregular. Her personal Wikipedia page had probably already been updated to reflect her actions.

As she stepped off the escalator, several journalists and camera operators loitering by the entrance and exit doors sprang into action; she was the topic of the moment. One journalist, a TV news presenter from a major network who had interviewed Helen a couple of times before, approached her quickly.

"Helen, that was quite a display. Are you willing to give an interview?" she asked, being the first to reach her, with other reporters waiting behind, eager to ask the same question.

With parliamentary privilege extending only to MPs when speaking inside the chamber, Helen knew she needed to be exceptionally cautious about what she said. She was aware that she had antagonised the Prime Minister, and that was probably enough for one day. She needed to get upstairs to her office, clear her head, and then head to the hospital to check on Alison.

"I have no further comments at this time, and I stand by what I said in the chamber. Now, if you'll excuse me, I need to get to my office," she replied.

"But Helen, this is your chance to express your thoughts. What you did was very courageous!" The journalist didn't let Helen escape and walked alongside her as they passed a restaurant, a coffee shop, and various seating areas. "Look, I don't think you'll know yet, but I'm told it has been confirmed as a targeted attack. There was an explosive device."

Helen immediately stopped walking and turned to the news presenter. "How do you know this?"

"I have a police contact at Scotland Yard. It will be officially announced in the next couple of hours."

Helen glanced behind her. It was lunchtime, and most seats were taken. Swathes of eyes were staring at her from every direction. "I need to get to my office. Maybe later, okay?" She left the journalist and her camera operator behind, striding towards the lift. With so many eyes upon her, she couldn't wait to escape the buzzing hive of gossip surrounding her. As she waited for the lift, she was distracted by movement to her right. Armed police officers, both in uniform and plain clothes, were heading toward the far stairwell, forming a protective barrier around the Prime Minister. When he noticed her standing by the lift, he briefly locked eyes with her and scowled before quickly disappearing.

Thankfully, the lift door opened, and she stepped inside quickly. As the door closed behind her, she turned casually to glance through the glass doors and noticed that many people were still watching her as the lift ascended to the second floor. Once briefly out of sight, she placed a hand against the side of the lift for support and took a deep breath, reminding herself that a camera was inside and that her actions were likely being monitored. Her thoughts shifted to Alison; according to the news presenter, what had previously been mere suspicion was now confirmed. When the lift doors opened, she stepped out and hurried toward the single-occupancy toilet, which was slightly to her right. Aware that the corridor was under surveillance, she locked herself inside the toilet, dropped her bag, closed the toilet seat, and sat down. Finally, she found a moment of peace, trying to run a hand through her hair, but stopping immediately when she noticed her fingers were shaking. The situation was spiralling out of control; it was only a matter of time before those responsible for the attack on Alison came for her. This was not something she could discuss with the police or any other government officials. Only Alison knew what was at stake, and they were trying to silence both of them.

Only a few weeks ago, Alison had visited her in parliament. The documents she presented were disturbing. As an executive at a major television channel, Alison confided that she lacked the confidence to run the story on their network, especially after they had lost a major lawsuit with The Beauty Beach and couldn't afford to face another one. Alison had sought out Helen because of the public support she had given Alison's campaign, as well as the fact that she possessed something money could not buy: parliamentary privilege. Alison knew she could make allegations and raise public awareness within the House of Commons without facing legal repercussions. So far, except for fifteen minutes ago, Helen had never named Alison in the chamber or discussed the sensitive information she held.

A whistleblower contacted Alison via email, and initially, she thought the messages were a hoax and chose to ignore them. However, the emails continued to arrive, and the subject lines grew increasingly incendiary with each new message, until she finally took notice. The informer claimed that a revolutionary cosmetic beauty filler was nearing completion. Along with these claims, he sent a scientific analysis that included a complete laboratory breakdown of the product's composition. More worryingly, he also provided schematics detailing how the filler interacts with and moves through the body, along with photographs that suggested human testing had already been conducted. This new filler breaks down more quickly than any other regulated filler, requiring users to seek additional applications more frequently. The whistleblower alleged that the product would never receive regulation in the UK or anywhere else. According to this source, the manufacturer shows little concern for compliance and plans to bypass the regulatory process entirely. This could lead to the production of large batches of contaminated products. By the time the contamination is discovered, it may have already spread too widely, residing in the skin and affecting the brain cells of those affected. The outcomes could result in a crisis unlike anything previously encountered; a product recall would likely be ineffective and could incite global panic and chaos. Medical insurance companies might face collapse, and the British National Health Service could be pushed to the brink of ruin. The whistleblower asserted that the pharmaceutical company responsible for this product is primarily motivated by their financial losses, placing the blame squarely on Channel 8.

Helen took a deep breath and shook her head. She was aware that two members of the House of Lords were being paid as 'consultants' by the pharmaceutical company that also donated a significant amount to her political party.

Helen pressed her lips together and rubbed her forehead, feeling a growing sense of anxiety. She had never undergone a cosmetic procedure before, and her stance on the issue was clear. The thought of having the new filler injected into her skin terrified her, mainly because it had a hidden property that required it to be reapplied every six to eight weeks. As the effects wore off, the user could experience a rapid decline in their overall health, leading to fatigue and other adverse effects. The whistleblower alleged, though lacking concrete evidence, that in their human experiments, the ageing process accelerated between applications, causing the body to weaken and develop a dependency on the product. These experiments resulted in one patient committing suicide, while others exhibited violent behaviour and showed unreasonable and untrustworthy actions. Initially, Alison approached this information with scepticism, believing that such claims could not possibly be valid. However, everything changed when a key scientist at the pharmaceutical company made a groundbreaking discovery. He found that as the filler broke down, a neurological component could be introduced to stimulate the brain. This compound would gradually release tiny, almost imperceptible amounts of stimulation, increasing serotonin levels in the brain. The scientist who developed this new compound referred to it as lipomorphilas, but its hidden property was diacetylmorphine, which, for many, is more commonly known as heroin.

++++

Dr John Farmer sat at his computer, carefully examining the map displayed on the screen. The information seemed unusual, and he began to wonder if there had been a mistake. He glanced at the card the security guard had handed him. According to the card, the venue for the board meeting was a three-star hotel just outside Bromley in Kent. Considering that most of the board members had a snobbish, old-money demeanour, this lack of luxury was sure to raise some eyebrows.

Aside from their annual general meeting, the board rarely convened unless there were urgent business matters to discuss. They had met just a couple of months prior for an emergency meeting at their UK headquarters in London, where the sole agenda item was the decline in profits. For three hours, they deliberated, hearing numerous points and interjections, but ultimately accomplished little. Their core income stemmed from cosmetic products, and over the past year, they had experienced a significant decline in consumption. The meeting's outcome was largely ineffective, and given that board members were from the United States, France, and the UK, the collaboration turned out to be an expensive non-achievement.

One comment from Darius Neith lingered in John's mind: an offhand remark about a new product that was supposedly on the way. Many board members, including John, were left in the dark about this comment, which was quickly dismissed and never brought up again. Darius often consulted with three other senior board members who sat beside him during meetings. All the board members, John included, were educated at private schools and were academically accomplished, except for one. This individual, an American in his early fifties, had benefited from his father's wealth, and there were rumours that he had purchased his qualifications rather than earned them. Additionally, the board was male-dominated, except for one woman who had risen through the ranks in the business world. She was assertive in her views on growth and never intimidated by the male members of the board, who possessed the same voting rights as the other junior members.

John's father had made wise investments and left everything to him in his will after his mother's passing many years earlier. Financially secure, John indulged in his hobbies and sought a stress-free life. However, despite his wealth, he often felt unchallenged and yearned for something more. He took a part-time role with a private medical company simply because he could, not out of necessity. He consulted for them and occasionally served as a professional witness in legal cases. There was no conflict of interest between his consultancy work and the board, although he still needed the board's permission to take on that role.

Holding a board meeting at a three-star chain hotel was an unusual choice. As the company's profits continued to decline, the board members became increasingly animated. The company had received numerous threats of legal action from cosmetic surgeons who had gone out of business. So far, the company's wealth had shielded it from lawsuits, while its lawyers made the difficulties of those who dared to confront it worse. Clinics had closed worldwide, and pharmaceutical companies specialising in cosmetics had become pariahs in the industry. Every town initially had one aesthetic clinic, but within a couple of years, there were many. It became a booming business, with their fillers being more profitable than cocaine. They had effectively become a new regulated cartel, with their products licensed in multiple countries and approved for the medical trade.

However, that was all in the past, as cosmetic practices now faced the next wave of decline in the high street economy.

The board meeting was just two days away, and no agenda of business had been provided with the invitation. This lack of information was as unusual as the meeting's location. John had always felt something was off about Darius from their first meeting. Darius seemed to be hiding something, revealing only the bare minimum and never disclosing the full facts. His contempt for board meetings was evident; he preferred to run the company without consulting the board. On several occasions, John had seen Darius accompanied by another man. They always kept their conversations out of earshot, stopping talking immediately whenever someone else got too close. This man appeared to serve as some form of security, not a bodyguard, but rather someone who listened attentively. He had a hardened, intimidating presence, suggesting a military background. Because of reasons like these, John didn't trust Darius. The secrecy surrounding the upcoming board meeting led him to suspect that Darius was orchestrating something significant, likely unrelated to the company's ongoing financial troubles.

++++

Ben parked in his reserved space in front of Channel 8's London studios and turned off the car engine. He scanned the ground floor and saw two uniformed security guards on the other side of the revolving doors. He felt a sense of relief that no journalists or TV cameras were waiting for him outside. Following the lawsuit, several procedural changes were implemented to update the internal quality management system, with a focus on security and staff well-being, both in and out of the workplace. The procedure for employees was clear: if they received threats or abusive messages that warranted action, they were required to report them immediately to the internal security and quality manager. This manager would then provide guidance and, with the employee's permission, contact the police.

Following the backlash directed at Channel 8, particularly towards Alison, the IT department was assigned the ongoing responsibility of moderating the channel's website, news stories, and social media accounts. The moderators were kept busy and have recently received strong support from a dedicated group of individuals. The channel's stance against cosmetic surgery, makeup, and any form of "beautifying" has sparked a polarising debate. There were social media groups where supporters expressed strong opinions, insisting that *"a person's body is their own business, and we do what we like, enhanced surgery or not. No media organisation should make that choice for them."* Consequently, the channel had to begin moderating its midweek live chat show due to incidents during phone-ins and audience heckling. Although advertised as live, the show now has a 180-second delay between filming and actual broadcast.

Several legal cases emerged at an early stage, with the applicants alleging human rights abuses by a media organisation. Channel 8, however, took a contrasting stance, arguing that society places excessive pressure on individuals to conform to specific standards of appearance and questioning why we should attempt to defy the ageing process. This perspective drew ridicule from other channels, both domestically and internationally, sparking heated debates on television and extensive coverage in mainstream print media. Weekly magazines, including several women's lifestyle publications, expressed outrage over the channel's position. However, their responses gradually became muted as lawsuits began to emerge in various directions. Megan Launders won her case against The Beauty Beach production company and subsequently against Channel 8 for negligence. Her victory empowered individuals of all genders to challenge the media's influence, creating an opportunity to voice their concerns. Predatory legal firms launched television campaigns promoting a "no-win, no-fee" basis, quickly shifting legal focus away from the media and toward companies involved in beauty product manufacturing. This upheaval transformed the modelling industry; suddenly, everyone was deemed beautiful and unique, countering the previous notions that labelled individuals as "flawed." Fashion houses were forced to adapt to a new reality as extensive social media campaigns emerged to boycott specific brands. Traditional catwalk events were gradually phased out, and what started as heckling quickly escalated to stage invasions. VIP guests seated in the front rows became targets and were doused in human fat. In several instances, the perpetrators were arrested and jailed for assault and theft of human fat. Only those involved in the cosmetics industry had the financial resources to mount a defence. Initially, the UK government supported large pharmaceutical companies and tried to resist this wave of change, citing concerns about potential losses in trade and employment. However, these concerns were unfounded, as people began to take control of their own beauty choices. This shift led to greater integration and a renewed appreciation for the human form, resulting in economic growth. All sectors of the beauty industry faced financial challenges, from hair care products to basic eyeliner. In response, the government and political opponents started to distance themselves from the cosmetic sector, realising that supporting it might cost them votes. Pharmaceutical companies in the UK, USA, South America, Italy and South Korea engaged politicians as consultants to attempt to gain influence and resist change.

Ultimately, Channel 8 was responsible for the upheaval, as it played a crucial role in driving this evolutionary process. However, nothing that transpired should have led to the tragic situation involving Alison.

Ben stepped out of his car, ensured that it was securely locked, and walked toward the revolving doors. As he pushed through them, two security guards approached him, their vigilance evident.

"I'm sorry, Mr Tasker, but could you please put on your lanyard?" one of the guards asked.

Ben glanced down at himself and sighed as he pulled his lanyard, which held his ID card, from his jacket pocket. "I guess this is how things will be from now on," he said, fastening it around his neck.

"Our head of security is insisting on it, Mr Tasker; no one is exempt, I'm afraid," the guard explained.

"Lead by example, I understand," Ben replied.

The guards stepped aside to allow him access to the lifts. As he passed the reception desk, he nodded at the staff and pressed the button for the elevator. The main recording studio, located on the ground floor, had a seating capacity of 400. When audiences were present, security was tightened for health and safety reasons; however, currently, only the two guards were stationed at the entrance.

Once the lift doors opened, he stepped inside and pressed the button for the eighth floor.

Upon arriving on his floor and stepping out, he immediately spotted his nameplate on the wall, just above Alison's. To his left was a small reception desk. This floor housed the channel's management offices.

"Ginny," he called to the lady behind the desk.

"Yes, Ben, how can I help?" she replied.

"Could you please ask Andrew from IT to meet me in my office immediately?" he requested.

"Of course," she replied promptly.

He noticed Ginny picking up the phone as he walked past the reception area. As he entered the corridor, he paused briefly outside the first door on the left, which had Alison's name plaque and title displayed in the centre. The Venetian blinds to the right of the door were slightly open, allowing him a glimpse of her desk, which had an empty chair behind it. Rubbing his eyes and forehead, he struggled to believe the situation Alison was facing. Shaking off his thoughts, he quickened his pace and headed decisively to his office at the end of the corridor.

The door to his office was unlocked when he entered. From now on, locking the doors when they are not in the building will become a new routine. He tossed his jacket onto the sofa to his right, walked behind his desk, pulled the chair forward, and took a seat. Pressing the space bar on his keyboard, his computer came to life and prompted him for a password. After entering it, he opened his email system and began scanning for any information that might provide answers. Just then, he heard a knock at the open door.

"Ben, you wanted me?"

He looked up to see Andrew, their head of IT, staring at him.

"Yes, I need your help," Ben replied.

"Sure, what is it? I heard you went to the hospital. What's Alison's condition?"

Ben leaned back in his chair and nodded. "Yes, I went. It's too early to tell. She's in the high-dependency unit and is not currently responsive."

"Christ," Andrew said, leaning against the door. "I don't know what to say."

"None of us do, and that's where you come in."

"What do you mean?"

"The internal computer system has everyone's passwords, right?"

Andrew nodded.

"Good. I need Alison's password. I need to access her computer, specifically her email system."

"Oh…look, Ben, I'd like to help; I really would, but I'm not comfortable doing that."

Ben flicked his head back and frowned. "You listen to me. An attempt has been made on our friend's life! Stop pissing around and get me access to her computer."

"Ben, I'm well aware of what's happening, but ethically, I don't think that's right. I could get into trouble…"

"Trouble? How much trouble do you think we're all in right now? A friend of ours may die. I need to find out if there's something that can help. I want answers, and we all need answers."

Andrew licked his lips, suddenly feeling concerned. His throat became dry. "Respectfully, shouldn't the police be handling this? From what you've told me, I'm surprised they haven't come here yet."

Ben nodded. "It's only a matter of time before they show up. Listen." He beckoned Andrew closer. "Something serious is going on here. This isn't just some angry person from social media with a grudge. She was targeted. Doesn't that tell you something? These things don't just happen. What if she were researching something or sticking her nose where it doesn't belong? We could all be implicated or become targets as well…"

"Alright, alright! You don't need to scare the shit out of me!"

"Good. So, you'll do it then?"

Andrew nodded as Ben rose to his feet. "Andrew, if it makes you feel any better, her contract clearly states that the internal email system and all IT belong to the company."

"Right," Andrew said, straightening up from leaning against the door. He pulled out his phone from his pocket.

"Is that the work phone?" Ben inquired.

Andrew nodded. "I should be able to access the secure database through this phone, so I don't have to go back to my office."

They both walked down the corridor.

"You look tired, Ben," Andrew remarked.

"Yeah, I feel it. I'm honestly bloody terrified," Ben admitted as they paused outside Alison's door. "But you can't tell anyone I said that. We need to keep a cool head for the benefit of the younger staff members."

Andrew glanced at Ben, who was pointing his finger at him. "It's not just the younger staff members you need to worry about," Andrew replied before opening the unlocked door. He pulled the chair away from Alison's desk and pressed the space bar to turn on the computer. "What do you think you're going to find here?" he asked as he settled into the chair.

"Well, I don't expect a professional assassin to have emailed her, but let's hope we can uncover some clues. No one acts without a reason; there must be a trail leading somewhere," Ben said, waving his hands in the air. He knew he was grasping for answers. "If there's something to find, I need to ensure we are informed. When the police arrive, I suspect they'll be taking her computer."

Andrew began tapping buttons on his phone. "Honestly, I'm still surprised they haven't been here already."

"I think they're busy elsewhere, searching her street, car, and house," Ben replied.

"Okay, I have access to our secure server on my phone. There's an encrypted file that contains everyone's passwords. Just give me a few seconds," Andrew said, moving the cursor over a box in the centre of the screen labelled with Alison's name. "Alright, here we go." He clicked on the box, and when the password prompt appeared, he entered her saved password. The password box disappeared, and her tabs opened up. "Alright, we're in. You said you wanted to start by looking at her email?"

Ben moved next to him, leaning down to see the screen. "Yes, please, let's start there."

Andrew clicked on her email icon, and it opened immediately. "Well, not surprisingly, there are hordes of messages coming in," he remarked. The inbox displayed over forty messages, with many more filtered into the junk folder. "Do you recognise any of these names?" he asked.

Ben nodded. "Based on the titles, it seems many people have heard about what happened."

"I recognise a few names too; there are some journalists among them," Andrew added.

"No doubt they're looking for a story. However, I'm not interested in today's messages. Can we scroll down to see if we can find something more relevant?"

"I don't want to rain on your parade, Ben, but there are over two thousand messages in the inbox."

Ben scratched his head in frustration. "Is there any way you can give me remote access to this computer? We could be here for ages otherwise."

"Sure, I can do that. I need to download a program so you can see her screen from your office."

"Great, can you initiate that? Also, could you search for any additional password-protected files?"

Andrew nodded. "That'll take a moment to scan," he said as he grabbed a pen and a piece of paper from the desk. "I should write down her existing password for you, just in case there's a file that uses the same access code she's using."

"Thank you," Ben replied.

"Here, this is her password. Not the best choice, is it?" Andrew handed Ben the piece of paper as he began downloading the remote access app. "Blimey, she's using her husband's name as her password. That's another area of security we need to tighten."

"Yes, it seems that way. If you want to go into your office, I'll send you the remote access code so you can access her computer."

Ben quickly left for his office. "Let me know when you are ready," Andrew shouted down the corridor.

Ben switched on his computer, opened his email, and saw the link come through. "Got it!" he exclaimed, following the link that had been accepted on Alison's computer. Soon, Andrew arrived in his office. "Is it working?" he asked.

"Yes, I can see her screen. I'll start fishing," Ben replied.

"I'm due to finish work in about an hour. Would you like me to stay on?"

Ben shook his head, focused on what he was seeing.

"If you're sure, I can keep my phone on all night if you get stuck," Andrew offered.

"Mmm, thank you."

"Ben," Andrew said.

Ben looked up. "What is it?"

"Given what has happened," Andrew leaned in closer to speak quietly, "if you find anything that directly affects any of us, I have a family. Just saying, will you let me know?"

Ben paused; the weight of what had happened and the implications of what might come next hadn't fully sunk in. He nodded, "Of course, I promise."

Andrew took a deep breath. "Okay, thank you. I'll be on the phone if you need me."

After Andrew left the room, Ben immediately returned to look through the emails.

Chapter Six

Ben was the only person remaining in the building, aside from the security guards downstairs. His eyes were bloodshot from spending the previous few hours sifting through emails on Alison's computer. After flagging several important messages and consuming four cups of coffee, he took a brief break to call his wife, letting her know he was okay and updating her on Alison's condition. He hadn't received any detailed news or heard from Alison's husband, but after receiving an alert on his phone, he decided to watch a police update on a news channel. The report, presented by a senior officer at Scotland Yard, confirmed that a suspicious device had been discovered. However, the reasons for its presence and whether it was related to a targeted attack or terrorism were still under investigation. The officer urged the public to refrain from speculation, stating that more details would be released later. As the waiting press attempted to ask questions, she turned her back and quickly returned to the police station. Ben's wife had also seen the news; he tried to reassure her, but he felt uncertain about the outcome.

Ben wrapped his fingers around the edge of the desk, aware that he needed to act quickly. It was only a matter of time before the police arrived at their offices, and it might not just be Alison's computer that would be seized. He minimised her email window on the screen and began examining the files on her desktop. Most of the titles were related to scheduling, along with several accounting documents and many development files. However, one file titled "personal" stood out like a sore thumb. He couldn't understand why a personal file would be on a work computer and hesitated about whether to open it. Rubbing his eyes, he found himself in a dilemma. As a personal friend, he felt that opening it would be an invasion of her privacy. Leaning forward, he rested his elbows on the desk and buried his head in his hands. He knew he had to do it; the police would open it eventually. Taking a deep breath, he grasped the mouse and clicked, hoping it contained nothing more than pictures of her family. When he opened the file, Ben felt a sense of relief upon discovering a handful of images of her family. However, he noticed another file titled "Upper House," which puzzled him. He hadn't realised she owned two properties. Curious, he opened the file and found just one document inside. As he opened it, a few words appeared in bold: **"If reading this, look in a safe place."**

Rubbing the stubble on his chin, Ben took a deep breath and leaned back in his seat. He sensed that the words held significant importance. Sitting up straight, he opened her email account and typed the word "house" into the search bar, wondering if he had overlooked something. A multitude of messages appeared, with "house" being a common term. He quickly skimmed the results; most were about a late-afternoon program focused on property renovations. After reading a few emails, he realised they were primarily exchanges between the show's producers. He then picked up his mobile and called Julie Bateman, the head commissioner and the woman who had brought Alison into the team. The call was answered immediately, and he could sense her anxiety in her tone. "Have you heard anything further? I saw the police statement on the news."

"The straightforward answer is no. I'm not aware of any information beyond what has already been broadcast. This might sound odd, but I'm reviewing Alison's computer, trying to uncover anything I can."

"Okay, what's your question? What have you found?"

"Well, nothing concrete, but I came across a document that mentions another house. It was in a personal file, but the message is cryptic. Does that mean anything to you? Was she considering investing in another property? Maybe she upset someone. I'm just looking for any clues."

There was a brief silence. "No, she's never mentioned anything like that to me."

"I know you two are very good friends. Can you think of anything at all? I found a document titled 'Upper House' that says, 'If you're reading this, look in a safe place.' Any ideas?"

"If she were buying another property, I'd know. Her relationship with Mike seems solid, as far as I can tell. I don't think she wants to move or separate from him."

Ben began tapping his fingers on the desk again. "Look, it's only a matter of time before the police show up here, and when they do, I suspect they will keep us in the dark. Our newscast is only reporting what everyone else knows. Something serious is going on, something deadly serious. Please try to think. I don't want us or the channel dragged further into this than we already are."

"Those words mean something, Ben, but she's not cryptic. You've seen how terrible she is at quiz nights. Wait, you mentioned a safe place; could she be referring to something, maybe in the basement? The old safe is down there, but I'm pretty sure it's broken. The last time I checked, it didn't lock at all."

Ben's eyes widened. "That seems a bit random, don't you think? But there are no other clues. I'm not finding anything here; I'll go take a look."

"Do you want me to come in? I'm just glued to the news channel. Journalists keep texting me, but I'm not responding."

"No, don't worry. If I find anything, I'll let you know."

"Okay. I'll keep thinking, but I don't know anything about a house, and she's never confided in me about any event that could explain what has happened to her."

Ben rubbed his eyes again. "No, neither do I. I'll be in touch if I find anything. If you think of even the slightest detail, please don't hesitate to call me. My phone will be on all night."

"Mine too. Talk to you later, then."

"Sure, bye for now."

Ben hung up the call and stood up. It was a long shot, but he decided to check the basement; he had nothing else to go on.

++++

It had been a while since Ben last visited the basement, and as he expected, it was a showcase of organised chaos. The vast space was filled with backdrops, props, clothing racks, and what could only be described as disused "vintage" lighting and sound equipment.

He recalled the old safe, a prop from a nineties television series from his younger days. It had been acquired cheaply; while it looked impressive and served their needs, the mechanism was damaged and couldn't be locked properly. He moved to the centre of the floor, placed his hands on his hips, and turned in circles several times. Some items had been rearranged since his last visit. Costumes from the nineties detective drama were now further down on the left. He recognised a backdrop from a key scene in the series, which had experienced declining ratings each week and had run for only one season. The central characters' clothing hung on a rail, each item sealed in a clear bag. For the actors who wore them, the big break they hoped for never came; press reviews labelled the show as crass and old-fashioned. As he moved some of the backdrop away from its propped position, he uncovered a piece of A4 paper with a crudely drawn arrow in the centre. The paper was secured to the wall with tape, and the arrow pointed to the right. He might not have paid much attention to it, but the initials "A.H." were scrawled next to the arrow. The 'H' had a curl at the top, and the capital letters resembled Alison's handwriting, as she always drew her 'H's that way. He shifted the rolled-up backdrops to the side and uncovered a stack of sheets and curtains resting atop a square container covered with a dust sheet. The container was about four feet tall and two feet wide, just as he remembered. Kneeling, he tugged at the bottom of the dust sheet, revealing a thick, exceptionally heavy green safe. He pulled the sheet up and tucked it under the old curtains. Ignoring the dials, he reached for the gold-coloured handle. As he pushed down and turned the handle slightly counterclockwise, he heard a firm click, and the door opened easily. Inside the safe, he discovered empty jewellery boxes, counterfeit banknotes, and a couple of old watches. The drawer at the bottom was empty. He pulled out the contents, still unsure of what he was looking for. The arrow symbol meant something; there had to be something hidden here. Shaking the jewellery boxes yielded nothing, but he noticed one box that was closed and seemingly tucked away. He grabbed it and opened it to find a small plug-in drive, no longer than half an inch. Quickly, he placed it into his pocket and reassembled the safe's contents. After closing the safe's door, he hastily pulled the sheet back down to cover it. Instinctively, he glanced around, feeling nervous about being watched. He was alone, aware that the basement was the only area not monitored by CCTV. He covered the arrow sign with the backdrop and made his way to the lift. Before stepping inside, he tapped his trouser pocket to ensure he hadn't dropped the drive. With a camera inside the lift, he did not want to draw any attention to himself. With little else to focus on, he was conscious that security would be monitoring him; they were likely positioned on the ground floor and would have heard the lift pass by.

He felt his nerves as he tried to appear calm while the lift ascended. Whatever was on this drive had been hidden away for a reason. Although he wasn't a computer expert, just someone who understood the basics, common sense told him not to leave a digital trail, especially given recent events. If he found something important that could help the police, he would share it with them. For now, though, his safety took priority. He decided against opening the drive on a work computer to avoid leaving a trace on the company network.

When the lift doors opened on his floor, he hurried down the corridor to his office and locked the door behind him. He grabbed his personal laptop from its bag, switched off the built-in camera, and disconnected from the internet. He scratched his head and let out a sigh, fully aware that he had no idea what he was doing. Taking a deep breath, he inserted the USB drive. His laptop recognised the device, and he clicked nervously, waiting to see what would appear. There was only one file on the drive, titled "Upper House." Relieved, he knew he had found a crucial piece of the cryptic puzzle. He opened the file, hoping to find some answers. A multitude of files appeared on the screen; he noticed several Word documents, one of which stood out, titled "Proposal," along with dozens of screenshots that seemed to be copies of email chains.

He opened a video file first and noted its poor quality; it resembled footage from a hidden camera worn by someone. He saw what appeared to be a female hand knocking on a door. Despite the low sound quality, he barely heard the word "Come" as the woman opened the door. Leaning closer to the screen, he recognised the person sitting behind the desk: Sebastian Hetfield, the Member of Parliament and the government's Chief Whip. As the woman took a seat, Ben, drawing on his years of experience as a political journalist and later as a TV producer, realised that this footage had been covertly filmed inside the Houses of Parliament. The Chief Whip was visibly angry, berating the woman sitting across from him. Their discussion revolved around issues related to the pharmaceutical trade. He referenced a specific company and the amount it had donated to the party, claiming she was "unbalancing their position." The woman defended herself, noting that a couple of members of the House of Lords were paid consultants to that company, mentioning that the Prime Minister was also involved. The Chief Whip looked furious. Ben was taken aback when he heard Alison's name mentioned in their conversation, as the Chief Whip told the woman to "distance herself from that bloody meddling woman."

Ben rubbed his head in worry, unsure of what he was witnessing. He paused the video, minimised it from the screen, and opened the first screenshot of the email chain. "Oh God," he muttered, rubbing his lips as he recognised who Alison had been communicating with. In an instant, he understood the term "Upper House." It referred to Helen Lord MP, and the Upper House meant the House of Lords. The email chain mentioned a source; whoever or whatever this source was, it remained unnamed, but the conversation hinted at a new cosmetic beauty filler that contained a highly addictive component. If he understood correctly, the notes implied that a drug was concealed within the filler. Puzzled, he scratched his head, trying to comprehend the situation. He browsed through a few more screenshots, and one in particular stood out: a comment about "no further communications." He guessed this was related to the source; the MP had been trying to contact them, but all communication had ceased. The email expressed concern about something that might have happened to the source. There was a reference to a location in South America and "the labs."

Clearing the previous image, he noticed another screenshot that appeared to be a diagnostic printout. He opened it, revealing a scientific breakdown of what he presumed were the core components of a substance. The image was crooked, as if it had been taken quickly. The printout was titled "Lipomorphilas Filler," and at the bottom, it featured the logo of a pharmaceutical company, with the company's name written beneath it. This was the same company mentioned in the covert video. Not being a biochemist, Ben had no idea what the schematic meant. It listed various chemical compounds and elements from the periodic table. It had been a while since he was last in a classroom, and he was none the wiser.

He continued scanning the screenshots. The conversations between Alison and Helen grew more urgent over time. There were gaps in the dialogue, suggesting they had been speaking on the phone as well as meeting in person.

He then opened another video file featuring a man talking to the camera. The quality suggested he was recording with his laptop. The man spoke alone, with no one responding to him; it was a recorded message, and his name was not displayed on the screen. The man was sitting outside, seemingly at a coffee shop. He nervously surveyed the road, constantly glancing over his shoulder. Whenever someone walked by, he would abruptly stop talking. Occasional cars passed in the background, their license plates clearly from a foreign country, and you could also hear snippets of conversation, possibly in Spanish. The man spoke excellent English, but he appeared anxious, his face pale and gaunt. Much of what he said was difficult to follow as he frequently referenced previous conversations or messages. Despite this, Ben seemed to grasp the main points as the man spoke closely to the camera.

"The product has been in development for over eighteen months. In the initial stages, we encountered complications that forced us to move to human trials." He looked pained as he carefully chose his words. "Our security team recruited individuals from the streets, those who would go unnoticed: drug addicts, prostitutes, and street kids without families who were desperate to survive." He turned to glance behind him again, his anxiety palpable. "Promises were made; they were offered money in exchange for their participation. They were required to attend the clinic every week for observations; that was the arrangement. However, the first batch was a complete failure. There was too much product, leading to rapid distortion of the user's facial features and an acceleration in their addictions. Many failed to attend their scheduled appointments, and several individuals were lost, later found dead in backstreets. Initially, the causes of their deaths were unclear. A couple of the cadavers were brought in for examination, while the others remained on the streets, their deaths attributed to drug addiction. We discovered that the victims suffered from bleeding in the brain, which led to catastrophic failures. Others experienced heart attacks, and some overdosed on the main drug component while on the streets. Their immune systems failed, and the distortions of their faces rendered them unrecognisable. After compiling the results, the bodies were disposed of. We also encountered challenges in the labs with the live subjects. They often arrived in an irrational state, sweating profusely and desperate for their next treatment. The situation became unmanageable and needed to be stopped." The man wiped the sweat from his forehead, took a sip of coffee, and took a deep breath. "The research and development team were well compensated; no one spoke up, and enormous pressure was placed on all of us. We were too afraid to leave. Most of our team members have strong academic backgrounds and come from respected families. Threats have been made against us and our families. I am the only one not from this country, but those making the threats have significant resources and can find anyone, anywhere. We also have another problem: new security forces, known as the Kaibiles, have been deployed. They are the Guatemalan Special Forces, and they are serious. Their motto is something like, "If I advance, follow me. If I stop, push me. If I retreat, kill me!" That is what I'm dealing with, and I believe they are onto me; they know I'm not married and have no children. I feel as though I'm being watched at every turn, and I'm worried they can access my communications. That is why this will be my last message. You must expose this before there are mass casualties." He paused again. "About four months ago, we had our first successful candidate, a woman in her early thirties who worked as a prostitute. She was brought in and paid for her participation. Unlike many others, she was a low-level drug user, street-smart, and willing to do anything for her family. This is where the project started to escalate. She had filler injections in her face, which were successful; they tightened her skin, and she claimed to look younger. Initially, we monitored her closely in the lab, noting that her mood was generally excellent. She was happy, ate well, drank well, and felt both physically and mentally capable. However, this positivity only lasted for about three weeks. After that, she began to crash, exhibiting symptoms similar to those of previous subjects. Filler is usually administered every few months, or even more frequently, depending on the patient's needs. But she craved more, so we provided it. Her mood would improve instantly, but it was a repetitive cycle, and she would attend the lab days before she was due, and her visits became more frequent every time. The core ingredient of the filler was feeding directly into her brain, and it began to take over. She became addicted without even realising it, becoming a slave to her own mind." He paused, his face showing immediate concern. "I've got to go." Ben saw the man's arm rise as the camera cut out when he closed the laptop. Ben leaned back in his chair, his hands shaking as he took a bottle of whiskey from his drawer and took a large swig. "Jesus, Alison, what the hell have you gotten yourself into?" He placed the bottle on the desk and began scanning through the other files. His cursor hovered over the file titled "Proposal." When he opened it, his heart raced, and beads of sweat formed on his forehead. After finishing the document, he immediately pushed the laptop away and slumped in his seat, panic stricken. His hands trembled as he processed what he had just read; it was something he almost wished he hadn't seen. The proposal revealed that an informer had exposed a deliberately contaminated cosmetic filler that was set to enter the market. This chemically altered product would be disguised within an existing approved product to evade detection. Ben buried his face in his hands, suddenly realising the gravity of the situation. The new filler contained a hidden property that was highly addictive. It would be contaminated with a derivative of heroin, and the whistleblower had worked in the lab where it was developed. The implications could affect tens of thousands of people, potentially triggering a new opioid crisis.

People would be unknowingly consuming heroin, and Helen and Alison were planning to make a documentary about it.

Chapter Seven

"Bonjour, frère. Peux-tu parler?"

"Yes, brother, I can talk."

David was pleased that Rubin had answered the phone so quickly. "It's been a while."

"That it has. I'm guessing this is not a social call."

"Just wondering if you're still working? I have something in your usual line."

"Yes, occasionally. I'm more selective with my projects now. I don't spend much time in the UK; I try to avoid it."

"I understand. Are you open to a meeting? I don't want to discuss this via these means. It's well-paid."

There was a brief silence on the other end of the line. "Is it in the UK?"

"Yes, just outside the capital for the first phase, and inside the capital thereafter."

"How long will it take?"

"Just an action, no longer than a week; it will require your complicated toys, though, as an area needs to be checked over."

"How many subjects?"

"Just one. Male. But before that, your specialist equipment is needed for room sterilisation."

There was another brief pause on the line.

Truth be told, David needed Rubin; he didn't have the specialised surveillance-detection equipment Rubin had. He had told Darius, his client, that he had contacts in this field, but for this specific task, Rubin was his first choice. Finding specialists in tactical surveillance countermeasures in the UK was challenging, and contacting others abroad, especially those outside his usual network, posed risks he preferred to avoid. Being skilled in the field was one thing, but ensuring that no information was leaked was entirely different. Confidentiality was expected to last a lifetime, often sealed with a simple handshake. However, there were occasionally rogues in the industry, typically those without military backgrounds, whom David didn't trust. In this business, personal recommendations were crucial; when you vouch for someone, your word is your bond. Despite Rubin's past failings, David had heard that, having found peace in his religion, Rubin could be trusted once again. The silence on the phone indicated that Rubin would need further incentive. "When you are outside the UK, the funds will enable a substantial donation to your cause."

"I'll pack for a week and come to hear you out. If I don't like what I hear, I'll walk away. Regardless, you will still be responsible for my time, so be prepared to have sufficient funds on hand. Those are my terms, agreed?"

"Of course. Those are the terms I was expecting," David replied.

"Alright. Is the old place still available for us to meet?"

"It is. Thank you, brother."

"We haven't worked together for some time, and my fees have increased since then. I trust that won't be an issue."

"It's not," David assured him.

"I'll be there tomorrow morning at seven."

"Seven it is. See you tomorrow, brother."

David hung up and put his phone back in his pocket. He had no idea where Rubin lived now; it could be Nepal, but he was glad to have caught him in the country. Rubin's tone and concise words indicated that he was back to his old self, focused and money-oriented. It was a relief that Rubin mentioned money a couple of times; that meant he could be bought. Although they had worked and fought together in the past, David wasn't keen on Rubin staying at his home or knowing his address. Both men respected their professional roles and each other's privacy. The meeting place in the morning was only about an hour from David's home, and he planned to pack for a week and bring his own equipment. He would also need to carry a substantial amount of cash.

++++

Dr John Farmer had finished his consultancy work for the day. As he opened his email account for Knightark Pharmaceutical, he noticed a familiar email subject line: *"Invitation to a Reception with Lord Gatesouth and Lord* Hawthorne a*t the House of Lords."* It had been many years since he received his first invitation to Parliament, before his involvement with Knightark. Back then, he accompanied his father, who relished the pomp and enjoyed being surrounded by "like-minded people." This would be the first of many evenings he spent either in the Lords or in the House of Commons. However, the initial enthusiasm for such invitations had long since faded. They were more of a tactic to drum up business, an opportunity to wine and dine investors. Distributors and a select few who were at the top of their profession were invited, including doctors, surgeons, and pioneers in the cosmetic industry. Their sales agents competed fiercely to secure these sought-after invitations. Their gatherings were glorified social events, filled with eloquent speakers and predominantly privately educated men. He was acutely aware that he fit some of that description.

He had a reasonable relationship with Lord Hawthorne, but he found Lord Gatesouth to be prickly and difficult to engage in conversation. John was under no illusions; for both Lords, it was primarily a financial arrangement. They served as 'consultants' to the company and were well compensated for their services. However, what they declared on the parliamentary register of financial interests did not accurately reflect their actual earnings. Since joining the board, John had gradually become aware of these issues, including undisclosed cash donations. It was simply a matter of creative accounting, and to be honest, he didn't have a strong opinion about it. This was how their business operated, and having strategic individuals in key positions was a wise investment to protect the company. They were consistently regarded as paid "assets," and as he spent more time on the board, he found himself gradually being drawn into their circle. He knew that Darius and both of their 'consultants' in the Lords had attended the same college, along with the current Prime Minister. He had been educated abroad, and despite having attended private schools, his presence made some of the others uneasy; he was seen as an "outsider." His father had to advocate for his appointment to the board since he was not part of their close-knit group. Along with three other senior board members, he felt that Darius and his privately educated friends withheld information from him. The bond among the four was strong and unbreakable. He couldn't quite identify it, but the company's financial struggles were not his only concern; he sensed that much was being left unsaid and that decisions were being made without his or the other board members' approval. He suspected that other board members felt similarly, but the subject was never brought up, and he had no close relationships with any of them.

With the upcoming board meeting just two days away, he decided to wait and see what was discussed there before deciding whether to accept the Lord's invitation.

✣✣✣✣

The television was turned down immediately. "It's fair to say you've attracted quite a bit of attention!"

Helen closed the door to her office in Portcullis House and smiled at Joanne, her most trusted research assistant. "What's being said?"

"What's not being said, I think you mean," Joanne responded as she turned the small television on her desk towards Helen. "You've completely dominated the news. The only topic of discussion is you, Alison Harwood, and the Prime Minister not answering your question."

This political TV program airs for thirty minutes following Prime Minister's Questions every Wednesday when parliament is sitting. In addition to the presenter, current and former MPs offer commentary. Most often, the show evaluates the Prime Minister's performance. However, today the focus has shifted, thanks to Helen Lord MP.

Joanne had been working as a researcher for Helen since the beginning of Helen's first term in office. She was one of the few people Helen trusted. Her other researcher, Tobias, was out of the office, likely during his lunch break. He had only been working with her for seven weeks, so Helen was careful about what she said around him. Parliament was filled with spies and gossip, and some researchers could switch allegiances more rapidly than the weather could change. Many did not stay loyal to a single political party.

"Can you turn that up, please?" Helen asked as she dropped her bag on the table, kicked off her shoes, and took a seat. "That media leech will do anything to get on TV." She was referring to a former MP who had lost his seat in the last election and had since found himself in a career crisis. She had heard that he spent thousands of pounds each month on a public relations agency to keep himself in the news. His political career was over, and it was only a matter of time before he appeared on a television show, such as one featuring dancing or ice skating, earning a new title: "celebrity."

Joanne increased the volume. The former MP was speaking, addressing Helen's behaviour in the Commons chamber. "Well, I just don't agree; the Prime Minister should be challenged, but being ambushed by one of his own MPs…" He shook his head. "You can bet that right now, the Prime Minister is surrounded by advisors figuring out how to handle her not following the party line. Her whole persona has changed; she has become some misplaced comedy character. This isn't the Helen that I remember."

Helen laughed, "You didn't even know me!"

"But what's happening is incredibly serious. A professional attempt on a public figure's life has taken place," the presenter stated.

"Indeed," the former MP replied. "The Prime Minister will likely need to address this matter in some way. However, challenging the Prime Minister in the chamber regarding something this serious is poor protocol. This is a highly sensitive case, and the police would be better off without MPs sharing their personal opinions. Let the professionals do their job, and we can comment once the facts are known."

Helen chuckled again. "That's rich coming from him. Can you turn it down? I've heard enough of that."

Joanne smiled and muted the volume. "What happens now?" she asked. "I've stopped answering the phones and turned off the ringer. Do you see the red lights flashing?"

Helen nodded in response.

"It's all journalists; my email is going crazy, too. Everyone wants to interview you. I've received a couple of messages from individuals claiming to live in the constituency, asking for appointments during your surgery this coming Friday. One message concerns the relief road, and the other is a complaint about fly-tipping. However, the emails are too polished in tone; they sound like professionals wrote them. I suspect they might be journalists trying to catch you off guard. I'm worried that anyone who meets with you now could be wearing a hidden camera to gather information for a story. I think it would be wise to revisit your security arrangements with the Serjeant at Arms Department."

Helen understood. "I appreciate your perspective; I truly do. You know that Alison has been in the office a few times."

Joanne nodded. "Of course."

"But given the nature of our discussions, I can't share everything with you."

"I figured as much. You always close the door when she arrives. Is there something you want to confide in me?"

Helen took a deep breath and leaned back in her chair. "I think it's best if I don't share anything right now, especially with journalists probing for information. There's no easy way to say this, but I want you to be careful."

"Me?" Joanne exclaimed, taken aback and looking perplexed.

Helen nodded, her face showing concern. "I mean it. We've worked together for a long time. I value your perspective; you are loyal and honest. However, could you listen to me for a moment? Alison and I are onto something serious, something that could be significant. You are known as my researcher, and that's a matter of public record. Please be careful about whom you talk to, and be cautious of anyone who suddenly comes into your life wanting to strike up a conversation..."

Joanne's jaw dropped. "What!"

"I'm serious. I believe what we know could explain what has happened to Alison."

"Bloody hell, are you serious?" Joanne replied, her tone filled with disbelief.

At that moment, the door opened, and Tobias walked in after his lunch break. The conversation stopped abruptly.

"Wow, that was brave!" Tobias said, smiling widely. At only seventeen and studying politics at Durham University, his work experience period was nearing its end.

Helen gathered her shoes and stood up. "Sometimes, you have to stand up for what you believe in."

Tobias nodded in agreement, but couldn't help but sense the tension in the room.

++++

THE FOLLOWING MORNING, 7 AM: DARENTH, KENT—THIRTY-FIVE MINUTES FROM CENTRAL LONDON

"I take it you're still wasting your time fishing?"

David turned, not hearing that he had been approached. He

quickly glanced around to make sure the anglers on the lake weren't watching. Satisfied, he stood up and shook hands with his old friend. "I haven't had much time for that lately."

Rubin placed a large work bag on the ground alongside a heavy, protected case. He removed his backpack and took a seat next to David on the bench.

"How did you get here?" David asked.

"Bus and taxi. I try not to use a car here; there are too many paper trails to follow, and there are cameras everywhere in this country now. I prefer to avoid the law."

David nodded in understanding, noting that his colleague had more scars than the last time they had met.

"I haven't heard from you in a long time. So, what do you have for me?" Rubin asked.

David smiled. "Straight to business, then."

"Time is money, and that's why I'm here. I don't enjoy working anymore, or even being in this country, for that matter. The job offers little satisfaction; I'm tired of cleaning up the mess created by others."

"It's that mess that pays our bills. But fair enough. This task is a bit outside my scope and more in your area. It's a two-part assignment: first, boardroom sterilisation, and second, surveillance on an individual."

Rubin looked surprised. "Surely you've cleaned rooms before; you've been in this game long enough."

David nodded. "Of course, but this requires extra assurance. My equipment is old, and I rely on trusted techniques, some of which many would consider antiquated."

Rubin nodded. "So, you're still searching by hand?"

"Mostly, yes."

Rubin laughed out loud and shook his head. "Very time consuming in this age, and there are no guarantees of success. A room remains sterile only until someone enters it. But of course, that's an outdated way of thinking. I've had to learn and adapt; I think outside the box, not just inside it. You suspect that someone wants to listen in on your client. Are there trade secrets involved? Is there a direct threat, or does their line of business conflict with others? I need to understand the methodology."

"Their business is definitely competitive. From what I understand, they are looking to bring a new product to market," David responded.

"Okay, so we're talking about brand and patent protection. But I need to know: do their competitors have people like us? Are we likely being surveilled, or do we need to counter-survey them?" Rubin asked.

"I haven't been informed of any such situation, nor have I seen any evidence suggesting it. They've been a client of mine for several years now, and I solve their problems," David replied.

Rubin nodded. "But you don't think you're capable of handling this?"

David didn't care for the tone of Rubin's voice; his disdain for the problem-solving business was evident. He looked his military brother in the eyes. "That's not what I'm saying. I'm just making sure there are no issues. Also, this matter is time-sensitive. The board wishes to meet this evening."

Rubin raised an eyebrow. "Sounds to me like someone is panicking; something has hit the fan or is about to. That's no time to plan, assess, or implement control measures. If I weren't here, you'd struggle to clean up in such a short timeframe."

"Trust me, I'm well aware. That's why I called you; your speciality lies within TSCM."

"Is the meeting at their headquarters or in a building they own?" Rubin inquired.

"No, that's the difference. They usually would use their own offices, but for some reason, they don't want to this time."

"You don't know why?"

David shook his head.

"It sounds to me like you're being kept out of the loop, which concerns me, but that's more your issue than mine. Conducting a thorough sweep of the room isn't a problem; that's not unlawful. However, the other matter you mentioned could be illegal, depending on the target and the actions required. Often, laws need to be bent to achieve a result, and I don't want any heat from it."

"Understood. For the first phase, they've rented the entire floor of a hotel. They've informed me that their internal security will visit later to monitor the floor and the surrounding area. The second matter is different altogether, a person who isn't associated with the company. A person putting their nose where they don't want it, we'll be looking for anything we can use against him."

"First of all, does your client's internal security team know about us and what we do? Secondly, can't they conduct a room sweep? Are they former military?"

"I don't know much about them; they handle property management and close protection services. I've seen a few of them from a distance, and they look military, but the client has approached me for this service."

Rubin nodded. "And thirdly, what is the profession of the subject you want to place under surveillance? Does he have a public profile or attract attention?"

"No, he's a family man. He's a former TV producer who worked his way up at a television channel."

Rubin's tone shifted. "Was he a former journalist? Many of them are."

"Yes, I've been running checks on him since I received his name."

"You know as well as I do that journalists are often surveillance aware; this could be tricky. It's not helped by the amateur who made a bollocks of that car bomb yesterday. Every dick and his dog associated with the media will be on high alert now."

David looked away. He had thought about informing his old colleague about what had happened, especially considering the close connection between Alison and Ben. Sooner or later, Rubin would piece it together.

"Let's address your boardroom problem first. I'm fine with that.

As for the other matter, I want to wait until I have more information. Where is the location? And I trust you brought cash with you?"

"The hotel is about fifteen miles from here, just outside Bromley in Kent. And yes, I have cash with me. If you agree, we need to go immediately."

"You need to coordinate with your client regarding their security. We'll go in and out. Once we're done, the room will no longer be my responsibility; after that, it will be up to them to take care of it, unless you plan to handle that yourself?" Rubin asserted.

"I'll check with my client to see what they want. How much do you need?"

"For complete room sterilisation for both passive and non-passive bugs that can transmit across all mediums, including FM, UHF, and GSM, I have a spectrum analyser, a thermal imaging camera, a non-linear junction detector, and other high-spec equipment. Additionally, I will secure the windows. The total cost will be six thousand pounds. I'll need to consider the other matter later."

David's expression was stoic.

"What did you expect, brother? This equipment costs in the tens of thousands."

Six thousand pounds for what would be less than a day's work seemed excessive. David looked around; in the distance, an angler stood on the opposite side of the lake. He couldn't see anyone else as he pulled out bundles of used twenty-pound notes from his jacket and counted out the amount Rubin requested. Rubin's charges were exorbitant, and he dreaded the costs for the other work, but he felt he had little choice.

++++

Ben woke up early and studied his reflection in the bathroom mirror. He had struggled to sleep the night before, his thoughts dwelling on Alison. His wife, Julie, had questioned him for over an hour about Alison and had also commented on the smell of whisky on his breath. So far, he had been economical with the truth.

His phone had remained silent beside his bed throughout the night; there were no updates on Alison's condition. As a friend, he hoped she would improve and pull through. He desperately wanted to talk to her, especially with the information he now possessed.

With tired eyes and dark bags beneath them, he brushed his teeth, wrestling with confusion. Alison would never be able to make a documentary about the contaminated filler; it didn't work that way. An exposé wouldn't just materialise out of nowhere, and she understood that. It would require financing and board approval. He had seen no evidence of financial backing or involvement with a production company. Even with a sponsor, whether private or commercial, programs still took months to get off the ground. Making such serious accusations would need to be reviewed by the board and require consent from their legal team. The mere thought of a heroin derivative being hidden in plain sight put everyone involved in the documentary at significant risk. The whistleblower, whose identity remained unknown, had vanished, leaving Helen, the MP, in a state of distress. The tone of their email communications had become frantic; perhaps they had taken on more than they could handle. Although they had used innocuous email addresses and fictitious names, their IP addresses could still be traced if someone chose to make the effort. From his experience as a journalist, he knew that MPs were often not very tech-savvy, and Alison indeed fell into that category as well. He wasn't entirely sure due to gaps in their communications, but it appeared that the source had initially contacted Alison. This was presumably because she had taken a public stance against the cosmetic pharmaceutical trade; her personal war on the beauty industry must have caught the lab technician's attention. Reading between the lines, it seemed that Alison had involved the MP, who publicly supported her campaign. Now, both of them had meddled with the wrong people, and their attempts to cover their tracks had likely failed. It was impossible to predict how this situation would unfold. As the senior executive at Channel 8, he wondered if he was next on their list. Until the night before, he had been unaware of any of this. Did these people know that?

He dressed as quietly as possible. It was just 6 a.m., and Julie was still sleeping in their bed. Aside from her concern for Alison, she lay blissfully unaware of the unfolding situation. He needed to keep her in the dark for now, not just for her sake but also for the children's. He would have to speak with their security company, as their home security measures were practically non-existent.

After getting dressed and wanting to avoid conversation, he unplugged his phone, put on his watch, and quietly left the bedroom. He checked on both children and felt relieved to find them sound asleep. He planned to grab a coffee before heading out, contemplating his next steps.

Downstairs, he let the cat out and turned on the coffee machine; he desperately needed an espresso, fully aware that today would be long and challenging. Feeling nauseous, eating was the last thing on his mind. He had to consider whether the evidence he found should be taken to the police. Common sense told him yes, but his former journalistic instincts urged him to hold off and think it through. He added a couple of large spoonfuls of sugar to his espresso and leaned against the kitchen countertop, relishing a rare moment of silence in a house with two young children. He grimaced after tasting the overly strong and sugary coffee. The only other person he knew involved in this situation was Helen. He had met the MP once before, and Alison often spoke of her; a friendship was developing between them. However, he had no idea that Alison had been going to the Commons to meet with Helen. He thought of Helen as a decent person, but, like many career politicians, he held a reserved opinion of them, often viewing many of them as turncoats. Initially, he had read Helen like a book. She was a backbench MP, but her drive and charisma suggested that she could rise through the government ranks if she chose to do so. This new revelation changed everything.

After finishing the terrible coffee, he grabbed his jacket and left a note for Julie, saying he had been called into work. He added that he loved her and would be in touch later.

He had made up his mind: he needed to go to the Commons to demand a meeting with Helen. Whether or not he would involve the police would depend on how deep the rabbit hole went.

Chapter Eight

"I've arranged for one of my client's security team to meet us outside the hotel," David said as he parked the car on a side road. "It doesn't look like there are any obvious cameras here."

Rubin laughed as he studied the side of the hotel. "Exactly what level of client are you dealing with, David? This place looks like a shithole!"

"They are meeting discreetly; they don't want to attract attention."

"And yet they booked an entire floor and brought their own security. That doesn't sound very discreet to me. We're all going to stand out like sore thumbs. I wouldn't even stay here."

David frowned and turned to look Rubin in the eyes. "I thought you'd found God or something and were leading a frugal life now, that's what I heard."

Rubin paused. "Well, yes… when I'm at home, but when I'm working, I prefer a nice place."

"Nepal, isn't it?"

Rubin ignored the question, nudged David's arm, and rolled down the window as a military-looking man approached them.

"Good morning, gentlemen. Is one of you David?" he asked.

David nodded in response from behind the window.

"Good. I'll show you to the meeting room, and then I'll leave you in peace to work. The elevators are ready to take you up," he said.

"Thank you, we appreciate that," David replied.

"Do you need a hand with your equipment?" he asked.

"No, we've got it," Rubin responded abruptly, causing David to give him a surprised look.

"However, David, you can help me with the main case; it's quite heavy. There are probably cameras out front," Rubin said as he leaned over to the back seat to retrieve a cap from his backpack. "I trust you have one of these with you?" he asked.

David unclipped his seatbelt. "Yes, I have one in the back," he replied as they stepped out of the car and out of earshot of the security man.

Rubin opened the back door, carefully placed his work bag and case on the ground, then put on his backpack. David grabbed a baseball cap from the back seat, put it on, and pulled it down as far as he could to shield his face from any cameras.

"Well, this isn't a great start, is it?" Rubin commented.

"What do you mean?" David asked.

"A rundown hotel and a guy who doesn't know us from Adam just asked if you're David. You could be anyone; it's not like he has your picture or knows what you look like."

David closed the car door. "I noticed that too, but we're here now, so let's follow him and get this done."

✢✢✢✢

Ben swiped his debit card at the exit barrier of Westminster tube station. Still underground, he ignored the public signs directing him to the Palace of Westminster and walked a short distance to the right. There, he found the private entrance for members of parliament and palace staff. Two armed police officers stood next to the revolving door. They were not always stationed there, but since the police had not released any further information about the suspicious explosion on Alison's road, a terrorist incident had not yet been ruled out. As a result, he expected to see an increased police presence around the capital's landmarks that day.

It was just before 9 a.m., and he hoped that Helen would be at the Palace today. Typically, on Thursdays, MPs were quick to leave Parliament to return to their constituencies for their Friday surgeries. He had read that there was discontent within Helen's constituency of Shrewsbury. Her involvement in the so-called "beauty war" had overshadowed the local issues she should be focusing on.

As he pulled his phone out of his jacket pocket, he noticed the police officers watching him closely. This was not a place to linger, and he didn't doubt that the surrounding CCTV was monitoring his every move. He walked past the officers and went up the stairway to ground level. Once there, he crossed the road, weaving through the gridlocked cars, and stood next to Westminster Pier. The Victoria Embankment was crowded at the start of the workday; even tourists were out early, taking pictures of the Palace and Big Ben before the rain that was forecast for later in the day. He looked up at Portcullis House, uncertain of the location of Helen's office within the vast building. Standing so close to the parliamentary estate, he knew it wouldn't be long before someone approached him if he continued to loiter. He walked to the corner, glanced at Big Ben, and dialled his office, knowing that his personal assistant should already be at work.

"Good morning, Ben Tasker's office," came the response.

"Hi, it's me. I'm glad you're in. Have you seen any of the others yet?" he asked.

"Jennie and Debbie are here somewhere. Do you need to speak to either of them? It sounds very noisy where you are," she replied.

"Yes, I'm in Westminster. I need to see someone."

"You know you have a meeting scheduled for ten o'clock. The PR agency wanted to meet with you online."

Ben rubbed his forehead. "Crap, I completely forgot. With everything that's happening, I'm surprised they still want to proceed. Please cancel it. If they want to improve their PR, they should start by watching the news!"

"Okay, I'll take care of that right away."

"I called to find out if anyone has heard any updates about Alison. Any news?"

"I asked Debbie and Jennie when they arrived this morning, and neither of them had heard anything. I'm assuming that means you haven't either?"

Ben glanced around. While he wasn't breaking any laws by standing where he was, he felt uncomfortable, deeply troubled, and paranoid about what he knew. "No, I haven't heard anything. Can I ask a favour? Could you text me the phone number for Helen Lord MP, specifically her London office, not her constituency office? It should be available online."

"Sure, I can find that for you now. She was mentioned on the news last night due to her actions in Parliament, where she referenced Alison."

"Yes, I'm aware. They were close to each other, apparently. I want to see if she knows anything."

"Okay, bear with me for a second... Right, yes, I have both numbers. I'll text you her Westminster number now. Will you be in later?"

Ben saw the number appear on his screen. "Look, I'm not sure. Can you cancel any appointments I had scheduled? I'm sure everyone will understand. Please also notify the senior team. Only contact me if it's urgent. I need to check on a few things."

"Of course, I'm certain everyone will understand. Are you going to see Alison?"

"I'm not sure yet. I'll try to contact her husband. If I get any updates, I will let you know."

"Thank you. I'm sure everyone, including myself, will appreciate that."

Ben turned around again. As far as he could tell, no one was watching him. "Look," he said, scratching his head, "this is going to sound odd." He immediately froze as a police siren blared beside him, and his hands shook with anxiety.

"Ben, are you there?"

He heard the words and swallowed with relief as cars parted to let the marked metropolitan police car through the traffic. "Um, yes… still here. Look, if you don't hear from me again…"

"What?"

"Yeah, listen, I know this is weird, and please don't repeat this to anyone. But something's going on. Just let people know that Westminster was the last place you heard from me, okay?"

"Um… God, are you okay? You're scaring me."

"Yeah, yes. I'm sure I'm fine, but… I have some concerns. What happened to Alison was hardly an accident. Anyway, thanks for the number; I have to go now. Bye."

"Um, okay, bye."

Realising he'd probably just frightened his personal assistant, he hoped she would keep what he said to herself. He also wished she wouldn't hand in her notice. He opened her text message and called the number. He glanced up at the iconic clock again, feeling a nervousness he hadn't experienced in years. He felt nauseous, as if he might be sick at any moment.

"Office of Helen Lord MP." The phone was answered by a young man, likely a researcher for the MP.

"Is Helen available, please?"

"What is this in connection with, please?"

"Look, if she's there, just put her on, will you? I don't have her mobile number. It's a private matter."

"Sir, we are currently inundated with people wishing to speak to Miss Lord."

"I just told you it's a private matter."

"Would you like to make an appointment at her constituency office?"

"What! No, can you please just put her on? It's urgent."

"Sir, I'm sorry, but I cannot confirm or deny whether she is here. GDPR regulations prohibit me from doing so, and I also do not know who you are."

Frustrated by the young man's condescending tone, Ben's patience wore thin. "Stop pissing around, you little prick, and put her on."

"Excuse me!"

"You heard me. Put her on; it's Ben, Alison Harwood's boss. I trust you know that name!"

There was a brief pause. "Putting you on hold."

Ben took a deep breath as he paced back and forth on the pavement. It was unlike him to speak to strangers that way; the young man was doing his job. However, with a dry throat, shaky hands, and an elevated pulse, he didn't have time for niceties.

"Ben?"

He recognised Helen's voice immediately. "Praise the Lord, I'm glad I got through to you."

"What is it? Have you heard anything further about Alison?"

He heard another police siren in the distance and turned around. He could feel himself perspiring. "No, nothing. Have you?"

"Not a thing. I'm in the office early, trying to find out what's going on. I'm liaising with the police as well, but I haven't heard anything yet, I'm afraid."

"I need to see you."

"Okay, of course. I'll only be at Portcullis for a few hours before heading to my constituency. Would you like to come in next week? My researcher can set up an appointment for you."

"No, I need to see you now. Right now."

"Ben, look, this is a difficult time, and I'm really worried about Alison. I'm doing everything I can from my end. I have a hectic morning ahead before catching the train back this afternoon."

"I don't think you understand. I need to see you right now!"

"Ben, I know how much you care for Alison..."

"I know!"

He heard a faint, unconvincing laugh from Helen on the other end. "Is there something I can assist you with?"

"No. I know! I'm not going into details over the phone."

There was silence on the other end.

"I know everything. I know what you two have been planning, and you will see me now!"

++++

David nodded at the security guard as he closed the door behind him.

"Alright, let's see what we have," Rubin said while assessing the meeting room and unzipping his work bag. "I need to set up my laptop and some other equipment. Here, catch this," he added, throwing a rolled-up utility belt to David. "Before you start your physical search, I want you to unscrew every plug point and switch in this room. It doesn't look like there are any adjoining rooms, and there's only one way in and out. The ceiling appears solid, which is a good sign, but we'll still need to verify it. Additionally, remove the brackets underneath the main lights. At first glance, it does not appear that there is a phone line here, which is unusual but will save us time since it is one less thing to check. The television set needs to be taken outside, along with any other items that could potentially contain a device. We are stripping this room down to the bare essentials."

David began to pull at the Velcro strips and took out a couple of screwdrivers.

"After you've done that, start at the top of the room and work your way around in circles, going clockwise and lowering your focus with each turn. You'll end at the bottom near the skirting boards, where we'll look for any cabling behind them as well."

David smiled but shook his head in annoyance. "I know how to search a room; you don't need to advise me."

"This is what you're paying for, David. I appreciate that it's your client, but if you don't mind, let me handle this phase," Rubin replied.

David approached the first socket and began unscrewing the wall cover. "Don't you need to be a qualified electrician to do this?"

Rubin looked up from his laptop. "It helps, along with an understanding of telecoms. I took a crash course in both subjects a few years ago. I'm qualified in what I need to know. You do realise that if anyone leaves this room, even for a moment, to use the toilet or something similar, the room will no longer be sterile. Will your client be searching his guests or removing their phones?"

"I don't know the answer to that. I will be discussing it and putting some standard operating procedures in place for the security team."

"Military or not, they haven't impressed me so far," Rubin said, taking off his cap and picking up his protective case.

David pulled the plastic fitting away from the wall and stood up. "Do you mind if I take a look at your gear?"

Rubin shrugged. "Be my guest. I know this isn't your area of expertise, so I'll give you a brief overview of what I have. There's one piece of equipment I want you to use."

David dropped the screwdrivers on the table as Rubin retrieved the spectrum analyser from the case.

"I'll be using this," Rubin said. "I just need to get the laptop sorted out as well. Here, slide my black bag toward me."

David dragged the bag along the table toward Rubin.

"Okay," Rubin said as he unpacked items from the bag. "In here, I have some radio frequency identification devices that use magnetic fields to identify and track what we are potentially looking for. Let me show you this separate bag. Inside, there's an infrared and heat detection camera. However, as technology advances, future bugs may emit less heat. This is a radio microphone detector that will identify various frequencies. What else do we have here? Oh yes, these are cable testers. We're looking for anything that could be mains-wired. By the way, I never asked you, do many people know this room is being used for this meeting?"

David shook his head as he examined the various pieces of equipment. "No, not to my knowledge. My best guess is that only the security team and the board are aware."

"Good," Rubin replied. "Hopefully, we can wrap this up quickly. We'll need to disconnect the air conditioning unit, and I want to secure the windows. They'll need to remain permanently closed, and I'll apply a protective film over them. Once you've removed all of the plug points from the walls and completed the physical search, I'll show you how to use this." Rubin took a detector out of his bag. “This is a non-linear junction detector. I want every piece of furniture in this room checked; anything unnecessary should be removed and placed in the corridor. Is that clear?”

David nodded, “Yes, I understand.”

Rubin glanced at his laptop screen. “Okay, let’s get started.”

++++

Nervous and with a very dry throat, Ben stood outside the entrance to Portcullis House, waiting impatiently for his meeting. Although only a few minutes had passed, it felt much longer. Members of parliament walked by effortlessly as they entered the building. With his laptop bag slung over one shoulder and an anxious expression on his face, he was attracting attention.

An unarmed, uniformed police officer approached him after stepping through one of the revolving doors. After inquiring about his purpose there, Ben explained that he had a meeting with Helen. The officer informed him that there had been threats made against her. Eyeing Ben and his bag suspiciously, the officer nodded and gestured for him to enter the outer perimeter of the building through the revolving door.

“Please place your bag on the conveyor belt and put the contents of your pockets in this tray,” the officer instructed.

At that time of day, a steady stream of people flowed into the building. Although they had to pass through the revolving doors, those with the correct accreditation were waved through the remaining security checks. Thousands worked on the estate, and it seemed like most had shown up for work that day.

“Please also place your jacket on the conveyor,” the officer added.

Ben complied, and while his belongings were being scanned, armed police stood ready on the other side of the conveyor.

“Do you object to being searched?”

Ben shook his head at the male police officer.

“Please proceed through the body scanner. Once you’re done,

collect your belongings and take a seat over there," the officer instructed, pointing to a seating area off to the side.

"Of course, thank you," Ben replied as he walked through the scanner.

"And stop there, please," The officer said.

"Is everything okay, officer? I didn't hear a noise from the body scanner."

"Do you have any items on your person that could harm you or me?" the officer inquired.

Ben shook his head as he was lightly patted down.

"Given who you are seeing, we just need to be sure."

"But of course," Ben replied, noticing the number of police officers and other official-looking individuals in the area. Some wore suits, likely working for the security service or another specialist department. One police officer sat by the scanner while another stood behind her, examining his items as they moved along the conveyor belt.

"Okay. You can proceed," The officer said as he stepped away from Ben.

The seated officer spoke to the one standing behind her. "Sir, please come over here and open your bag."

Ben nodded, retrieved his bag from the conveyor, and opened it. "It's just my laptop, charger, and reading glasses," he explained.

"Can you open the laptop for me?" the officer requested.

Ben complied as she looked him in the eyes. "What is your purpose for being on the parliamentary estate today?" she asked.

"I have a meeting with Helen Lord, MP," he replied.

The officer nodded, her expression still sceptical. "Are you okay, sir?"

Ben felt beads of sweat forming on his forehead. The plug-in drive was inside his jacket pocket. He forced an uncomfortable smile. "Yes," he shrugged. "I'm fine, thank you. How are you?"

The officer picked up the laptop and noticed that an "Enter Password" box had appeared on the screen. "Please input your password," she said, handing the device back to Ben.

He typed in his password. "What are you looking for?" His voice was tense, and he could feel sweat running down his lower back.

"Threats have been made against the mentioned MP. I would like to see what's displayed on your home screen. I won't look through your files. What is the nature of your business?"

"I see. Um, I work in television. I'm a TV executive."

The officer nodded, clearly aware that television executives and journalists were eager to meet her at the moment. "You can close your laptop, sir. Please collect your belongings. What time is your appointment?"

"Now. I believe she is on her way," Ben replied as he closed the laptop and placed it back into its bag.

"Please see my colleague over there for your temporary ID. Your photograph will be taken. Do you consent to this?"

Ben nodded, feeling the sweat trickle down his brow. "Of course."

"If you are still here in ten minutes, we'll need to call upstairs to check on her whereabouts. MPs can cancel meetings at the last minute."

Ben offered a weak smile. "I completely understand."

"Sir."

"Yes," Ben replied nervously.

"Don't forget your jacket."

"Oh yes, silly me." He sighed and leaned over to retrieve his jacket.

He walked over to the area where his photograph needed to be taken. Afterwards, he was given a lanyard with a printout displaying his image, the time, the date, and the information that he was there to see Helen. He put the lanyard around his neck, took a seat, and finally wiped the sweat from his forehead. As he sat, he nervously tapped his right foot on the floor, watching as the police checked people through. Eventually, a young man approached him, dressed smartly in a shirt and tie. He ran a hand through his floppy dark hair as he got closer. "Are you Ben Tasker?"

Ben immediately stood up. "Yes, I'm here to see Helen."

"I'm Tobias, her researcher. We spoke on the phone."

"Oh, I apologise if I came across as rude," Ben said, adjusting the laptop bag on his shoulder.

"You were, but it's not the first time I've been spoken to like that. When you work for Helen, it becomes commonplace. Come on through. Have you been here before?"

"A little while ago."

"You'll need to swipe your pass over the scanner to get in."

He followed the young researcher as they passed through the barriers.

"Is Helen not coming down?" Ben asked.

"No."

They walked across the floor of Portcullis House toward the elevators on the far side. "You're going upstairs to see her. After yesterday's... erm... indiscretion in the chamber, every journalist wants to speak with her; this place is flooded with them. They're constantly watching who comes and goes, who sees whom, etc., looking for titbits for a story."

"You call it an indiscretion, but she had an important point to make in the chamber. It's very brave to address the Prime Minister like that."

"Oh, right." He stopped walking. "You're a friend of the lady who was blown up, aren't you?"

Ben's expression soured at the crude way his friend was referred to. "I'm her employer as well as a friend."

"Oh, right. Shocking business. This way." They resumed walking toward the elevators.

Ben stared at the back of the researcher's head. He was right about how he had described him on the phone; he really was a little prick.

✢✢✢✢

Rubin stretched his arms over his head and rubbed his eyes. A few hours had passed. "I'm done here. Unless we're dealing with someone I've never heard of, this room is now sterile. I'll take no further responsibility for it. You know the drill, David: when a window or door is opened, the room is contaminated. Are you going to stay in this room until it's used?"

David shook his head. "No, I hadn't planned on it."

"Are you confident that the security outside will protect it?" Rubin asked as he stepped closer to David.

David frowned and scoffed in disgust. "No idea. I didn't recommend them. Their company had a contract in place long before their former problem-solver vouched for me."

Rubin leaned in, maintaining his intensity. "Well, listen, and I mean this. I know you're experienced in this business, but here are my rules: You've engaged me today, and I don't want to know who your client is or what's happening in this room. Once I leave, my part is over. There will be no comebacks. If anything, like a conversation, leaks from this room and things go haywire, that's your problem. You do not contact me. You never reveal my name to your client, the police, or any asshole lawyers. Clear?"

"Crystal, I'm surprised you even brought it up. I'll call my client to let him know the room is clear and remind him of the rules regarding access to this room and the entire floor. I'll implement a standard operating procedure for the security company: no unauthorised access to this floor."

Rubin glanced at his watch. "Good, the afternoon is ticking away, and I'm starving." He put on his jacket and cap, pulling the cap down to conceal his eyes. There were CCTV cameras in the hotel lobby area, so he planned to dip his head as he passed by them on his way out. He began to reorganise the contents of his work bag and placed the spectrum analyser back into its case. "I noticed a rundown café just down the road. It probably won't have cameras, and that's as good a place as any. I want to limit how often we're seen together on camera. Does that work for you?"

"Of course, I'll RV with you as soon as I can. I'll call my client, speak with security, and inform them of the SOPs."

Rubin nodded, put on his backpack, grabbed his black bag and opened the door, "I'll walk to the café. Can you bring my case with you when you leave, as you have the car?"

David nodded. As Rubin left the room, he switched on his phone and called Darius Neith. Darius answered quickly. "Are we all set?"

"The room is prepared as you requested. Members of your security team are on the hotel floor," David replied.

"Good, we'll be there soon. I appreciate you arranging this so quickly."

"My colleague has just left. He was expensive, and I've already paid him."

"I'll handle that for you as per our usual terms, so you don't need to worry about it."

"Darius, I cannot stress enough the importance of ensuring that no one enters this room under any circumstances until you arrive. The other board members will need to wait in the lobby or in their cars until you provide instructions for entry. This room must remain secure until that point. If you have any concerns about internal issues or staff, you should be the first to enter the room. I will leave the master door key with the guard outside, but I don't know this security team personally. They appear capable, but I want to be cautious. To that end, my colleague has set up a temporary CCTV camera in the corridor; it's motion-activated and will serve as a deterrent. It's a good piece of kit and focused on the door. The suite has only one entrance and one exit."

"I don't want the board members being filmed!" Darius responded.

"They won't be. The camera is positioned outside the room, and I will monitor it on my phone. As soon as I see you, I will turn it off and instruct the room guard to remove it upon your arrival. If your team is competent, they should already be familiar with these protocols. I assume they are well-acquainted with all board members, including their identities and appearances?"

"No, they only know some. I've already arranged with the security team leader that anyone I don't recognise must be removed by force. They will be made to feel... uncomfortable. Since only the board is aware of this meeting, it is unlikely that anyone else will show up. However, if anyone does arrive, the meeting will be cancelled immediately, and we will reschedule."

"Roger that. I need to go now. Your team leader is now responsible for the room and your safety. Also, remember that during the meeting, the windows must remain sealed and not be tampered with. No windows are to be opened at any time. Additionally, the air conditioning unit has been disconnected and covered. I assume there won't be a presentation requiring a screen, as there was only one TV in the room, and that has been removed. Furthermore, all power outlets have been checked and covered."

"No, we will only be discussing important work matters. In that respect, is your colleague ready to move to the next phase?"

"I've briefed him, and I'm about to meet with him again. We'll discuss it, and I'll get back to you. After your meeting, I need to return to the room to reconnect the air conditioning, uncover the power outlets and windows, and collect the camera."

Darius nodded. "Thank you, David. I'll speak to you later and keep you updated on our progress." Darius sat down, placed his phone on the table, and began flipping through the front pages of the newspapers on his desk for the second time that day. Most of the tabloids led with the attack in London, questioning the current state of Harwood's health. Many speculated about her anti-beauty campaign, implying that it was the reason for the attack. One tabloid featured a crosshair from a weapon, which even Darius found to be in poor taste. However, there was no mention of his company, and at least the woman had been silenced.

Darius had paid David a substantial amount for his services, but David had failed to complete the task. Although David was a professional and highly recommended by Darius's former problem solver upon his retirement, the facts remained undeniable. The involvement of the security service, anti-terrorism units, and the police was always inevitable; however, Alison's survival was not. Regardless of the outcome, if David left even the slightest trace that implicated him, it would have serious consequences.

Chapter Nine

Tobias knocked on Helen Lord's private door.

"Yes, come in," she called.

He opened the door and peeked his head inside. "Helen, Mr Tasker is here for you." He noticed Helen take a deep breath, and she appeared worried for some reason.

"Send him in, please." She rubbed her lips with concern as Ben entered her office. Like most offices for backbench MPs in Portcullis House, it was small, barely enough room to swing a cat. Knowing that a barrage of questions was coming, she felt uncomfortable being so close to him. She lifted her right hand to shake his. "Ben, it's so nice to see you again." Her words were upbeat, accompanied by a beaming smile that she put on for Tobias's benefit. "Would you like a coffee?"

He nodded. "A coffee wouldn't hurt; thank you," he replied, ignoring her gesture to shake hands.

"Tobias, please take care of that. How do you take your coffee?"

Ben glanced at the arrogant upstart. "Strong and black, please."

Tobias nodded. "It will be a few minutes." He disappeared, leaving the door open.

Helen motioned for Ben to close the door. "I wish he'd stop doing that. He's far too nosy for my liking."

Ben closed the door gently and turned to her, his face a mix of anger and worry. "Maybe that's because you have something to hide!"

Helen coughed slightly under her breath. "Please, take a seat."

"If I must!" He pulled a chair closer and set his laptop bag on the floor.

They sized each other up for a moment, but Helen spoke first. "So, tell me what you know."

"What do I know? Christ, where do you even start?" He leaned forward in anger, spittle flying from his mouth as he spoke. "Contaminated fillers, a source, heroin, what the fuck are you two playing at?"

"That's enough! Lower your tone; remember where you are and who you're addressing," she replied.

"Oh, piss off! You're a backbench MP at best. We voted you in; it wasn't gifted to you." He waved his hands in frustration. "I've met enough of you over the years to know you're full of self-importance and self-gratification instead of actually fighting for a cause."

Helen emitted a faint chuckle. "Now you do sound like a journalist!"

Ben scoffed. "This anti-beauty campaign you're running is nothing more than a publicity stunt for you. Do you want to be elevated to the Lords in the future? Become Baroness of some such place?"

Helen took a deep breath. "Look, I understand you're angry and worried. So am I. However, what you don't understand is that Alison brought this to my attention. There's no way either of us could have anticipated how things would pan out. Have you had any updates on Alison?"

Ben crossed his arms. "No, not a thing. What about you?"

Helen shook her head. "Look, she came to me..."

They were interrupted by a knock at the door, and Ben's phone vibrated in his pocket.

"Come in," Helen called out.

Tobias walked in with the coffee, which had been prepared much quicker than they had expected.

"Thank you," Helen said, gesturing for him to set it down on the side table. "Could you please close the door behind you this time?" She noticed the concern on Ben's face as the door clicked shut. "What is it?"

He was reading a message on his phone and sighed, his eyes slightly watery as he put it back in his pocket. "The police have a search warrant. They are raiding our offices." He collapsed into his chair, staring at the steam rising from his coffee. He shook his head and dabbed at his eyes. "I found the folder."

Helen looked confused. "What folder?"

"Upper House."

Helen's expression showed that she still didn't understand.

"It refers to communications between both of you and names two members of the House of Lords."

She shook her head, her confusion deepening. "I still don't follow."

"There is a folder on Alison's computer called Upper House."

Helen blinked in disbelief, her voice incredulous. "You what?"

"It led me to everything that you two have been up to."

Helen bowed her head in despair. "Oh, for God's sake."

"You didn't know about it?"

She shook her head, groaning. "I guess that means it's only a matter of time before the police show up here as well."

"You don't need to worry. I've saved you from embarrassment."

Helen looked up, intrigued. "How?"

"The file only contained one Word document, and the only words in it said, 'If reading, look in a safe place.'" He fiddled with his jacket pocket. "This is where your troubles lie. This is your safe place." He pulled a flash drive out of his jacket pocket and held it up. "And I'm afraid to carry this, especially around here."

Helen felt a surge of tension as she focused on the small plug-in device in front of her. "What's on that?" she asked.

"Enough... enough for me to know what you've been up to," he replied. "There are photographs and emails between you and a scientific diagram of something; I'm guessing it's this 'enhanced' beauty filler." He decided not to mention the covert footage he had seen featuring Helen... at least not for now. "And now, here we are. I'm in your office because my friend is lying half-dead in the hospital!"

Helen rubbed her temple. "She is also my friend."

"You know, incredibly, I thought she'd just pissed someone off, someone influential, someone with resources, but still just a person. The truth is that since that bloody Beauty Beach series, we have been under tremendous pressure; the channel nearly folded, and lawsuits have been flying everywhere. She fought back; she was trying to change things, and that's what I initially thought it was about. I couldn't have been more wrong. This is what it's really about!" He waved the drive in his hand at Helen.

Helen swallowed and looked away, trying to gather her thoughts.

"You two have pissed off some serious people in the pharmaceutical industry. Between the two of you, you've probably cost them millions in lost sales due to your online campaign. Did it never occur to you that they might be a little upset when their shareholders lose money?"

"Ben, we are trying to promote natural beauty; this isn't about feminism. Many people of all genders choose cosmetic surgery. This has always been about ageing naturally and not conforming to social media pressures. As I understood it, you supported Alison in her campaign."

Ben looked away from the MP. He had raised his concerns about the vitriol in the debate and the online arguments; they were aimed more at Alison than at the channel, but he had always supported her.

"Look, as I mentioned earlier, she brought this to my attention." Helen stood up and handed a cup of coffee to Ben before sitting back down with her cup. "At first, she called me to introduce herself. I recognised her immediately because I had been following her stance on the issue. The debate surrounding it was both polarising and fascinating, and social media was buzzing with activity. Many of the barbed comments were directed at her. Honestly, I admired her and what she was trying to achieve. Why shouldn't we promote natural beauty and encourage people to age gracefully? There is too much pressure on both the young and the old alike. Initially, most commentary was overwhelmingly negative toward her views, but this shifted when the legal profession became involved, leading the country to become more lawsuit-centric. We're not naive, Ben; we know how much we've cost big pharma. They are part of the problem, profiting from people's insecurities, but that's not our concern."

"It is now!" Ben said nervously as he sipped his coffee. "What exactly did she bring to you? I've read some of the emails, but there are gaps."

Helen raised her hands. "Okay, here's what happened. She received a message through one of her social media accounts requesting her private email address. At first, she ignored it, but the messages kept coming. Each one included more details, yet it was clear that whoever was sending them was risking their safety if the claims were true. However, she wasn't naive; it could have been someone trying to mislead her, so she didn't take it too seriously. But when photographs of vials from a lab in South America began to surface, along with chemical analysis breakdowns, Alison had to take it seriously. She created a personal email account with a random address that didn't link to her identity. When the messages appeared and seemed credible, she brought them to me. She didn't know what else to do. No crime had been committed, the product hadn't been distributed, and we had no idea where the lab was located. She could hardly go to the police with this, could she? So, she turned to me, knowing I had researchers at my disposal. I never provided my researchers with specific details, but extensive research tools are available to members of parliament. Here, we are protected by firewalls and have our digital services staffed by exceptional technicians. We needed to gather facts before deciding on any course of action, if we were to take any at all."

"But she mentioned a proposal, a documentary series, or something similar. It defies all logic; she would need our funding to produce it, which would require a decision from the board!"

"Well, that wouldn't be necessary. She anticipated your response, but she believes in the cause. Consider what we're discussing here: a filler that is being used by thousands of people across multiple countries, contaminated with heroin! People could become drug addicts without even realising it, and they would have to return to their clinics for more filler because, sooner or later, their brains would link the use of filler with feeling good. This could create a new breed of drug addicts from all backgrounds and professions. Even within this place, some MPs use fillers, Botox, undergo facelifts, and who knows what else. It could spread like wildfire, and where would it end? Addiction masked by the desire for beauty; only the darkest souls would pursue profit through this. Before we know it, we could face an epidemic as significant as the opioid crisis in the United States. And, of course, it wouldn't be limited to just this country; the informant believes they plan to target the UK first."

"Why, why here?"

"Because of your TV channel and the campaign spearheaded by Alison," Helen said forcefully as she pointed at Ben, "all of you have played a role in this! The idea wouldn't have even emerged if it weren't for you and that initial lawsuit won by the woman on The Beauty Beach show. That's why they want to target us first: to prove a point and create chaos. Someone high up in this situation wants to laugh at our expense and revel in our suffering. It's personal, and this needed to be exposed!"

Ben rubbed his throat anxiously. "Oh my God, I feel sick."

"You and me both," Helen replied. "And now poor Alison is paying the price. Only a company with serious resources could have orchestrated an attack on her in such a way."

"But you still haven't answered the question. We would never have approved a program that exposes this without solid scientific evidence. We wouldn't have created a program like that."

"Wouldn't you? Just think of the ratings if you could pull it off. As a journalist, this is the story of a lifetime, so yes, you would have. The problem is that your processes take too long, and we've run out of time. The whistleblower has disappeared; we suspect he was discovered, and if so, it was only a matter of time before they started investigating. If they find out who he was communicating with, it would lead right back to here. In that regard, the proposal was accurate; it just didn't involve you."

Ben's eyes widened in shock. "Wait, she was taking this elsewhere? Who was she going with?"

"No one. It had to be quick and cost-effective. We were putting it together ourselves. I can only guess they found out about our plans." Helen sighed and rubbed her eyes. "We were going to put it on YouTube."

"Oh my God!"

"It was the only way that didn't involve bureaucracy, and we could make a quick broadcast to the masses. It was meant to protect our safety, not compromise it."

Coffee sloshed over the sides of Ben's cup as his hands trembled. He set the cup down and rose to his feet. "I can't believe this, or what you've done!"

"Well, you better believe it, because it's happening right now, and I may be their next target."

Ben looked directly at Helen. For the first time in this meeting, he saw fear in her eyes. "But what about the source, your informant? If you broadcast this, you risk his life."

"He's gone! We can't prove it, but those behind this have invested too much; he disappeared, and we fear the worst for him. If he is still alive, the broadcast might protect him. That's why we had to move quickly. I'm afraid to say, I suspect they just got to us first. Last night, we were scheduled to meet with people who could help us put everything together. It was supposed to be the first time Alison's husband would be informed, too. He knows nothing about this; she values his opinion and wants him to hear the facts."

Ben started pacing back and forth in the small office, then suddenly stopped. "You know, I've seen the video."

Helen shook her head. "What video?"

"The one featuring your whistleblower. He appeared to be sitting outside a coffee shop in another country, somewhere in South America, I guess."

Helen nodded. "I see. I have no idea why Alison kept that footage. The plan was that if we could go to broadcast, we'd then try to get him out. But, of course, it isn't as easy as that. He was still involved in this. He may not have been when he started working at the lab, but that's the direction the powers that be were taking."

"But a crime has been committed! He spoke of human experiments, of people discarded and left to rot in the streets! These aren't jokers; they have serious resources. Between all of you, you've pissed off a legalised drug cartel! If they find out that a film like that exists on this very drive, they'll pop us all off! People like that have networks everywhere. Do you understand? I have a family!"

Ben's voice had risen considerably. Helen suspected that her overly eager researcher might now be listening at the door. She lowered her voice in an attempt to instil some calm. "I know; that's why we had to meet with people. If we took this to air, the next step would be to go to the police. But that was never going to be easy; there's no tangible evidence, and no proven crime has been committed. We're talking about international relationships involving a company that financially supports not just the two members of the House of Lords you mentioned, but also serves as a major party donor and directly invests in the government. What could we possibly do? Scandal doesn't even begin to cover it, and they would come for your channel. That's why we were considering the other route."

"But making accusations like that without any tangible evidence means the film you create would likely be taken down."

"We understood that, but we also knew it would be copied around the world by the time that happened, and the global press would cover it. This would likely attract the attention of authorities in South America, specifically in Brazil, where the lab is located. It would significantly complicate big pharma's operations and progress. It was a scare tactic, but it had a chance of working."

Ben scratched his head and said, "Hold on, they'd never get away with that. Heroin in cosmetic products? It would never pass; it wouldn't get approved."

"Wouldn't it? I wouldn't be so sure. Imagine taking an existing approved product, obtaining clearance, and simply replacing the batch with a similar product; no one would ever notice. They have people in the right places to make that happen. From what we understand, the heroin remains in the patient's system; it has to, or it wouldn't be effective. It provides a steady, drip-fed effect to the brain, creating a constant high that is completely different from what people use on the streets. This substance may remain undetected in individuals who have innocently received it during a cosmetic procedure for an extended period. By the time the issue is identified, thousands of people could be affected without even knowing they are taking a class-A drug, individuals from all walks of life. Let's face it: many beauty enhancements are used by those in the middle class and above. Who would have imagined that they could develop an addiction to heroin? This isn't some upper-class cocaine party; we could be witnessing a new wave of drug addiction among those who can afford it. These individuals make ideal clients, distinct from those on the streets who have lost everything. Regardless, they would keep coming back for more. Over time, any contaminated product could be taken off the market. By then, it would be too late, sales would have increased, and shareholders would be pleased. How could anyone possibly prove that an addiction began with a cosmetic filler?"

"Well, you'd need to have a sample from the contaminated batch."

"Exactly. We suspect they plan to log every batch and keep track of where each one is distributed. It could remain on the market for months, even a couple of years, before anyone discovers it. By that time, they would have switched back to the originally approved vials, which are tested and confirmed to be safe. After that, they would switch again, repeating the cycle. If they sensed that any official testing of their products was underway, they would intercept the batches and bribe the relevant individuals. Proving anything would be nearly impossible. Even if something did come to light, they would manage to cover it up. The narrative would likely suggest a contaminated batch, sacrificing some of their staff as scapegoats to protect the company, and then they would start over."

"But these vials are going to be contaminated with a heroin derivative!"

"Yes, but it would never be labelled as such, would it? Imagine the fallout if that information were to get out. It's more likely they would apologise, claim you had an allergic reaction to their product, and then offer you vouchers or a similar gesture. Trust me, there is so much money at stake. They could easily get away with it, and they have connections right here."

"Do you know who is actually behind this?"

"Not exactly. We know it's Knightark Pharmaceutical, but we don't know the individuals involved or who is funding them. I'm afraid it goes deeper than that. The head of the board is Darius Neith; he's the key player, and that concerns me."

"Why is that?"

Helen took a deep breath and stood up. "Because I'm worried about who is involved in this, and if it gets exposed, who might step in to cover it up." She looked out the window at the people below. "As you know, two members of the House of Lords serve as consultants for the company."

Ben nodded in acknowledgement.

"But Darius worries me." Helen turned back to face Ben. "The fact that he attended the same college at the same time as Alix Gregory, our Prime Minister, only adds to my concern."

Chapter Ten

Ben slumped in his seat, feeling the weight of the situation bearing down on him. His throat grew drier by the moment. He buried his face in his hands and exclaimed, "Oh my God! What have you done?"

Helen's face was as pale as a sheet, and recounting the facts filled her with dread. "I know. When Alison started communicating with the whistleblower, we had no idea it would lead to this. This situation could topple an entire government and undermine trust in politics. As politicians, we already face too many scandals; it seems like every month brings something new. Cash for questions, secret payments, and party donors from questionable backgrounds; if they then stay at a luxury villa belonging to those donors, well, you know how that goes, it's endless. An MP goes on a rant on social media, it backfires, and they end up having the whip removed. It just keeps going. But this… this is so much bigger than any scandal I've encountered, if what we suspect is true. Right now, it's just speculation. There's no solid evidence proving anything. But I can tell you this: we are onto something, and they want to silence us!"

Ben's eyes were fixed firmly on the floor, overwhelmed with worry.

"And they are accelerating their plans quickly, which began with what happened to Alison yesterday."

Ben shook his head, cradling it in his hands. "I don't know what to do!" He looked up, scanning the artificial ceiling tiles. "Are we safe to talk in here? Have you checked for any bugs?"

Helen nodded. "I'm not an expert, but I've done my best to check for listening devices. I researched them online."

"Blimey, you didn't do that from a computer in here, did you?" Ben asked with a note of concern in his voice.

Helen snorted in response. "No, I'm not a complete fool. I've made it a point to leave the estate several times, turn off my phone, disconnect the SIM card, and go to an internet café. It's the best I could do. I can't trust anyone."

Ben took a deep breath. "The police are currently at our offices. They're trying to find any information that could explain what happened to Alison."

Helen nodded. "I know, and I suspect they'll be here soon if they can establish a link. But searching an MP's office is not straightforward. In this place, sooner or later, everything comes to light. They will be cautious about coming in here; they need something substantial. They may also want to speak with me because of my connection to Alison."

"But this is now a police matter. We need to provide them with what we can," Ben insisted.

"That's true, but what you have on that drive is pure speculation and one person's opinion. What are the British police going to do with such findings? You can bet the pharmaceutical company will want that drive if they find out it exists. It certainly implicates the whistleblower, wherever he may be."

"But you were going to broadcast this using the same speculative evidence you have," Ben pointed out.

Helen nodded. "Yes, we had little choice. The difference is that, with this information in the public domain, the court of public opinion would then be able to judge them."

"But they will issue a statement denying it. Both of you will be labelled as scaremongers and become subjects of public ridicule."

"Better that than allowing another opioid epidemic to unfold in plain sight. It would give people a choice."

"Conspiracy theorists would latch onto this. You'd be laughed out of office and expelled from the party."

"Don't think I haven't considered that, but this is bigger than me, bigger than you, and bigger than Alison. We had to do what was right."

Ben started turning the plug-in device between his fingers. "What should I do with this?"

"I don't know."

"You don't know?"

"No. We're caught in the middle of something. I'm meeting with the Serjeant at Arms department in about an hour to discuss my personal security. However, I can't disclose what I know because we have no idea how deep this goes."

"Well, can I attend that meeting? I need guidance on security as well," Ben said.

"That's not possible, I'm afraid. You do not work on the estate. I expect I will only receive general guidance, nothing more."

They both jumped when their conversation was interrupted by a knock at the door. They exchanged nervous glances.

"Who is it?" Helen called out.

On the other side of the door, Tobias frowned slightly as he sensed the tension in Helen's voice. "It's me," he replied.

"Yes, come in," she said.

Tobias entered, holding a padded brown A4-sized envelope. "Something unusual has come in. You've received a delivery, and the postal mark indicates it's from South America."

Ben and Helen exchanged a panicked look immediately.

"Do you routinely check Helen's mail?" Ben asked sharply.

"No, that's okay, Ben," Helen replied. "Tobias is justified in doing so, even though it's marked private and confidential. What makes this envelope stand out, and why have you brought it to my attention?"

"Judging by the internal stamp, it has been here for a few days and was opened and searched in the mail room, likely because it was considered a suspicious package," Tobias explained.

Helen stood up. "The mail room must have flagged it. But it has been cleared, right?"

"As far as I can tell," Tobias replied, handing the envelope to Helen.

She nodded and carefully took the package from him. "Thank you, that will be all. I'll check it later."

"Okay, I understand. Would you like any more coffee?" he offered.

Ben shook his head without saying a word.

"No, we're fine, thank you. Could you please close the door behind you?"

As soon as Tobias left the room, Ben got to his feet while Helen placed the envelope on the table.

"What do you think it is?" he asked.

"We need to check this immediately."

Helen examined the package, noting that it bore Brazilian postal markings. The mailroom had placed a protective seal on the reverse side, where it had been opened, indicating that the internal mail scanners had detected something unusual.

"It must be safe to handle and open if it's made its way up to here," Ben said.

Helen nodded in agreement. "Yes, I suppose so." She turned the envelope over and gently pulled at the protective seal. As it came away, she set the envelope aside and peered inside. There were four small boxes. She placed them on the desk and immediately recognised the logo of Knightark Pharmaceutical, along with the name of their widely distributed filler, 'Hydra-Fillixir'. Carefully, she opened one of the boxes and found a vial inside. Puzzled, she shook her head and said, "This is the product we've been talking about."

"You're kidding! Is there anything else?" Ben replied.

Helen reached back into the envelope and pulled out a small piece of paper with a few handwritten words. She read them aloud: "Following our conversation, this is what you've been looking for."

Helen and Ben exchanged nervous glances, their expressions filled with intrigue.

"My God, I think we've got it. Look, the note is signed by Alexandre."

"Is that the whistleblower's name? I've never seen it mentioned before."

Helen nodded. "Yes, it was only referred to once at the beginning of this investigation. For his safety, we kept his name out of our communications. Alison told me his name." She placed the piece of paper on the desk and picked up one of the unopened boxes. "I believe we have them. This proves production!"

"Okay, so what are you going to do? Shouldn't we go to the police?"

Helen raised her hands. "Let me think."

"Helen, this is the smoking gun; it has to be!"

"It could be," she replied, scratching her head. "But the post date is from nearly ten days ago, and we were still communicating with Alexandre then."

"Well, let's take it to the police."

Helen sat down and leaned back in her chair, contemplating her options. "No, not yet. I can't trust anyone. Recently, I contacted a private lab in Kent. If the opportunity presented itself, I needed clarification and indisputable evidence. I'll contact them, and I'll take one of these samples to the lab myself. I'm willing to pay for the testing. If the results confirm our suspicions, then we'll be in a position of power."

Ben began pacing the room. "Okay, that kinda makes sense, but please do it quickly. I'm worried about this bloody drive. I don't want to carry it."

"Leave it with me. I'll store it in a safe place here."

"Inside your office?"

"Absolutely not. I have another location on the estate where I can hide everything. We'll obtain the lab results first and then determine our next steps. I need to make a call. We will figure this out and expose the truth."

++++

After briefing the security team, David left the hotel carrying Rubin's case and headed to his car. He couldn't recall the café that Rubin had mentioned. Since the hotel was at the end of a cul-de-sac, finding it shouldn't be difficult; Rubin had said it was "down the road," and he was on foot. David felt pleased that the briefing he provided to the security team leader was well received. The team leader was experienced, with a definite military background, and was accustomed to following procedures. David was confident that the sterile room would remain intact.

Although Rubin had exhibited arrogance and instability in the past, his supposedly reformed nature seemed to be slipping away, as evidenced by his recent behaviour. He clearly expressed disdain for the work, and his pricing reflected that attitude. If he charged six thousand pounds for a debug service, the costs would be high for surveillance on the television executive. Rubin's prices were non-negotiable, which might have been a tactic to price himself out of the work he no longer wanted to do. If accounts were to be believed, since returning to the private sector, Rubin had likely donated thousands to his temple in Kathmandu. However, his attitude today suggested that his willingness to continue making those donations was waning.

David had driven along two roads before finally spotting the café. Rubin had been right; it looked unkempt. The absence of cars outside suggested it wasn't a place for fine dining. He passed the café and parked nearby. Inside, Rubin was sitting with a mug of tea. David sat opposite him; aside from someone behind the counter, they were the only people in the café.

"You took your time," Rubin remarked.

"I needed to ensure that my brief would be carried out properly. Have you ordered yet?" David replied.

"No, I was waiting for you." Rubin turned and raised his arm toward the counter. "By the way, the menu is terrible."

David glanced around the café and didn't doubt it.

"Hello, gentlemen. What can I get you?" the young lady asked.

"I'll have another tea and a tuna sandwich, please," Rubin said.

David didn't bother reading the menu. He noticed on a chalkboard that they served breakfast all day. "I'll have the full breakfast, please," he said, nodding at the lady as she wrote down their orders.

"And a mug of tea?" she asked.

"Sure," David replied.

She smiled politely. "Back in a few moments."

"Your body is a temple, then," Rubin scoffed. "I don't eat the living anymore."

"The tuna you ordered would have lived at some point," David pointed out.

"True, but it's more about the meat for me; I just don't believe in it."

David considered the tuna's meat and noticed Rubin had milk in his tea, but he decided not to pursue the topic further.

"Did you remember my case?" Rubin asked.

David nodded in response, "It's in the car."

"That's an expensive piece of kit to leave in a car. I suppose we'll have to hope for the best. By the way, who does this TV guy work for?"

"Channel 8 television; he's the boss."

"Okay. It's not my concern, but do you know why he's the target? That information might be helpful."

"No, it's just a fishing expedition. The client wants us to find out anything he might be involved in that we can use. If we can't uncover anything, we may need to create a compromising situation for leverage."

"You mentioned he's a family man with kids."

"Are they his kids?"

"I don't know much about that. With everything happening and this suddenly dropping on my plate, I haven't had the chance to do thorough research."

Rubin nodded in acknowledgement. "This all sounds highly disorganised. Without proper planning, we could get burnt. If that happens, what potential fallout could there be?"

David leaned back in his seat, signalling a pause in their conversation as two mugs of tea were placed in front of them. Both mugs were filled with black tea; milk and sugar were available in sachets on the table. David noticed that the mugs weren't particularly clean.

"Here we go; your food will be ready shortly," the server said.

David smiled briefly as she left.

Rubin noticed David examining the mug and smirked. "Kent, the so-called Garden of England. What a shithole."

David laughed as he tore open a couple of milk sachets and added some sugar.

"Do you know where to find this guy?"

"I have his work address and phone number; we can trace him from there. I know he's in London, around the South Bank area, not far from Waterloo."

"Alright, we need to do some workups first," Rubin replied.

"Here we go, gents." Two plates were placed in front of them. Neither meal looked appetising, but one appeared healthier than the other. "Can I get you anything else?" the server asked.

They both glanced at their food: David's plate was swimming in grease, and the baked beans looked like they had been sitting on the heat for hours. They both shook their heads in response.

"Okay then, I'll be over here if you change your mind," she said, walking away.

Rubin watched as David cut into the overcooked sausage. "I don't know how you can put that in your mouth," he commented.

"Your sandwich looks stale. You haven't fared much better," David retorted.

Rubin grunted and took a bite. David was right; the bread was indeed stale. "Tell me, what is the endgame with this job?"

"The reasons for this, I don't entirely know. All I know is that my client wants to use him to secure something for his TV channel."

Rubin laughed, "You can't be serious." He turned around, realising he had raised his voice; the young girl was still behind the counter. He lowered his voice, "It's not about money, right? He hasn't witnessed anything, nothing like that?"

"No, they just want a program or some ads to be aired, something along those lines. It's a strange one."

"Strange it is," Rubin nodded. "But if that's all it is, it might be doable. Do you have someone who can track the phone?"

"Yeah, I have a guy here. I need to give him some money from time to time. He's great with IT, bank info, car info, all the suchlike, classic geek material, but he's useless directly in the field."

"Well, okay. If we can find the guy tonight..."

David's phone started vibrating in his jacket. He pulled it out and saw Darius's alias on the screen. "It's the client. Give me a second." He turned around to ensure no one else had entered the café. They hadn't, so he answered the call.

"David, there's a slight change of plans. We've been monitoring the other one; she just called a private lab. I need to see you immediately to explain."

"I'm still with my colleague at the moment," David said.

"Can you ask him to hold on? This new development could involve him as well."

"I can ask him once I know the facts. Can you make your way to Kent? I'm not far from the hotel."

"I can do that," Darius said, "but what's happening takes immediate priority."

"Understood. I'll send you a map reference for a safe location in this area. Also, my colleague only works for cash, if you could bring some."

Rubin nudged David. "Try to avoid £50 notes if possible."

"Lower denomination notes, if you can," David added.

There was a grunt from the other end of the phone. "I'll see what I can do. If traffic is reasonable, I can reach you within the hour."

"Good. I'll send you the meeting location as soon as I have it."

The call ended, and David picked up his knife and fork again, deciding to take a risk by eating some of the fried egg. It may be a while before he eats again.

"So, what's going on?" Rubin asked.

David only knew that a private lab had been contacted; Darius must have been referring to the member of parliament. Rubin didn't need to know this yet, if he did, he might make the connection between David and the explosion from the day before. Looking at his long-time colleague, he lied, "I'm not sure. Something must be happening. He's on his way here, and I need to see him privately. He mentioned that something has come up that takes priority over the other job. If you're okay to wait, I'll find out more details. The good news is, he knows to bring cash."

Rubin grunted, "He needs to, otherwise I'll be pressing you for more information about who he is."

Chapter Eleven

David checked his watch; just over an hour had passed since Darius called. He had found a quiet place for them to meet, not far from the hotel where Darius would be holding his board meeting.

While he waited, he began researching. Darius had asked him to investigate Ben Tasker, and there was plenty of information available online. A former journalist, Tasker had risen through the ranks at Channel 8. The only negative aspect of his career appeared to be his association with The Beauty Beach, which had resulted in considerable fallout for the channel. As the head of the TV channel, Tasker had also overseen and supported Alison Harwood's appointment, and David found many photographs of them together. When he checked records at Companies House, he discovered that Tasker was listed as a director of the channel, but his home address was not publicly available. An industry database also did not provide a home address. However, Tasker was open about his personal life, presenting himself as a typical two-up, two-down character, nothing particularly remarkable or noteworthy. He claimed to be happily married with two children, but such statements are often found on professional databases, and their accuracy could be questionable.

Whatever Darius had planned, Rubin would have no problem conducting surveillance to determine Tasker's home address; that would be a matter of process and cost. If necessary, the children might serve as useful leverage. In this moment of calm, he reflected on his early years working with Rubin, before Rubin went rogue. Rubin's references to his beliefs sounded like clichés from an old movie. It was not uncommon for mercenaries to seek peace in the later stages of their lives; most had to find their own way to come to terms with their past actions. Some chose to block those memories out completely, erasing them from their minds, but as they aged, many began to experience a growing fear, fear of their own demise and a need to reconcile with their past and their makers, whatever that might mean. In David's case, he held no such beliefs. If the time came when he felt the fear, he would know it was time to move on and retire. This line of work required the ability to walk away at any moment while maintaining alliances with like-minded individuals who understood and had similar experiences. As time went on, some in the business had fallen apart, often turning to alcohol. In doing so, they became liabilities, bringing up matters that should have remained private in inappropriate settings. It was no surprise that a few had taken their own lives while struggling to find peace with what they had done.

David put his phone away as he recognised Darius's car pulling up behind him. This time, he decided to stay in his vehicle and let Darius come to him. Whatever was happening was serious enough for the multi-millionaire to visit him urgently. As Darius parked and exited the car, David noticed that he was holding a cool bag and was wearing gloves.

David pressed the button to unlock his car as Darius got in.

"Here you go," Darius said, handing him the small green cool bag.

"What's in here?" David asked, taking the bag.

"Something I need you to do urgently. I must warn you, it won't be pleasant."

David glanced down at the bag resting on his lap.

"It's quite safe to open, I assure you," Darius added.

Tentatively, David unzipped the bag and peered inside. He saw a folded piece of paper and a small, unmarked white box.

"Go ahead, read it," Darius urged.

David felt an instant wave of suspicion. "Why are you wearing gloves?"

"Because I don't want my fingerprints on anything. If you read what's printed here, you'll understand."

David retrieved the paper, which contained a few words printed from a computer rather than handwritten. "What does this mean?" he asked, confusion clear in his voice.

"It's an address, a name, and a photograph, specifically, the address of a small, independently funded research lab not far from here. We know our friend, the MP, has been in contact with them before and contacted them again earlier today. If she isn't there by the end of the day, I'm confident she'll go there at some point tomorrow. Fortunately, the lab isn't far from here."

"Okay. What do you need me to do?" David inquired.

"She will be taking one of our products with her. My concern is that the product may have been contaminated, so she's going there for testing."

"Do you need it intercepted? How did she get it in the first place?"

"You don't need to worry about that. No interception is required. The last thing we need is for her to get spooked any more than she already is. She talks too much and could cause us problems. Let her deliver the product she has and try to find out to whom she has delivered it."

"And switching it out with this product? That won't be easy in a lab," David pointed out.

Darius looked out the window, admiring the tranquillity of the lake down the road. "No, I'm afraid it's a bit more complicated than that," he said, turning to meet David's eyes. "First, the product in the bag must be kept cool. Our products are fine as long as they are stored at temperatures below twenty-five degrees. This time of year, I'm not taking any chances. It's a vial, and I need that specific one to be tested instead. I want the person conducting the test to contact the MP with the results of that vial, whether by phone, email, or any other necessary means. She must receive the results for the vial you have."

David examined the small box before removing it. Inside, he found a single vial and nothing else.

"They can break, so be careful with it," Darius warned. "They usually come with a syringe, but since this is a lab, they will have plenty on hand."

"Darius, I still don't fully understand how I'm going to do this. What are your expectations?" David asked.

"My expectation is that the MP will request an urgent inspection of the vial she'll be carrying. We can't take it from her for the reasons I've explained; I don't want her to be tampered with, at least not for now. Therefore, we must let nature take its course. The outcome will depend on how quickly they run the test, so you'll need to keep a close watch on it," Darius explained.

"If the building is secured, it may not be possible to do this," David replied.

"I understand, and that's why this is a test. However, I have faith in your professionalism. Do you have scopes or long-range vision capabilities?" Darius asked.

"Yes, I have a scope with photographic capture, but I have minimal surveillance equipment and clothing with me," David responded.

Darius nodded. "That's okay. If you can determine whether a test is being conducted, then you need to get to the person who performed it."

David frowned at this suggestion.

"I've looked up the lab online. It's small, but other staff members will be present, so you won't be able to walk in and switch the products. I know this will require your persuasion skills. From the communications we've intercepted, it seems she has been in contact with a man named Dr Ryan Dobey, the lab's owner and its most senior staff member. I'm confident she will only deal with him, and he will likely conduct the test himself. I've checked him out; he is well-qualified, financially stable, and appears to be a family man. He'll probably appreciate having a member of parliament as a client."

David looked at the picture of the man in a lab coat, which seemed to have been taken from a website. "Are you suggesting an abduction?" he asked.

“Oh, I wouldn’t use such terms, my friend, but he must be persuaded to test that vial instead. How you choose to go about it is up to you.” Darius noticed that David’s expression was one of perplexity. “Here, this should help,” he said, pulling out two bundles of notes from his pocket. One bundle consisted of £50 notes, and the other of £20 notes. “This is the best I could gather on short notice,” he added.

“Darius, this type of work requires weeks of planning. I need to assess every possible outcome. We should surveil this man first to determine how to get to him.”

“We don’t have the time!”

It was unusual for David to hear his client raise his voice so forcefully.

Darius pointed at the picture of the lab technician. “Get to him by any means necessary. He must contact the MP with the test results from your vial. Furthermore, he needs to fully understand the consequences if he reports any of this to the MP or the police.” His stare intensified as he looked David in the eyes. “I suspect you’ll need to meet with his family to ensure he comprehends the seriousness of the situation. I trust this won’t be a problem?”

David glanced at the picture of the smiling man in the lab coat and shook his head. “No, that won’t be a problem, as long as it can be done.”

“Good. We have an accord. This is why I pay you what I do. Is your colleague still in the area?”

“Yes, he’s not far from here. I’ve also been researching the other target, Ben Tasker. What do you want to do with him?”

Darius took a deep breath as he weighed his options. “For now, let’s save him. We can pick him up another time. This takes priority. Given the recent developments, your colleague may be useful for this new task.”

David nodded. “That shouldn’t be a problem.”

“Good. I need to go; I have to meet with the other senior board members before the main board meeting. Make sure it gets done,”

Darius said as he opened the car door and stepped outside. He leaned down and added, "Don't forget to keep the vial cool."

David acknowledged him with a nod as Darius closed the car door and walked back to his vehicle. Shaking his head, David reflected on how rapidly events were changing. He glanced at the bundles of money before putting them into his pockets. He didn't like the situation; there was no clear plan in place. Darius always expected results, but actions like this rarely ended well, and mistakes were a real possibility. David watched as Darius executed a three-point turn and sped away toward the main road. Once Darius was out of sight, David rubbed his forehead, feeling trapped and committed to something he would rather avoid. Holding up the piece of paper, he read the address and name of the target. Studying the picture of the lab technician, he realised there was a good chance they would meet before the end of the day.

++++

Helen had decided to cancel her meeting with the Serjeant-at-Arms department at the palace. She knew that security was something she needed to take more seriously, but the vials had landed directly in her lap. This was an issue she couldn't ignore and needed to act on immediately.

Having taken public transport for granted her entire life, she found it more challenging recently. Her involvement with Alison had thrust her into the media spotlight, making her a public figure who faced both criticism and support. As a politician, public opinions were freely expressed, without being asked for; for her, this had become a daily occurrence. If people couldn't capture her attention online, they wouldn't hesitate to confront her in person.

She had taken the tube from Westminster to Charing Cross station. Now, sitting on the train heading towards Dartford in Kent, she was careful about where she sat, always trying to avoid groups of people. Those engrossed in books typically offered her a sense of security, as they were less likely to pay attention to her. In contrast, newspaper readers, flipping rapidly between stories, could be much more unpredictable.

The envelope she received from Brazil was both exciting and concerning, compelling her to investigate on Alison's behalf. Given the circumstances, she frequently scanned her surroundings on her way to the train, stopping periodically to check if anyone was following her. As a backbench MP, she had never received proper security training, only the occasional briefing, and instead relied on her adrenaline and instincts.

The train journey would take about forty minutes, and she would need a taxi to reach the lab. After Ben left her office, she called Dr Ryan Dobey, the lab's director, to explain the urgency of her need for a test. Now, in the middle of the afternoon, she hoped to arrive in time to have the test completed that day. Dr Dobey had mentioned that the lab was under pressure from a private medical client due to a heavy workload, so he advised her to wait a few hours before departing from Westminster. All she needed from him was confirmation that the vial in her possession contained the heroin derivative. The vial and its packaging indicated it had been produced in a Knightark Pharmaceutical laboratory. If this were proven to be true, she would have a major story on her hands, one with profound implications not only for that specific pharmaceutical company but for the industry as a whole. This was what they had fought for; positive natural beauty would finally have its day.

The carriage shook as the train pulled away from the platform. She anxiously scanned the list of upcoming stations, eager to reach her destination as quickly as possible. The automated display overhead, illuminated in orange, flashed the message: the next station was Waterloo East, followed by London Bridge and others, before arriving in Dartford.

Before leaving her office, she had tried to reassure Ben, although she suspected she hadn't succeeded. However, taking the drive from him had eased his nerves slightly. Now that she had cancelled her constituency meetings for the following day, she considered the possibility of going for a drink, especially since she might need to spend the evening in either London or Kent, depending on the turnaround of the test results. She knew her local newspaper would likely run another story about her; cancelling her constituency surgeries was not wise, especially if the polls were to be believed. She was aware that her support was declining locally. This situation needed resolution; after all, it was in the national interest. When her constituents found out what she had uncovered, she would be vindicated, the sleuth who cracked the case. Of course, it wouldn't be that simple; there was the small matter of two members of the House of Lords being on the payroll of the pharmaceutical company, along with the fact that the Prime Minister was close friends with a top executive on the board. Realising there was still much to be done, her thoughts wandered.

They had only been moving for a few minutes when the train arrived at Waterloo East station. Hardly anyone left the train; a few passengers joined, but she found herself mostly alone. Nevertheless, she kept a watchful eye on everyone who boarded, searching for anyone who seemed out of place. It wouldn't be easy; whoever attacked Alison was a professional who could blend in anywhere. It was too early to determine whether this was the work of a lone wolf or a coordinated effort. As the train pulled away, she closed her eyes. She had lied to Ben, claiming she had a safe place to hide the drive and the three remaining vials. With much of the estate under surveillance and a constant police presence, she resorted to hiding them in the only place she could think of: a single-occupancy toilet just down the hall from her office on the second floor of Portcullis House. This floor was off-limits to the public, and the toilet was used only by staff. It was one of the few locations without any cameras. Although the toilet was cleaned regularly, she had chosen to take a risk. Standing on the toilet seat, she pressed on a lightweight panel directly above her and slid it to the side. She pushed the envelope as far down between the other panels as she could reach.

The fact that she might not be able to retrieve it was of little concern to her. If the vial tested positive, she would return to the toilet with a stepladder in hand; by then, being observed by the CCTV in the corridor would matter little.

Joanne, her trusted research assistant, had called Helen's constituency office to cancel her appointments for the next day. However, Joanne was curious. She had helped collect research data on the pharmaceutical trade and had spent considerable time compiling information using the Commons Library's vast resources. Joanne sensed that something significant was happening with Knightark Pharmaceutical, but Helen had chosen to keep the main investigation from her for the time being and tried to reassure her. After her controversial outburst in the Commons, both of them suspected that Helen would soon be contacted by the Chief Whip again. While the Prime Minister would not get directly involved, she was sure that behind the scenes, he would be discussing her, though from a safe distance and hidden behind others. With no other allies, Helen needed to tread carefully, particularly as the police might still arrive at her offices in Westminster and at her constituency office. She had staff working in the constituency office, and under the current circumstances, it was important for her to consider their safety as well. When the Chief Whip summoned her, and he would, she might need to consider recording their conversation. Protecting herself was vital. Her hidden pin camera, although well-concealed in her jacket, had poor picture and sound quality. She had purchased it online from a generic website, not a spy shop, and had avoided mentioning her title of "MP" to prevent drawing attention.

As the train approached London Bridge station, Helen realised that in just a few hours, they would have a clear understanding of their situation with the crucial evidence they needed. She hoped that when the successful test results came in, her friend Alison would be awake and well enough to receive the news.

++++

In addition to his hand-delivered instructions regarding the emergency board meeting, Dr John Farmer received a text message directing him to travel alone. This was unusual, and the abruptness of the message made him uneasy; something was amiss, and it didn't bode well for him. Although he typically preferred to drive himself, other board members used their own chauffeurs and security drivers. For reasons he could not understand, this time the information was being kept tightly controlled. This secretive approach was something he had never encountered before. During his father's tenure on the board, he had no recollection of receiving such cryptic instructions. The choice of venue was odd: a lacklustre hotel just outside Bromley in Kent. While this suited him because it was only eight miles from his home, it was an unusual location, nearly seventeen miles outside London. Board meetings typically took place at their central offices. When the board convened, it received only minimal coverage in broadsheet newspapers, primarily those focused on financial news. No one was particularly interested; their profits had been well publicised over the years, and their current financial troubles were the only reason they garnered any attention at all. This further fuelled his curiosity, suggesting that their head office was not a safe venue for whatever was to be discussed.

Darius, their key director, was someone he didn't trust. There always seemed to be something held back when he was around, along with his three cronies, creating an uncomfortable atmosphere whenever everyone gathered.

About three years ago, William De La Roche, the senior American board member, was eager to establish a new research lab. At the time, this proposal raised concerns among some board members, but not among the core group of four; they quickly raised their hands to vote in favour, suggesting that a decision had already been made and construction might have begun. Although the vote was not unanimous, the majority consent allowed the project to proceed. In subsequent board meetings, presentations were given about the lab to be located in Brazil. The country's economic uncertainties made it a more cost-effective place to operate. Dr Guilherme Aranteses, the leading scientist and head of product development, was flown in to present to the board. He discussed various new product developments and filler configurations he was working on, aiming primarily to reduce overhead costs to counteract dwindling profits. However, over the past year, there have been no further presentations or communication from Dr Aranteses, only vague assurances that "things were on track" and "products were still in development." The core group of four never asked any questions; only the other concerned board members, primarily worried about their financial interests, dared to inquire. The four's dismissive attitude, especially Darius's, made other board members feel they had little control over the company. Board meetings became mere formalities, and for Darius, they seemed like an inconvenience. Darius was an intelligent man who could sense the mounting discontent around him. To quell the unrest, he authorised large bonuses for all shareholders, despite lacking the financial figures to justify them. This action effectively silenced many questions, particularly from less senior shareholders.

He parked outside the Fairline Hotel in Bromley, rolled down his car window, and waited. In addition to being instructed to drive alone, he was also told to remain in his car until he was called. He couldn't be the only one suspicious about these secretive instructions.

Turning off the engine, he looked around at the other parked cars. The car park was generally quiet, though he wasn't the first board member to arrive. While he couldn't spot any senior board members, several junior members were already present. He noticed Harry Whitney, a fellow junior board member, and nodded at him. Harry responded by waving his arms in confusion, grinning and shrugging; he seemed bewildered by the unusual protocol they were expected to follow. Given their regular invitations to the Palace of Westminster and charity events attended by VIPs and celebrities, it felt quite unprecedented to be sitting in a line of cars like this.

He heard the roar of a fast car speeding down the road behind him. As the car pulled into the parking area, he recognised it as the black Gran Turismo Maserati belonging to Lisa Wellings, the only female board member. Lisa consistently outshone what John called "boys' toys" with her unique flair. He held her in high regard; she did not tolerate the male-dominated board's condescension and, for him, represented the company's future. John believed that the old boys' network would eventually fade away, and he had wholeheartedly admired and supported Lisa since she joined the board three years ago.

As she parked, the sound levels returned to normal when the Maserati's engine shut off. John instantly recognised the security guard who appeared at the front of the hotel; it was the same military-looking man who had delivered his 'invitation' to be there. Two other men flanked him. They were casually dressed but exuded an air of authority. One of them held a phone and glanced over the parked cars. He nodded, and the three of them split up as they approached the vehicles one by one. The man John recognised approached his car. He nodded at John, who noticed that his window was already open.

"Dr Farmer, the senior board members are already here. Would you mind following me, please?"

John rolled up the window and grabbed his keys. As he stepped out of the car, he noticed the other board members also exiting, standing in a line like students awaiting a reprimand from the headteacher. He couldn't help but smile as he watched Lisa strut past the security guard, clearly wanting to avoid any fuss and procedure.

John nodded at the serious-looking security guard. "Well, after you, then, I guess."

The guard lifted his arm and said, "This way."

As John turned, he noticed the flesh-coloured earpiece the guard wore; it suggested heightened security wherever they were headed. "I don't suppose you can tell me why we are going through this rigmarole?" he asked.

The security guard replied, "What do you mean by 'this rigmarole,' Dr Farmer?"

"This! What's going on at our central offices? Why are there so many of you here?"

"I'm sorry, Dr Farmer, but I'm not privy to that information."

"Then can you at least tell me where we're headed?"

"Of course. Your board meeting is on the second floor. My colleague has already reserved both elevators for you and the other board members. You will go straight up when we get inside."

"I see," he responded cautiously.

"It's quite warm in the meeting room; the air conditioning is not working. I thought it best to forewarn you," the guard added.

John surveyed the hotel's exterior. It looked dirty and neglected, so it was no surprise that the air conditioning was out of order. "Well, there are always windows," he said.

"There are, but I'm afraid they are locked," the guard replied.

"What?" he exclaimed.

"For security reasons," the guard explained.

John shook his head with a smile, though his curiosity was only growing.

As they entered the hotel, the former military security personnel caught the reception staff's attention. Four of them stood behind the counter, taking turns staring as each board member was escorted to the elevators.

"This is not exactly discreet," John muttered to his security escort.

"It was the best we could do. We considered using the back doors, but that would have meant escorting you through the kitchen."

John blinked in surprise. The whole situation felt unusual; the reception staff likely seemed disappointed, expecting to see famous figures instead of suited board members.

The eight board members were divided into two groups of four, with each group assigned to a separate elevator. John entered one of the elevators and stood next to Lisa, offering her a slight smile. She shrugged in response as the doors closed. Not a word was exchanged between them during the short ride. When the doors on the second floor opened, they were met by another security guard, who led them to their temporary boardroom.

"I think I'll sit next to you," John said.

Lisa nodded and leaned in closer. "Do you have any idea what's going on?"

"Nope, not a clue," he replied.

She continued to whisper, "Don't you think this is a bit odd? It seems like overkill for a meeting."

As they entered the room, they saw the four senior board members seated at the head of the table, with Darius positioned among them. The security guard who had escorted them exchanged a few words with Darius before moving to the corner of the room.

John took a seat next to Lisa and loosened his tie; the room was stuffy and humid.

Darius stood up and addressed the group. "I can only apologise for the temperature in this room. The air conditioning isn't working."

"Can't we open the windows?" Lisa asked reasonably as she tied her hair back into a ponytail.

"No, I'm afraid not. We have to make do," Darius replied.

John noticed that the curtains were drawn. He stood up and approached the trolley with refreshments. Grabbing two bottles of water, he glanced at the windows and saw that a protective seal had been affixed to the glass through a gap between the curtains. He returned to his seat and placed one of the bottles in front of Lisa. She smiled and said, "Thank you."

As John leaned forward to grab a glass for his water, he whispered to her, "The windows have been sealed." Lisa frowned, took a glass for herself, and looked around the room. It was sparse, lacking a television, presentation equipment, and furniture, which gave it a stripped-down feel.

"Alright, now that we're all here, we can begin. I'm sure you're curious about why we're meeting here. This is a very competitive industry, and walls have ears," Darius said with a grin. "This is as good a place as any for this extraordinary meeting, and it will not be recorded. In that respect, please take your phones out of your pockets or bags and place them on the table or hold them up." A few board members exchanged glances, clearly unsettled by this unusual request. "My colleague, who escorted you into the room, will be collecting them. They will be returned to you once we've finished."

Lisa looked at John with concern.

"Is this really necessary, Darius?"

"I understand your concerns, Dr Farmer, but we must proceed and needs must."

Unimpressed, John let out a deep sigh and took his phone from his pocket, only to have it snatched away immediately by the security guard. The guard walked around the room collecting phones, gathering eight devices and placing them into a sealed bag. Judging by the expressions on some of the board members' faces, it was clear they noticed that the phones of the four senior executives had not been collected.

The door closed behind the security guard as he left with the sealed bag.

Darius began, "Alright, now that we are alone, we can start. Lady and gentlemen, you are all aware of our declining revenues in the current climate. If we do not address this issue, we foresee no change in our fortunes. Big pharma, particularly in our beauty-related specialities, will continue to be plagued by lawsuits, benefiting only the lawyers involved. This situation must change, or we will dwindle into oblivion. Our experts and advisors are advocating for a focus on innovation. The relentless campaign led by the Harwood woman, assisted by the crusading MP, seeks to eradicate the beauty business; if that happens, it would bring us to our knees. We must either diversify into new fields or concentrate on what we do best: cosmetic beauty. Over the years, our industry has provided you all with exceptional lifestyles, and I, along with the senior board, have no intention of changing that. However, we must evolve."

He sat back down and took a deep breath. "The senior board

members and I will not allow this great company to fail, and you will be rewarded once again. As you know, we have established a new laboratory in Brazil. Dr Guilherme Arantes has been, and continues to be, the lead on this project. Over the past few years, he has been experimenting with new fillers and compounds, utilising state-of-the-art technology that has not been seen before."

Darius glanced at the senior board members beside him, and it was clear they anticipated what was coming. "What if I told you about a new compound that not only performs its intended function but also helps clients feel... well, how should I put this? Better."

Harry Whitney, seated across from John, leaned in. "Darius, what do you mean by 'better'? Our products provide empowerment and confidence; that's the very nature of cosmetic surgery."

Darius gestured in agreement. "And that's true. Touché. But what if I said it makes them feel genuinely better?" He looked at Harry, confident he had everyone's attention.

John took a sip of his water and loosened his tie further. "Can you clarify what you mean by 'genuinely better,' please?"

"I'm glad you asked, Dr Farmer. Our lab has developed the ultimate filler. We've created a filler that produces a natural high, if you will. This compound gradually stimulates serotonin levels in the brain. We're talking about a beauty product that provides a positive experience."

Lisa quickly surveyed the other board members' expressions, noticing that only John looked concerned. "But that sounds like a drug," she stated.

Darius shrugged. "It's a matter of semantics, Lisa. Just imagine how groundbreaking this could be. There's nothing like this on the market…"

"Probably because it wouldn't be approved," Lisa interrupted sharply.

Darius turned to his left to look at William De La Roche, the American board member, who then took the lead. "What if I told you it could be approved, Lisa? It's simply an enhancement of our core product, the one we supplied worldwide until social networks turned against us."

"William, what is this key property that creates this high?" John asked.

"It's complicated," William replied.

"I'm a doctor; please try me."

"This compound is called Lipomorphilas. It has taken months of design, and trials in South America have been very successful."

John took a pen from his pocket to write down the name.

"Ah, no notes, please. This is a confidential meeting," Darius asserted.

"We need to know what this is. Are you saying you've already conducted human experiments?"

The senior board members exchanged glances. Ronald Ward, who hadn't spoken until then, tapped his fingernails on the table. "Well, we can't use monkeys, can we?"

A few sniggers rippled through the room. Lisa and John exchanged concerned looks.

Darius smiled and continued, "We are in the people business, Dr Farmer. We ask that you trust our judgment. The senior board has never received complaints from any of you regarding your bank balances."

"I never supported this lab; I thought it was odd at the time," Lisa responded.

"Yes, we remember, you hadn't been with us for very long. Why do you feel so strongly about this, Lisa? We always need to innovate. That's the nature of business; if you don't innovate, you get left behind. As someone successful in business, you must understand that more than anyone else."

"But it sounds like you're discussing a drug. How could this ever be approved by the OPSS in this country, the FDA in the States, or other regulatory agencies around the world?" Lisa asked.

"Because we have it on good authority that it will be approved. We require your approval to proceed to the next phase. That is the purpose of today's meeting," Darius explained.

"Darius, why couldn't we do this at the main office? Why is there so much security? Are we trying to hide something?" Lisa pressed further.

Darius laughed. "Come now, we're not the only players in this industry. We cannot risk our competitors discovering our revolutionary product. This is just a precaution, nothing more. You should feel confident that I take the security of this company very seriously."

A brief silence fell across the room.

Andrew Dutton, a board member for over fifteen years, wiped the beads of sweat forming on his forehead. "Look, if approval can be granted, I see no harm in it. This company needs to improve its performance. If not, we could face mass redundancies."

Darius smiled and nodded. "There you go, that's the spirit. And that's my role as the head of this great company: to innovate and adapt to the times, always leading from the front."

John noticed Darius fiddling with what might be one of his trouser pockets under the table. He observed Darius looking down, his body language suggesting he was pressing buttons on his phone.

"I'm uneasy about this. Aren't the rest of you?" Lisa asked, glancing around at the other board members, but most of them avoided her eyes.

William, frustrated by her statement, snapped, "What do you expect us to do, Lisa?" This crisis isn't going away. The social network will continue to gain momentum. In this country, there is a blanket ban on one of your Brit TV channels. No one with any enhancements is allowed on screen, and this is severely impacting us! Personal freedoms are being stripped away, and that's never a good thing."

Darius raised his hands in a calming gesture. "Okay, okay, let's all stay calm here. This is good; it's a debate, and it shows passion. Passion is what I invest in every day to safeguard our livelihoods. Our forefathers would be appalled to see this company declining. John, your father was a crucial member of this board for many years. You must understand that, right?"

"I understand, Darius, but like Lisa, I have concerns. What if this product, along with the positive feelings it generates, becomes addictive? That could lead to all sorts of consequences. I've never heard of such a thing or the name of the compound you mentioned," John replied.

Darius leaned back in his chair and crossed his arms. "I hear you, I do, but your father would have done whatever it took to support this company. It was his life."

John shook his head, displeased with how his father's name was being used. "I'm not blind to what's happening. Surely you all saw what took place in London yesterday. There was an assassination attempt on Alison Harwood, a senior executive at the TV channel you just mentioned."

"Ha," Darius laughed loudly. "That bloody woman."

"That bloody woman, as you just referred to her, was blown up!" Lisa exclaimed. "I know she has caused us immense damage, but this situation is spiralling out of control. I believe someone targeted her." Lisa threw her arms in the air in frustration.

William grinned widely. "Not anymore."

The room fell silent as Lisa noticed the sinister look on the American's face. Darius stood up.

"I understand that passions run high in business, but today we need your vote to proceed with the new filler. There are costs associated with this, not just in production but also in shipping and storage in the UK. We plan to start here before rolling it out globally." Darius then looked at John. "If we receive the approvals I mentioned, we can move to the next phase of distribution and put this business back on a profitable track. That's all we're asking of you."

The heat in the room intensified Darius's persuasion; a couple of board members were sweating and likely eager to leave. "If our forecasting is correct, within two years, your dividends could yield a few million pounds. I am highly confident of this."

"I haven't seen such forecasting," Harry Whitney questioned.

"That is correct; those figures will be submitted to you securely in due time. However, for now, based on what I'm presenting, I am seeking a majority vote to proceed." Darius looked around the room.

"I'm sorry, Darius, but I cannot vote on something I don't fully understand. As a doctor, I need to see the precise scientific breakdown and the testing results you mentioned. Are there any complications associated with this product?"

"I respect your request for further information, Dr Farmer, and I will ensure your questions are answered. However, we must proceed because this is a time-sensitive matter. I hope you all agree that we cannot afford to stagnate."

Darius received a few nods, but also some concerned looks.

"Can I speak with Dr Guilherme Arantes, the lead scientist?" John asked.

Darius shrugged. "Of course, but not right now. I've given him an extended leave. He has worked incredibly hard, and when he returns, you can speak with him then."

John glanced at Lisa; she looked very uncomfortable.

"So, there are twelve of us present, and we will go by majority rule," Darius said. "Please raise your hand if you support this innovation. And yes, I will provide you with the information you've requested, Dr Farmer."

Darius raised his hand, followed by the three senior board members, including Hugh Darlington, who had remained silent until then. One by one, the other board members raised their hands in support, except for Lisa and John.

Lisa and John exchanged glances as the senior board members stared at them. The other board members quickly joined in, collectively trying to persuade Lisa and John to support the initiative. It was clear that the prospect of receiving additional funds had swayed the votes of the other board members.

Darius nodded. "So be it. Ten hands have been raised, indicating that we will proceed. John and Lisa, your lack of support is disappointing and duly noted, but it will not be logged. We will remember," he said with a smile, placing his hands in his pockets.

"Lady and gentlemen of the board, that concludes our meeting for today. The senior board members and I appreciate your time. We will keep you updated on developments, and now, I'm sure we could all use some fresh air." He walked to the door, opened it, and nodded at the two security guards positioned on either side. One of the guards pressed his earpiece, instructing his colleague to summon the elevators. At the same time, the other entered the room and unzipped the sealed phone bag, carefully placing its contents on the boardroom table.

The overweight, perspiring board directors were the first to grab their phones. They shook hands with each other and exited the room, leaving John and Lisa feeling alienated as the other directors passed by without offering a handshake.

As Lisa reached for her phone, she whispered, "Let's talk outside." John discreetly nodded as he collected his phone. The senior board members remained seated, their eyes fixed on them. John managed a brief smile, but it was not returned. "See you both soon," William remarked, the only comment given.

John left the room, uncertain if he had just received a veiled threat. The offhand comment from William about the TV channel lady weighed heavily on his mind. He hoped, for God's sake, that they were not involved.

Chapter Twelve

After the junior board members left the room, Darius leaned back in his chair. "I didn't expect them all to agree. I expected decent from Lisa, but John surprised me, especially considering his father's background."

"They could become a problem. If they make waves and interfere with our plans, we'll need to silence them," William replied.

Darius glanced at William. "Don't worry; I've got it under control." He picked up his phone, opened his recent call list, and dialled. The call was answered almost immediately. "Please come into the room."

They waited only a moment before there was a knock at the door.

"Come in," Darius said, looking at the senior board members. "This will only take a moment."

A security guard entered the room. "Yes, sir?" he asked.

"I trust you received my text?" Darius inquired.

"Yes, sir, I did."

"Where are board members Farmer and Wellings?"

"They are outside in front of the hotel, sir."

"Did you place trackers on their cars?"

"Yes, sir, we have a strong signal on them."

"Monitor their activities. If it appears they are scheduling a meeting together, immediately assign someone to keep an eye on them, someone they haven't encountered before. I trust you have a suitable candidate in mind?"

"Yes, sir. I have a reliable female asset whom they have never seen."

"Excellent. Assign her to them. We must ascertain what they are discussing; this information is crucial. If you can accomplish this, you will be well rewarded. Your findings must be reported to me in person, only to me. Is that clear?"

"Yes, sir. I understand."

"Your assistance is appreciated."

"Thank you, sir. I'll get right on it." The security guard nodded to the board members and left the room.

"Do you trust him?" Hugh Darlington asked.

Darius nodded. "He's a professional. While he may not be the right choice for our more specialised work, I know he will stay on top of things. Speaking of which..." He lifted his phone. "We need to put this room back together. I'll call the others back, and then we can discuss privately the real reason why we implemented the security measures in this room."

Ronald Ward, the oldest member of the senior board, looked concerned. "This worries me, gentlemen. They need to be on board with our plans. Farmer is a doctor. If he's not satisfied, he'll investigate; it's in a doctor's nature to dig deeper. I suggested from the beginning that we be transparent, which would have left no room for questions. Alternatively, we could have proceeded without involving them at all."

William chuckled, leaned back, and placed his hands behind his head. "Come on, Ronald. A filler laced with some form of natural high? Heaven forbid they discover the truth, that it's a derivative of heroin. It was never going to pass without scrutiny from a couple of them. Just look at how few questions the others have; they only care about money. They don't care about the people using the product; to them, those users are just collateral damage. All they want to know is that they will get paid and face no repercussions. If it weren't for company protocol, none of them should have known about it in the first place. We should have just gone ahead as you suggested, Ronald."

Darius nodded, "And we are moving forward, my friend. I'll green-light it shortly. Please hold on while I speak with our asset; his phone is ringing." The phone was answered quickly. "Ah, good.

David, we've finished in the room. I'll be here with the senior board for another ten minutes or so. Before you move on to your next assignment, could you and your colleague come back to clean up the room?" Darius added, "I appreciate that it will be tight, but I don't want anyone else coming in here and seeing the measures you've implemented." He leaned back while David responded, "Okay, I understand. We'll probably be gone before you get here. Thank you for your assistance." Darius hung up the phone and began, "Right, gentlemen, here's the state of play: I've asked one of our assets and his colleague to handle something. I'll share those details if necessary, but for now, here's where we stand. Although the board voted today to proceed, as you know, production is already well underway, and the first batch has departed from the Spanish coast. We have nine thousand units on the way. This will serve as our starting point, and they will be integrated into our existing inventory. I'm also considering donating some of the upgraded filler to leaders in the private cosmetic industry, with the hope of reintroducing the product to the mainstream. Ideally, they will offer cheaper procedures initially to encourage business."

"Darius, how can we differentiate between the two products?"

Darius grinned. "That's an excellent question, Hugh, and it takes a keen eye to distinguish them. Each vial is presented just as it normally would be, complete with the same packaging from our Hydra-Fillixir range. However, if you look closely at the small print on the side of every box, you'll notice that an extra full stop has been added where it shouldn't be. That's how we manage to bring them into the country. They will all be sealed and surrounded by our existing fillers. I don't anticipate any issues at the borders, and I'm not expecting British Customs and Excise to pose a problem."

"Nine thousand, that's a great start," Ronald added.

"It is, and unless there are any interruptions, I'm planning for immediate distribution. Once they arrive, they will be separated and stored in a secure, undisclosed location. If our warehouses and cool rooms are inspected, I've already arranged for another nine thousand original vials to be flown in via a private airstrip, so the numbers will match in case we get checked."

William and Hugh nodded in agreement.

"Impressive," Ronald remarked.

"However, speaking of potential problems, on Saturday evening at our event at the Palace, I'll address our two supporters in the House of Lords. I'll also have a word in the ear with my old school friend, the Prime Minister. I think it's time to call in some of the favours we're owed from him, starting with dealing with the rogue MP in his party, Helen Lord. I want her out."

++++

Lisa nodded at the last board director as he drove away. Standing by her car, she and John were the only ones in the car park. "Well, he nodded back at me," she said.

"They were pretty eager to leave, and I don't think it was just the heat in the room. None of them stayed for questions, did they?" John replied.

Lisa smiled briefly as she glanced toward the front of the hotel, where two security guards stood at the entrance, watching their every move. Out of earshot, she turned her back to the guards and cautiously covered her mouth as she spoke. "I can't believe what I heard in there. You're a doctor; have you ever heard of a product called Lipomorphilas?"

John turned away from the security men as well. "No, that's why I didn't push it. I need to do some research. But considering the name, it sounds like Morphinan, and for this kind of application, I'm very concerned. The dismissive comment about yesterday's explosion in the city has sent shivers down my spine."

Lisa looked him directly in the eyes, her hand still cupped over her mouth. "That's my concern, too. Are we involved in something here?" She lowered her hand and straightened her jacket.

"I don't know; that's the honest answer. I don't trust them and haven't for some time. Decisions are being made without our consent."

"Don't turn around; I know those military types are still watching us," Lisa added. "Do you fancy a drink? I don't know my way around here, but there must be a place nearby. We need to talk."

John sensed her worries and felt concerned as well. A chat couldn't hurt; it was rare for them to see each other, and they still knew very little about one another. "Sure, why not? I don't live too far from here, so I know my way around. It might be best to move a few miles away to get some distance from this place. There are a couple of pubs in the Bickley area, just a few miles away. Would you like to try one of those?"

"Okay, that sounds good. I don't know where to go, so I'll follow you," she replied.

John glanced at Lisa's car. "I'm not a very fast driver, but I suspect you can keep up," he said with a grin.

"Trust me, that won't be a problem. I'll call you if we get separated on the way."

John nodded and walked to his car. The sound of Lisa's Maserati starting echoed through the empty car park. As John started his Mercedes, he noticed one of the security guards speaking into his radio. The other security man quickly left his side and disappeared from view. For the first time in his years on the board, he felt worried. As he drove away, he glanced in the rearview mirror and saw the security guard watching him intently while tapping at his earpiece. John had an overwhelming feeling that he needed to stay alert.

++++

As the train approached Dartford station, Helen swallowed, feeling her mouth go dry in an instant. It was a warm afternoon, but not sweltering. The anticipation of receiving her test results filled her with both excitement and fear. If the result was positive, she knew what that would mean: she would have to disclose the information to the press or engage with the media immediately. After what had happened to Alison, Helen understood that such media coverage would be essential for her protection. If something were to happen to her, there would be a motive, making her a much harder target for the influential figures involved. The public outcry would lead to a scandal, and the key to it all was in her jacket pocket.

The train announcer's voice filled the air, informing passengers that it was the end of the line and advising them to exit the train. Helen rose to her feet and gathered her bags as the train came to a stop. Stepping off the train, she took her phone out of her handbag and texted Dr Ryan Dobey, hoping he would have some time available for her in the lab. The message let him know she would be there soon, depending on the availability of taxis outside the station.

✢✢✢✢

After picking up Rubin from the café, they had to work quickly as time was short. It was a hurried race to the hotel to dismantle the anti-surveillance measures and reconnect the air conditioning. The room had been stifling, and they felt relieved to reopen the windows as they worked. David collected the surveillance camera from the security guard, and after explaining they were in a rush, the guard agreed to reset the room to its original state.

As they drove towards Dartford to locate the research laboratory that Darius had instructed them to visit, David tried to adhere to the speed limit. "What have you learned so far?" he asked.

"According to Google Maps, the lab is part of an industrial unit," Rubin replied.

"That won't be easy to survey. Do you know if the other units look occupied?"

"I'm checking that now," Rubin said, pulling up an image on his phone. "That's interesting, though."

David glanced over. "What did you find?"

"It looks like there's some green space behind the building, with plenty of trees for cover. It might be doable."

"I don't know what's in your backpack or the contents of your other bag. Do you have kit with you to do this?"

"Some," Rubin replied. "I noticed you didn't bring much."

"I didn't expect us to end up in this situation. The day has already taken a different turn."

"You know how this works, brother; you always need to be prepared."

David rolled his eyes internally; he could do without the lecture. "What do you have with you?"

"The usual gear. I have a ghillie suit packed in case we need it. It's been a while since I've worn one. I've also got scopes and other equipment. What weapons do you have?"

David laughed. "Weapon is more accurate, singular. As you know, it's not so easy to possess one in the UK anymore. Just a Glock 17, short. I take every precaution. If you're caught with a firearm, you face a minimum seven-year sentence. That's why this car has a cloned number plate; all the serial numbers have been filed off. I can dispose of this vehicle without a second thought; there are no consequences."

"True, but there's also the small matter that cameras are everywhere these days. That's another reason I prefer working abroad," Rubin replied.

"Speaking of which, I was fortunate to catch you here. Were you working or was it a personal matter?"

Rubin paused before answering, "Just a quick action, nothing to write home about or stress over. I keep my gear in a self-storage unit here in the south. Inside that unit, there's a motion tracker connected to my phone in case of any compromise. One of our brothers helped me put together the documents so I could secure the unit in the first place. It's a purpose-built, five-story building. I rent it under a different name and have to change my appearance every time I go in and out, with a wig, fake beard, the whole works. You should consider getting one too. It's great because it's always unmanned, which makes things easier when you have a lot to hide.

However, they do have cameras at the entry and exit points, mostly for general security rather than for anything specific."

David glanced at his phone after noticing a quick flash on the screen. "Keep an eye out for the police while I read this," he instructed. After scanning the message, he quickly replied, "The MP has arrived at Dartford station. She texted Ryan Dobey, the senior technician, to let him know she's on her way. We need to hurry. Make sure you find pictures of Dobey online so you can recognise him. Once you are dug in, I'll try to obtain the senior technician's home address. I suspect that one of us will need to pay a visit to his family."

++++

John felt a sense of relief after leaving the stuffy, makeshift boardroom at the hotel. With the windows down on this warm summer evening, he enjoyed the refreshing breeze flowing through the car. Although they passed several pubs and eateries where he and Lisa could stop, the presence of security guards at the hotel made him uneasy. The flippant comment he had heard about yesterday's assassination attempt continued to haunt him, making him eager to find a place away from the hotel where he and Lisa could talk privately. After driving for about twenty minutes, they followed signs to Chislehurst. Lisa kept pace with him as they passed Chislehurst Station and made their way up a large hill. The pub he had chosen was called the Rambler's Rest. He anticipated there might be some evening commuters returning from London, but he hoped it wouldn't be too busy. As he turned left off the main road, he saw the pub nestled down a lane, with parking available outside. The green area in front of the pub had a few people sitting on benches and lying on the grass, along with some children playing, but it wasn't too crowded. It seemed perfect for their needs.

John parked outside the pub and noticed Lisa pull into a space next to the green. The engine roared one last time as it was turned off, drawing immediate attention.

He removed his suit jacket, locked his car, and waited for Lisa to join him. John smiled as she approached and said, "Looks like you've got a fan club."

Lisa glanced back at her car and laughed when she saw a couple of people gazing through the glass at the Maserati's interior. "I guess it always attracts attention," she replied.

She looked at the white timber-framed building with a sign outside that read, "Traditional hospitality since circa 1684." "This looks like a nice place," she remarked as she walked through the open front door. Inside, there were two bar areas: a smaller bar at the top with a seating area and a television screen, and a larger area down a few steps with multiple sports playing on various screens. Lisa selected the top bar as it was quieter. "What will you have?" she asked John.

"Thank you, I'll have a gin and tonic," he replied.

Lisa nodded. "Good choice. It's strange; we've been on the board for a while, but we rarely socialise outside of those bloody VIP marketing events. I know very little about you. I prefer rum."

"Likewise, I don't know much about you either," John agreed.

At the quieter bar, Lisa was served immediately.

"Shall we sit outside?" John suggested. "It's a lovely afternoon."

Lisa looked around. Inside, several tables were occupied, and they needed to talk privately. The outside option seemed better. "I didn't check outside, and I don't want to sit on the grass. Can you see if there's a table available?" she asked.

"Sure," John replied as he stepped outside while Lisa paid for the drinks. The server handed her the change, and she carefully held both glasses. John soon returned and said, "There's a table further up on the bank. Do you need a hand with those?"

"No, but you can take yours," Lisa replied.

"Thank you," he said, accepting the glass she offered him.

People lounged on the grass and sat at tables scattered throughout the area. The men wore shirts but had removed their business ties, while some women had taken off their heels. Nearby, children played, creating a reasonable amount of noise, but that was fine; it helped drown out their conversation. They sat opposite each other on pub benches with a circular table between them, taking in their surroundings. Positioned near the top of the bank, they could see a game of cricket being played in a field further down, across the road.

John lifted his glass. "Well, cheers then."

"Cheers to you, too," Lisa replied, clinking her glass against his before taking a sip. "Oh, that's good! I wish I weren't driving now."

John smiled and took a sip of his drink. "I know exactly what you mean."

After exchanging the initial pleasantries, Lisa paused to assess their surroundings. She was the first to express her concerns. "What do you think we should do? We were outvoted, but I'm not surprised, considering the money hoarders on the rest of the board."

John took another sip of his gin. "I completely agree. I'm surprised that some of the board members didn't ask more challenging questions, or hardly any questions at all, now that I think about it. It worries me. It feels like the top-tier executives had already made their decision; they knew what was coming and likely approved this so-called *'innovation'*. This issue doesn't just rest with Darius; they are all equally complicit."

Lisa nodded in agreement. "Yes, that's how I feel, and it has been for some time. Also…" She was immediately interrupted when a football was kicked under their table, and a toddler, probably around three years old, stumbled nearby. "Oh, I'm sorry! Let me get that," the mother said as she rushed over. "I apologise; he's at that age." As she bent down to retrieve the ball, her phone slipped from her shirt pocket. She picked up the ball, gently tossed it back to the child, and then retrieved her phone. "Do you two have kids?" she asked.

John and Lisa exchanged a glance and laughed. "No, we're just friends," Lisa replied with a smile.

"Oh, right. Anyway, if you want my advice, don't have any!" The woman laughed, turned away, and started kicking the ball around with the toddler.

Once the ball-kicking mother was out of earshot, John and Lisa exchanged glances and laughed.

Lisa ran a hand through her hair, looking concerned. "That comment about what happened in London yesterday was so dismissive. You must have seen William's face; he looked almost pleased about it."

John took a deep breath and studied the ice cubes melting in his drink. "Do you think they were involved? This is the pharmaceutical business, not the mafia."

"Isn't it? Consider the impact of our activities and the millions in revenue our products generate globally. We've taken a major hit; our stock value has been steadily declining." Lisa glanced around before leaning in toward John. "Do you know who was targeted in that explosion yesterday?"

John nodded. "Yes, I saw it on the news."

"Good. Then you know she played a major role in our downfall; her campaign created the divide between what she referred to as the 'plastics' and the 'real.'"

"I'm aware of her and her campaign, but I avoid social media. I lead a private life and have no interest in such things."

"John, I lead a private life too. As I mentioned before, I know very little about you, and you know very little about me. Furthermore, I know very little about the other board members, especially the senior four. When we meet at charity fundraisers and try to persuade others to support our business, we always discuss work and never share anything personal. Don't you find that strange?"

"I never really thought about it, to be honest," John said, stopping to take a sip of his drink. "As a private person, that arrangement has always suited me. I've never considered forming friendships with the board members. It was different in my father's day; he was close to some of them. When I was younger, he often left me alone when he wanted to speak with the hierarchy. Now that I think about it, whatever was discussed, he never mentioned, and I never questioned it. I suppose I understood my place back then."

Lisa nodded, "Regarding these so-called consultants, when you review the accounts, you can see the thousands paid out each month. It's brushed over, just like the financial entries for security services, but I've never questioned it. Have you ever seen an invoice?" she said.

John put down his glass and rubbed his eyes in concession. "No, I haven't."

"That's my point; to my knowledge, none of the other board members have either. As long as the money comes in, we all give it our approval. We have been inattentive as directors, and that's a fact! We don't communicate enough."

John nodded. "I think you're right. I must admit that, in my case, this was my father's legacy; I've never sought to take an active role."

"You mentioned that we are a pharmaceutical company and not a mafia. Are you sure about that now? If we start probing into things in more detail, I'm telling you, they're not going to like it. And what about those shady military types who keep appearing? What are their backgrounds, and where were they recruited from? Security is supposed to make us feel safe, but it feels more like intimidation to me."

John was aware of his surroundings as he spoke. "Who has the skills to execute what happened yesterday? The police haven't indicated that it was a terrorist attack." He lowered his voice. "It must have been someone with a military background or connections to an obscure government department."

Lisa nodded. "Exactly. Look, I know you don't closely follow these matters, and given the nature of our business, I avoid using my real name on social media. However, I keep track of things through a couple of accounts set up under other people's names. You may not know much about her, but the woman who was targeted yesterday is named Alison Harwood."

John replied, "Yes, I was aware of that."

"Although, to my knowledge, she has never directly named us, she has certainly targeted us and our competitors. Do you think it's just a coincidence that we're paying a couple of members of the Lords as consultants? They aren't genuinely consulting for us. What services are they actually providing? I'm convinced it's all about having the right people in key positions. Harwood was a problem, and no amount of her complaints and campaigns about the so-called 'death of beauty' would justify how she was silenced. This was the work of professionals." Lisa swiped at her glass and took a large mouthful. "I'm worried we're getting involved in something dangerous. She needed to be silenced."

"Oh, come on, are you serious? Yes, she upset a lot of people, and I agree that the whole situation is suspicious and toxic," John replied with a shrug. "Maybe she angered someone in the government."

Lisa nodded. "It could be related to the new enhanced filler that was just approved today. Your decision not to vote for it suggests you're concerned."

"Yes, and by doing so, it also alerted them."

Lisa glanced at her watch. "I need to leave soon."

John instinctively glanced at his watch. "We need to gather more information. Perhaps we can talk to the senior board members privately; we have very little to go on."

"I agree, but a filler that provides the user with a natural high? What exactly does that mean? It sounds unethical to me. I suspect the company might have entered the drug business, and that was the plan all along. That's why William was advocating for the lab in Brazil; they could facilitate the distribution of South American drugs."

John shook his head and sighed, "It's mind-boggling that the other directors are so dismissive and unconcerned."

"They're only interested in the money. No one seems to care about the end user. Are we on the verge of pioneering another opioid epidemic? Ask yourself that! What is actually in this filler?"

"Well, we need to come up with a plan. I agree; we have to take some form of action."

Lisa nodded. "We can work on this over the coming weekend."

John raised his eyebrows, a slight smirk on his face. "Oh yes, the Lord's reception. I wasn't planning to attend."

"Neither was I; those events bore me to tears. But this changes things. We should be there. Let them enjoy some of that House of Lords wine, and then we can start pushing for answers to see where things stand."

John laughed, "I like the sound of that. I usually tune out at these events."

"But not this time. Look, I think it's best if we don't communicate beforehand. I'll meet you there at seven. We'll typically be greeted upon arrival. If I don't see you, I'll be on the terrace behind the Lord's bar."

John finished the last of his drink and said, "Okay, I'll see you there. Sounds like a plan."

Lisa smiled as she stood up. "It's all we have for now. Between you and me, I've always admired Alison Harwood; she was principled and stood by her beliefs."

John took his car keys from his pocket. "And look where that got her. Well, I'll see you Saturday night."

Lisa finished her drink and slung her bag over her shoulder. "See you then," she said as she walked toward her car. Once inside, she watched as John drove away and headed back up toward the main road. She entered her home postcode into the sat-nav, realising she had quite a drive ahead of her. As her car roared to life, it caught the attention of several people who would be staying at the pub much longer. She reversed from the edge of the green and drove off in the same direction as John.

The road wound to the right until she reached a junction on a hill, where she waited behind another car. Glancing across the green to where they had been sitting, she frowned as she noticed the toddler had wandered over to their seats again while the mother was bent under the table retrieving a football.

Chapter Thirteen

"So, you're local then?" the taxi driver asked.

Helen knew he was only being polite, but with so much on her mind, she could do without a conversation. "No, I've never been this way before; I'm just visiting a friend." She chose not to mention where she was from. Noticing that he kept staring at her in the rearview mirror, she turned to look out the window to avoid his eyes.

"I recognise you from somewhere!" he continued.

Helen's heart sank.

"You're an actor; I'm sure I've seen you in something," he said.

Helen laughed nervously. "No, definitely not." There was a time when she enjoyed the notoriety of being an MP, but that was not how she felt today.

"Oh well, you must have a doppelgänger," he replied.

She smiled and glanced at his sat nav display. The lab was only about a mile away. As they drove, she observed that the area was heavily developed. With London just a short train ride away, it was more affordable to have businesses and homes here than in the city. She pulled her phone from her bag to check if Ryan had responded; he hadn't yet, which concerned her. She kept a close eye on her surroundings, aware that she might have to stay here overnight. Thankfully, the taxi driver had stopped talking while she searched for the latest news stories on her phone. When she checked Channel 8's website, she immediately saw a picture of Alison, who was the lead story, but the accompanying text provided little additional information. As she scrolled through her various social media platforms, she noticed that her inboxes were flooded with messages. Generally, she avoided reading direct messages because they were often abusive. If her constituents needed her, they knew to contact her through the proper channels. However, Alison was trending, particularly under the tags #LondonExplosion and #DeathOfBeauty. Against her better judgment, Helen decided to take a look, more concerned for her friend than anything else. Selecting the "latest" setting, she hoped to find updates on Alison's condition. There was a post from the metropolitan police, but it didn't name Alison; instead, she was referred to as a "woman in serious condition." The post focused more on the investigation than on other specific details. The police were trying to prevent the public from jumping to conclusions about the incident being related to terrorism, emphasising that there was no evidence of terrorist activity at this time. The broadsheets offered their own interpretations of the events, and some comments appeared speculative at best. Helen rubbed her head in dismay at the surge of posts that followed. Many were laden with rhetoric, and some remarks from pro-surgery supporters were only a short step away from stating that Alison was "asking for it" and that "it was only a matter of time." Helen switched off her phone, anger swelling within her. In her job, she had learned not to take things personally and that freedom of expression shouldn't be suppressed unless it is harmful. Alison was making a point and fighting for what she believed in. What those making hateful comments didn't understand was the true nature of the situation and why Alison lay in the high dependency unit at the hospital. This needed to come to an end.

"Here we are, is this the place you are looking for?" The driver announced.

Helen rubbed her temple in annoyance, placed her phone in her handbag, and gently patted her jacket, feeling the reassuring presence of the box containing the vial inside.

The estate they had pulled into featured multiple buildings, including a children's nursery, fabrication companies, and a car workshop. It was an unusual location for a laboratory.

"It is, thank you. How much do I owe you?" she replied.

He quoted the price, and she handed him a couple of notes. "Keep the change."

"Oh, thank you! That's very kind," he replied.

She exited the cab and closed the door. The driver nodded and smiled as he drove away.

Helen looked up at the sign in front of her: Geographica Pathology Services.

Standing outside the building, Helen scanned it from top to bottom. In front, there was a small patch of neatly cut grass. The windows were tinted, and it appeared that shutters could be pulled down to protect them at night. A couple of CCTV cameras were mounted above the windows. To the right of the building, a small stream ran alongside a pathway. Behind the building, grassland extended, with woods visible in the distance.

Taking a deep breath, she walked toward the front door, hoping that inside, she would find some answers.

++++

"We're only a few miles away. Have you been able to find out anything else about the surrounding units?" David asked.

"Yeah, Google Maps lets you look at the site on Street View, but not enter the actual estate as it's private property. A few businesses are listed, and the industrial estate website provides details on the occupied buildings. It looks pretty standard: there's a kiddies' nursery, a mechanic's shop, and others. If that garage is ringing cars or anything dodgy is going on, they'll be eyes open and surveillance-aware. From what I can see, there's nothing to indicate they're not operating. I could check all of them on Companies House to see if they're still in business, but we don't have time for that since we'll be there soon. We need to talk through the plan."

"Yeah, we do. Here's how I see it: for reasons I don't fully understand, the MP has a vial in her possession. She's having it tested..."

"A vial of what?" Rubin interrupted. "David, what is it?"

"I'm not entirely sure. Some kind of beauty filler."

"Beauty filler?"

"Yep. The client is in pharmaceuticals."

"That woman who was blown up yesterday was against all that shit. I read about it."

David avoided looking at Rubin and ignored his comment. "The plan is for the vial I'm carrying to be tested, not the one the MP has. We need to encourage the technician to cooperate if we can't switch them."

"How the bloody hell can we possibly swap them? He might be testing it right now if she's already there."

David nodded. "I understand. I'm thinking on my feet."

Rubin let out a frustrated sigh. "You'd better think quickly because I'm telling you, if it can't be done, it can't be done. I'm not risking a compromise and a night in the cells for your client."

"A night? It'll be much worse than that with what we're carrying. In any case, I agree; if it can't be done, we'll pull out. All I know is that this is vitally important to them."

Rubin shook his head, recognising the routes he'd seen while researching on his phone. "This is not a plan, brother. How do we know she is in there? If you go in and put a gun to his head, and she's there, this will all end in disaster."

"I know."

"She's a bloody Member of Parliament. If you do that, it will be worldwide news. There's no leverage or way out of this unless you take them both out."

"I know, I know, I know." David glanced at his sat nav; they were only a mile from the unit.

"Look, as I mentioned, if it can't be done, it can't be done. It is what it is. We'll take a look and see what happens. If he has already run the test, then it's all fubar anyway, and end of operation."

Rubin scratched his head. "In this business, we only need to know what we need to know. But I've got to ask you, what do you think this test is searching for, and do you have any idea what you're carrying?"

"No, is the short answer. "I haven't got a clue."

++++

Helen pressed the entry bell, and a voice from the speaker quickly responded, "Geographica, how can I help?"

"Good afternoon. I have a meeting scheduled with Dr Ryan Dobey. It's Helen."

"Please hold."

Helen turned around, realising that it was the end of the workday. Cars were leaving the estate, and mechanics were pulling down and securing a nearby shutter. The nursery appeared to be closed, with no cars parked outside. A couple of units had their shutters down, possibly indicating they were vacant. Just as she observed, a vehicle with two occupants pulled into the estate.

The speaker came to life again. "He's expecting you, Helen. Please make your way to reception."

A buzzer sounded, and the door catch released. She pushed it open, making sure it closed behind her. The reception area was directly in front of her. A well-presented young lady stood behind the desk, wearing an outdoor coat as she placed papers into a large handbag. The unit was medium-sized, with a few staff members in lab coats sitting at their computers. There were five other desks, all unoccupied.

The lady smiled and said, "You've just caught me. I'm off for the day, but I'm sure he won't be long."

Helen nodded with a smile.

When a door on her right opened, Helen immediately recognised Dr Ryan Dobey from his online picture. This was the first time they had met in person; their previous communications had been through phone, email, and text.

"Helen, it's so good to meet you finally," he said with a warm smile.

She returned the smile and extended her hand. "And you."

He took her hand, and they shook briefly. Nodding toward the door he had just come through, he said, "My lab is in the back."

Curious, she followed him and asked, "Aren't there many people here at the moment?"

"No, most of the staff have gone home for the day. It's just me working late; the others will be off soon," he replied as he pulled open the door. "After you."

"Thank you," she said, stepping into a short corridor lined with a few doorways.

"My lab is the first door on your left; it's open." Once they entered, he secured the door behind him and followed her into his lab. Helen placed her bags on the side and walked over to the windows to look outside. "Is it just because we're in the building that I can't tell, or are these windows not tinted?"

He laughed and gestured for her to take a seat. "You MPs are always so curious, but you're right. We are a private facility, so the front windows are covered, and as you can see outside, the rear is just scrubland. The area has a high water table, so nothing can be built on it, which is why the glass remains unchanged. Shutters come down at night with the press of a button to protect the windows."

Helen took the offered seat with a faint smile.

"Look, I need to be honest with you, Helen. I currently have a very heavy workload. I appreciate that you are an MP, and it's great to have you as a client, but I'm concerned that this may not be strictly legitimate."

Helen frowned, clearly shocked by his words. "It's completely legitimate!"

Ryan raised his hands in an effort to clarify his point. "What I meant to say is the urgency you've mentioned. As it is, I already have to work late into the night. Our work is confidential, and I assure you that our conversation today will remain so. However, I've never encountered a member of parliament requesting something to be tested before. Additionally, you've been a bit vague with the details. I understand it's a type of cosmetic filler that needs testing, but could you specify what exactly you are looking for?"

Helen retrieved the box from her jacket and placed it on the work surface beside her. She gently tapped the box with her index finger a couple of times. "This is what needs to be tested. I conducted my research a little while ago, which is why I approached you. I needed an expert opinion from a private laboratory, conducted by someone with whom I have no connections. From what I've read about you, it seems you have no political party affiliation. Are you tied to politics in any way?"

"As it happens, I am not. Even if I were, I wouldn't necessarily disclose it; it's not good for business. My client base spans various industries, and politics is irrelevant to my work."

Helen smiled. "Politics is always relevant, but I understand your point."

Ryan smiled back. "You still haven't answered my question: what do you think you have there?"

Helen rubbed her eyes. "It's complicated, and I hope I'm not mistaken. If what I've been told is correct, it is indeed a cosmetic filler. It's widely used and distributed around the world, manufactured by one company that holds exclusive rights to this type of filler." She crossed her arms and looked Ryan directly in the eyes. "However, we suspect this might be a new or possibly different strain, and it may contain addictive properties."

"Wow!" Ryan exclaimed. "That sounds like something I'd read on a conspiracy website." He grinned, but his expression quickly shifted as he noticed Helen's seriousness. "Okay, okay. What kind of addictive properties are we talking about?"

Helen hesitated, not wanting to jeopardise any potential outcome or to answer him honestly. "We don't know for sure. All we can say is that if it does contain addictive properties, it would be highly illegal."

Ryan leaned back in his seat, disbelief written across his face. "But that would never be allowed."

"I know this is an unusual request," Helen replied.

Ryan blinked in shock. "You're not kidding! What do you plan to do with it if it contains what you suspect?"

"I'm not sure," she lied.

"I understand, but I need to proceed with caution. Whoever the company is behind this, you are making serious accusations."

"I know, but I have to do the right thing, and I've been entrusted with overseeing this."

Since the initial communication with Helen, Ryan had researched her background. She was a polarising figure in the public eye, drawing criticism even from members of her own party.

"Do you have any more of that product?" Ryan asked.

"Yes, I do. Why do you ask?"

"Because I need to consider our reputation. We're a small, specialised lab. If I find evidence to support your claims, it should be confirmed by a second opinion. I can recommend another company for that."

Helen needed to make progress and didn't want to waste any time. "We can deal with that later."

Ryan rubbed his chin thoughtfully. "Okay, but as I mentioned, I have other work to do, so I won't be able to complete this until later this evening. When do you need it?"

"As soon as possible."

Ryan rolled his eyes. "I figured you would say that."

Helen smiled. "Can it be done?"

"Well, yes, it will be ready later this evening, but I can't give you an exact time. I need to explain that this is a scientific process, and I need to know what I'm testing. If I don't have this information, the testing could take hours, or in some cases, even days. I understand it is a filler, which helps me speed up the process. However, the other property you are looking for may take some time to determine. If the results come back blank and I only find components associated with a cometic filler, please be aware that the time spent will still be chargeable. I want to be clear about that."

Helen nodded. "I completely understand, and this is what I expected."

"Where will you be? Would you prefer that I call or email you the results?"

"Either method works. However, depending on your findings, I may need to come and collect the results from you. I'll find a place nearby to stay."

Ryan nodded. "There's a pub with a carvery about half a mile from here. It's probably worth calling them first to check if they have a room available."

"Thank you. I'll look into it," Helen replied as she stood up. "I can't stress the importance of this enough. Please be careful with the vial."

"Oh, Helen, one more thing. Do you know where this has come from? I don't mean the manufacturing company; I mean, do you know where it has been?"

"Why do you ask?"

"Because filler should be stored in cool areas. You just took this out of your pocket, and it's been warm today. That could affect its properties and diminish the quality of the product."

Helen nodded, understanding the importance of maintaining a stable temperature. Ryan was right to raise the concern, and honestly, she had no idea what temperatures the vial may have been exposed to since it left the laboratory in Brazil. "I'll be honest; I don't know, and I can't testify to the temperatures the vial may have experienced."

Ryan offered a slight smile but felt uneasy. He hoped that the product was normal and that Helen's suspicions, though seemingly outlandish, were incorrect. He knew Helen was media-savvy, and he preferred to avoid the spotlight. "Well, I guess that's it for now. I'll see you out, and regardless of any findings, you should seek a second opinion," he said.

Helen went to the side and grabbed her bags, grateful that he agreed to run the test. "Thank you for your time. I really appreciate it," she replied.

Ryan led her through the corridor back to the reception area. Before she left, she extended her hand. "I look forward to the results."

He shook her hand. "I'm sure they'll be interesting. I'll be in touch. Just press the green button on the left to unlock the door."

Following his instructions, she made her way outside.

After ensuring the door was securely closed, Ryan returned to his lab. The MP's request was unusual, but if Helen was right, he understood the urgency of the situation. He glanced at his watch, realising it would be at least a couple of hours before he could begin working on it.

++++

"Christ, that's her," David exclaimed as he pulled the car into the estate.

"Do not use the Lord's name in vain," Rubin replied.

Seeing the MP standing outside the unit directly in front of them, David quietly reversed out of the estate, noticing that she had glanced over at them. He merged onto the main road, quickly took a right turn, and then turned around to park. "We've got an eyeball from here to see when she leaves," he said.

"Okay, Sherlock, what's your plan?"

David frowned at Rubin, finding his jibes tiresome; he pulled down his sun visor for some cover. "We can't go in until she's gone, if we go in at all. Once she leaves, we'll recce the place."

"But what if the test has already been conducted? That would make all of this a waste of time, wouldn't it?"

David nodded. "Yes, it may. I doubt it, though. As you've seen, she just went in. If she comes out quickly, my guess is that the test hasn't been run yet. If she's there for several hours, it suggests she's waiting for it to be done."

Rubin tutted. "And that's the plan?"

David shrugged. "Well, neither of us is an expert, but I imagine you can't test a product in just a few minutes. It's not like a standard blood test looking for something expected; it must be more complicated than that."

"You said it," Rubin said, crossing his arms. "You are not an expert. This could be an unnecessary risk with no real results."

"This is how it is, okay?"

Rubin smiled, noticing that David was becoming agitated. He decided to hold off on sharing any further opinions for the moment.

"Look at the time of day; that whole estate seems quiet. Most of the units have closed for the day. However, I think there's still someone in the lab. Do you see the two parked cars?"

"Yeah, I see them," Rubin replied.

"If one of them belongs to him, then there might only be one or two others inside, which makes things easier for us."

From the side road where they were parked, hundreds of cars passed by as the evening rush hour was in full swing.

"Just to confirm," Rubin said, pulling down his sun visor, "if she comes out quickly, you want me to go around to the back and dig in somewhere?"

David nodded. "Yes, if you can do that. I don't like the look of the front windows. They appear tinted from here, and if it's the same in the back, you might not be able to get a visual anyway."

"Alright. We'll sort out comms when we're ready."

"Roger that," David replied, keeping his focus on the front of the estate.

"Look, the front door is opening," Rubin said as they both observed a woman leaving the building.

"That's not her," David remarked, watching a well-dressed woman exit the estate and walk down the road.

"At least that's one less to deal with."

"Yep," David replied, keeping an eye on her until she disappeared from view.

They sat quietly for a few minutes.

"I wish I had brought a flask of tea now."

David nodded. "We may be here for a while. So, how much did you pay for this lockup where you keep all your gear?"

"About a hundred pounds a month. It's well worth it for what we get paid. Are you thinking of getting one, then?"

"Wait, wait, she's out!"

Both men froze as the MP exited the building and made her way to the foot of the estate. "She's calling someone," David said, watching the MP as she spoke on the phone. "If it's important, we'll hear about it."

"Is she bugged?" Rubin asked.

David nodded. "The client has an enthusiastic nerd for these things; it's not something I can do."

They waited for a couple of minutes, keeping an eye on Helen Lord until she finished her call. Still holding her phone, she left the estate, walked left, stopped, glanced at it, then turned and began walking right.

"She's lost; she's reading a satnav on her phone. She's looking for somewhere," Rubin observed just as David's phone rang.

David answered, "It's the client."

"Okay, let's see if he has a plan."

David answered the call, noting Rubin's patronising tone. A few words were exchanged before David said, "Yes, we are here; we are currently watching her."

Rubin kept a close watch on the MP while David listened to what Darius had to say.

"Yes, it may be doable. We still need to recce the area; we've only just arrived."

Across the road, the MP moved away from them, still engaged with her phone.

"She's moving and looking for the place now," David informed Darius. "Yes, I understand."

Both men observed Helen as she walked until the road bent to the right and disappeared from view.

"Okay, I'll be in touch as soon as I have more information." David disconnected the call.

"Do you need her to be followed? I can go foxtrot and keep my distance," Rubin offered.

"No, there's no need to track her; we know where she's headed. There's a hotel and a pub just around the corner. She's booked a room there for the night, so she's housed. No need to pursue her."

"Understood. I noticed she had bags with her, so I figured she might be staying in the area. But what does your client want to do? What's he thinking?"

"In his opinion, she hadn't been at the building long enough for the test to be completed. He based this on the fact that she was staying overnight. If she had the results, she would have already been on her way back to Westminster. It all makes sense."

"Roger that, but the question still stands."

David started the car. "I just want to take a quick look at the outside of the lab. There are binoculars in the glove compartment; Take them out, will you?"

Due to heavy traffic, they had to wait a couple of minutes before David could merge onto the main road. Once he did, he quickly pulled to the right and stopped at the foot of the estate. "Tell me, what do you see in front of the building?"

Rubin glanced around to ensure they weren't being watched before looking through the binoculars. "It looks like the windows are shuttered. They probably come down when the building is vacant; the fact that they are open now suggests someone is still inside. Two CCTV cameras cover the front door and possibly part of the surrounding area, so we shouldn't be seen from here."

"What kind of cameras are they, old or new?"

Rubin adjusted the binoculars to their maximum focal range and tightened the central focus ring. He took a deep breath to steady the image.

David watched as Rubin focused on one camera and then the other. "Well?" he asked.

"You may be in luck; they appear to be older, mains-wired models," Rubin replied.

"Do you think there's a central recording unit inside, rather than having the recordings backed up remotely or monitored from another location?"

Rubin set down the binoculars and nodded. "It's possible."

David tapped the steering wheel, considering their options. "Okay, here's what I think: it will have to be a pressure test. I suspect that someone, or perhaps just a couple of people, are still inside that building. However, I need confirmation on the number of individuals we're dealing with. You know what the senior guy looks like, right? You've seen pictures of Dobey online?"

"Yeah, I'd recognise him," Rubin confirmed.

David paused briefly. "Okay. It appears that there are no cameras on the right-hand side of the building; however, a gap in the treeline may indicate a stream or similar feature. You mentioned scrub land out back. Can you dig in there? If no one is around, you won't need the ghillie suit. But using your scope, I need to know if you can see inside the back windows. If you can head out back, dig in, get an eyeball, and let me know. We can plan our next steps from there. If you identify him, one of us will need to go in and apply some pressure to him to test what I'm carrying instead."

"And then what?"

"While you are dug in, I'll research the guy to find any weaknesses. My client mentioned he has a family; if that's the case, we can use his family as leverage to apply pressure. I'm okay with either option: if one of us goes in, the other will have to do a home visit."

Chapter Fourteen

Darius sent a message to his three senior board members. At home, he connected his laptop, and as it powered up, he added a few drops of water to a generous measure of whisky. He placed a hand over the top of the glass to gently swirl the expensive malt before bringing it to his nose to inhale the aroma. When his phone chimed twice, he decided to wait for the third alert before starting the conference call. Knowing that David and his colleague were in Dartford, Kent, he contemplated the potential outcomes. The vial test had to be completed, no matter the cost. He took a sip of whisky, set the glass down, and carefully removed the painting from the wall above his drinks trolley. After placing it gently aside, he dialled the combination to his safe. He knew that David's legionnaire friend would need to be paid in cash, and it would undoubtedly be expensive. Darius didn't mind paying professionals; they valued their freedom, were skilled, and well-prepared, much better than hiring loud-mouthed tough guys from local pubs. Such men could never be trusted; they would inevitably fail, get caught, and, despite any reputations they might believe they had, most would talk when faced with pressure. The cost of professionals would always be high, but it came with a sense of security. He examined the bundles of notes inside the safe just as his phone chimed for the third time. He left the safe open, deciding to count the money later. After grabbing his whisky, he took a seat at his desk and quickly read the messages on his phone. The senior board members were ready for his call.

His laptop was ready as he inserted his encrypted USB drive into the port. This secure laptop was synced with the USB drive, ensuring that no other USB device would work; similarly, if this USB drive were lost, it would not function with any other machine. This private network acted as their defence gateway, where he and the senior board members shared plans. Their conversations on this network were encrypted, ensuring they would never be detected or backed up by any retrieval system. He entered his password, activated the internal camera, and waited for the three others to join the network.

Ronald, the elder board member, was the first to connect, followed by William and finally Hugh. Hugh was in his car, William was still in the country, possibly in a hotel room, and Ronald's residence was familiar to him; he recognised it from previous visits.

"Gentlemen, thank you for joining me promptly. It was good to see you all at our board meeting earlier. The in-person meeting, along with the presence of the junior board members, was crucial for gauging reactions. With that in mind, I have a significant update to share with you. At the close of our meeting, a concern was raised. As you are aware, I take the security of our company and our safety very seriously. You will recall that two of our board members did not vote in favour of our new initiative. After our meeting, they had a private rendezvous just a few miles from where we gathered."

"What have you been able to find out?" Ronald asked.

"I have obtained a recording of their conversation, and I regret to inform you that what I heard raises immediate concerns. They met at a pub only a short distance away from the hotel where we held our meeting. Their discussion was brief, but I've heard enough to bring this to your attention. I arranged for a listening device to be placed under the table where they sat. The sound quality isn't perfect due to background noise, but it's clear enough for us to evaluate the situation."

William looked worried as he rubbed his chin. "Do you have a course of action? What are they trying to accomplish?"

"I'm not sure yet, my friend," Darius said while sipping his whisky. "However, they have been discussing the lab collectively and are trying to link it to what happened with our nemesis."

"Even communicating through these means makes me cautious

about what I say. But have they explicitly suggested a connection to the events in London?" Hugh asked.

Darius shook his head. "No, but they are attempting to piece it together. They both mentioned having no intention of attending our evening at the palace on Saturday night, but now they have changed their minds. They will be snooping around and listening to everything." He noted the concerned nods from all three. "Just be careful about what you say and who is around."

William nearly spat his words in anger. "We cannot tolerate this level of dissent. If there are any concerns, they should be removed from the board!"

"I agree with you, my friend, but it's not that simple. They were elected to the board, and if we push them out, it could lead to even more problems. I suspect they will only dig in deeper. I'm warning all of you to be on your guard." Darius took another sip of his whisky. "As you know, we have guests attending, so let's try to engage them in conversations that avoid board matters. This is supposed to be a social evening with some of our biggest supporters and clients, so let's keep them occupied."

Hugh nodded. "We can do that. However, what should we do if they start asking direct questions? What if we hear anything that raises suspicions? What should we do then?"

"We'll have to cross that bridge when we come to it. As you know, one of them has a pedigree; his father was once one of us. If things start to escalate, he's the one we can negotiate with. I'm confident he'll see reason before the end."

"And what if he doesn't?" William asked.

Darius nodded. "Well… that would be a great shame."

There was a brief moment of silence.

"That's all for now. I just wanted to inform you. I trust you will all be in attendance on Saturday."

All three confirmed.

"Good. I'll see you all then at 7 p.m. sharp. Thank you, gentlemen." Darius disconnected the call, removed the USB drive, slid the shutter closed over the built-in camera, and shut his laptop. He placed the USB drive in his desk, locked it, and went to the safe. He took out the sealed bags of notes inside and began counting.

++++

Rubin peered under the sun visor. "Just in case those old cameras out front can see us, can you move back to the spot across the road? I need to change clothes."

David started the car, reversed, and turned around, stopping to let cars on the main road pass by. "All I need to find out is how many people are in that building," he said as he spotted a gap in traffic and merged onto the main road, heading up the side road on the right. "Keep an eye out for cameras on the surrounding buildings, will you?"

"I'm already doing that," Rubin replied. "It looks like this isn't a huge industrial area any more; many of the units on this road seem vacant. Just pull over there and turn around."

After turning the car around, David kept the engine running while Rubin got out and walked towards the boot. He glanced around before removing his shoes and jeans, replacing them with green trousers and a worn pair of boots. After tossing his jeans and shoes into the boot, he put on a green jacket, grabbed his scope, and took a pair of radios from his bag. Once he closed the boot, Rubin returned to the car and handed David a radio. "This is on my channel; it shouldn't have any interference, and the battery is fully charged."

"Good, do you have everything?"

"Yeah, this will work here. I don't need to go fully green, and besides, there are too many people around." He put on a dark-coloured hat. "Can you drop me across the road? I think you're right; where there's a gap, it's probably a stream. Could you pull over a bit further down? I'll make my way to the back of the trees, so no one in the building should see me. I estimate we have another forty minutes of light left. I'll move closer if I need to after that."

"Okay, let's do a quick comms check." David picked up the radio. "What channel are you on?"

"Channel two."

Rubin fed an earpiece through his jacket and placed it in his left ear. They both turned on their radios.

"Radio check, receiving?" David asked.

"Received. Over," Rubin replied as David drove the car back to the main road. "I won't have much cover if I sit out front where we were. I'll quickly recce the estate to see where I can lie up."

"Okay," Rubin said as he handed David an earpiece. "Just in case you need to go walkabout."

"Thanks," David replied, as he manoeuvred in behind a moving car.

"Anywhere along here should do."

David turned on his left indicator and pulled over to the side of the road.

"Alright. See you in a bit. I'll make for cover as soon as there's a gap in the traffic."

"Okay, I can't stop here for long; I'll cause a traffic jam," David replied.

Rubin opened the door, got out of the car, and began walking slowly along the road. Seeing a gap in the traffic, David immediately pulled away and drove past Rubin. When he reached the end of the road, he turned around and headed back toward the industrial estate. By the time he arrived, Rubin had already disappeared. If the rear windows of the laboratory had closed shutters or tinted glass, this would be a pointless exercise. He drove into the estate, pulling the sun visor across to the right to shield his face as he passed the testing lab and its security cameras. The other units in the estate seemed to be closed, with no obvious cameras, and the buildings relied on physical security measures. Most windows were secured with grills, and many had alarm systems. Steel gates and bars were across the entrance doors, suggesting that crime had occurred here in the past. He drove to the corner of the estate, performed a U-turn, and parked in front of the vehicle workshop. He backed up to the shutter door; his old, nondescript car could easily pass for a vehicle in need of repair. He switched off the engine. From this position, he had a clear view of the front of the lab. It was uncertain how long he would have to wait here, but unless he heard from his client that the MP was on the way back, he would probably have to force his way into the lab after dark.

++++

Rubin quickly navigated across the scrubland, making his way towards the trees. Until he reached cover, he felt exposed. David's initial observations were confirmed; there was a small feeder stream, and due to the recent lack of rainfall, the mud banks on either side of the stream had dried out from the heat. The ground was uneven, but that wouldn't deter determined dog walkers, which meant he might have to deal with them later if he was spotted. He slid down the short bank, ensuring that his scope was clear of any debris, and crossed the stream, which was only a few inches deep. Once on the other side, he placed the scope on top of the bank and pulled himself up. Going to ground immediately, he found himself directly in front of the rear of the lab. Still without cover, he crawled toward the trees ahead. In the sparse scattering of small trees, he concealed himself as best as he could and raised the scope to his right eye. The shutters were open, but the glare from the sun on the glass made it difficult to determine whether they were tinted. The setting sun hindered accurate viewing. "Alpha 1, receiving?"

"Send."

"In position. Location viewable. Shutters open, received?"

"Received. I'm inside the estate. No movements here. Can you see anyone? Over."

"Negative, too much sun glare. I will have to remain here. Received?"

"Roger. Out."

David set down the radio and picked up his phone. He opened Google and searched for information about the lab technician. He quickly found his details on a networking site. While the professional qualifications were of little interest to him, the family details and personal interests were what he needed. "Okay, looks like he's into fitness," David muttered to himself. Hillwalking was listed as a hobby, even though they were in the wrong part of the country for that. David soon found social media pictures of the lab technician in Snowdonia, Scotland, and the Peak District. He examined the kit the scientist was using. It was high quality, and the scientist appeared competent. Some of the peaks he had climbed were challenging; he was not one of those "all the gear and no idea" types; he took this pursuit seriously. David quickly discovered tags linking Dr Ryan Dobey to a hillwalking group, and a visit to their website confirmed that he was indeed a member. Nodding to himself, David recognised that this was his key piece of information. However, Ryan's personal phone number wasn't listed. In this quick search, David could only find the work number for the lab right in front of him. It was a long shot, but he was willing to take it. Although the phone David was using was unregistered, he didn't want his number displayed on a screen that could be accessed later. He had no idea what would happen that evening and suspected that, by the end of his task, both the phone and the SIM card would need to be destroyed. From the photographs he had seen, David realised that Scotland was as far as the doctor had travelled for his hobby. Having spent many hours in the Scottish landscape, David knew that the Cairngorm Mountains could be very challenging, especially when covered in their winter coat. He searched for hill walking clubs in the Cairngorms and found a few options. He clicked on the third club he discovered, and its website provided details about its senior members. The head of the club appeared to be Neil McCloud, who had an impressive background in mountaineering, with the website revealing a lot about the Scotsman. David was aware that his Scottish accent was not very good, but he decided to give it a try. He made a few notes and then dialled the lab's phone number. Knowing full well that it might not be answered at this time of day, he added the necessary prefix to ensure that any screen would display "call withheld."

Dr Ryan Dobey took a sip of what was probably his eighth cup of coffee that day and sighed in dismay as his mobile phone began to ring. For the time being, the main office number was being redirected to his phone outside of regular working hours. He planned to turn off call forwarding after completing his current workload for his key client. He set his mug down and picked up his phone. The caller's number was withheld. His key client didn't contact him this way; in fact, he often declined to answer calls from withheld numbers. However, since the MP's number had always been withheld during their early communications, he wondered if it might be her calling. Tired, he rubbed his eyes; he hadn't even started running her test yet. He exhaled in frustration, knowing how impatient she could be. Realising she would keep calling if he didn't answer, he reluctantly decided to take the call.

"Good evening, Geographica," he answered.

"Oh, good evening to you!" David replied, sounding pleased. "I'm fortunate to reach you at this hour."

Ryan frowned as he detected a strange accent, possibly Scottish, and likely spoken by someone who hadn't been to Scotland in a long time. "How can I help you?" he asked.

"Is this Ryan?"

"Yes, what are you selling? I'm very busy."

There was a hearty laugh on the other end. "Oh no, you misunderstood. I'm Neil McCloud, the president of the Highloch Mountaineering Club. You've probably heard of me!"

Ryan hadn't heard of him, but he had come across the club online while researching a climbing trip to the Highlands. "Well, yes, of course, I have," he lied.

"Well, it's great to meet you. I've been speaking with Steve Dollard, the president of your hill walking club. Has he mentioned anything to you yet?"

Ryan shook his head. "No, he hasn't mentioned anything, but…"

"Have I caught you at a good time? You're not in a meeting, are you? Or do you have others with you?"

"I'm at work; you called my work number. But no, I'm the only one here, except for one other person."

David nodded in satisfaction as the information was presented to him voluntarily.

"My apologies; I must have dialled the wrong number. However, now that I have you on the line, I have some grand news for you! We want to invite your club to join us in the Cairngorms. As you are aware, this area features extensive ranges and numerous Munros. This is a new initiative, and our group has decided to collaborate with another group and vice versa. The great part is that, aside from your travel expenses to us, there are no additional fees involved. Our members are also willing to provide accommodation for you. What do you think about that?"

"That sounds like a fantastic opportunity, and I'd love to discuss it further, but I'm under a deadline at work…"

"That's okay. No worries at all. We have some literature to send you. Just take a look when you can, my contact details will be included. Let me know your thoughts."

"Sure, that sounds great!" Dr Dobey responded enthusiastically. "Do you have a pen handy?"

"I do! I'm ready when you are."

"So, my email address is…"

David quickly interrupted, "Actually, it's print literature. We are an old, traditional club. We also have some exceptional photographs of the ranges that we can send you. They capture our mountainscapes much better than a picture on a screen."

Ryan glanced at his watch. It was a generous offer, but he didn't have time for this right now. "Um, okay. Would you like my home address?"

"Yes, that would be very helpful," David's grin was ruthless as he listened to the technician. "Thank you, I've made a note of that. Just before you go, will you be bringing your family?"

"Well, my wife, Andrea, is really into hill walking; she's an amateur mountaineer. However, since our kids are both very young, we would need to make some arrangements."

"Oh, lovely! Do you have a boy and a girl?" David inquired.

"No, I have two girls, Sophie and Annabelle, aged four and seven."

David leaned over to the glove box and removed the vial from the cool bag, nodding in satisfaction at a job well done.

Chapter Fifteen

Natural light was beginning to fade. From his position in the car, David noticed a light turning on inside the lab behind the front door. He knew there were two people inside the building and hoped that the unwanted one would leave soon; more people meant more problems. For now, they would have to wait it out.

He picked up the radio handset. "Alpha 2, receiving?"

"Receiving."

"How's your position? Over."

"All is quiet. A dog walker passed by at one point. Lights are on inside. No protective screens. I have eyeball. Over."

"Received. There are two inside the building, including the subject. Receiving so far? Over."

"Roger that."

"I have further info, will send to your other means. Received?"

"Roger."

"Out."

David set down the radio and texted Rubin.

Nestled between three small trees, Rubin felt his phone vibrate in his pocket. He set down the scope and checked the message from David. It confirmed there were two people in the building, the subject's address, and indicated that he was married with two young daughters. Looking through the scope again, Rubin found his viewing position perfect with the fluorescent lights turned on. He could see the subject, wearing a white lab coat, as he re-entered the room with a mug in hand. Rubin took nothing for granted in this line of business; he needed facts to complete his work, and everything else was secondary. However, his mind was racing. He was spying on a scientist, and David had mentioned that the client was in the pharmaceutical industry. Although Rubin didn't care much about it, forcing someone to perform a vial test on a beauty filler was unprecedented. He was aware of the assassination attempt in London, where the target was against the entire cosmetic business. He also knew that the woman targeted had a relationship with the MP he had observed earlier. As he lowered the scope, he realised there was much more happening than what he had been told, and this assignment involved more than just his bug-sweeping services. Rubin had previously described the London incident as amateurish, but as his suspicions deepened, he began to think that David might be involved. The more he reflected on the situation, the more he felt certain there would be a lot more to clean up before it was all over.

++++

"Alpha 1, receiving?"

David replied, "Send." Thirty minutes had passed since he and Rubin had communicated.

"There's a second person in the room. He's dressed as if he's leaving. Stand by, stand by."

"Roger. Out."

As darkness began to fall and the shutters at the front of the lab descended, David prepared himself, knowing that the last non-critical person was about to leave. With the electronic shutters securing the facility, the only light visible came from behind the front door. As soon as the other worker departed, he would need to make his move.

"Alpha 2, receiving?"

"Go ahead."

"Sitrep. Do you still have a visual? Over."

"Yes. They are still talking. Wait... he's just left the room. Out. Out."

"Received."

David's fingers tapped on the steering wheel as anticipation built. The light at the front door dimmed as someone emerged. Judging by his attire, it was reasonable to assume he was leaving for the day. The man took keys from his jacket pocket, and the car lights flashed as he unlocked the vehicle. After placing a bag on the passenger seat, he closed the door, got into the car, and started the engine.

David watched as the man reversed, straightened up, and left the estate, without so much as a glance in David's direction. David was confident he had not been seen.

"Alpha 2, are you receiving?" he spoke into the radio.

"Receiving you."

"He has just left. Can you confirm sight of the subject? Over."

"Roger that, have eyeball."

"Okay. The shutters are down here. Standby."

David knew they needed to move to the next phase. He didn't want Rubin to enter the estate and risk being caught on one of the security cameras. It was a gamble, but he needed to pull away for a moment. "Alpha 2, can you make your way to where we parked earlier? Over."

"Roger that. On way. Out."

David waited for two minutes before starting the car, making sure the lights were off. He quickly drove past the lab; the heavy traffic from earlier had cleared on the main road. Confident that he was out of sight of the cameras, he turned on the car's lights, pulled onto the main road, and took the first right. Once he was out of view, he turned off the lights, made a U-turn, and parked in the same spot where they had been earlier. It didn't take long for Rubin to arrive. David unlocked the car doors as Rubin got in.

"So, what's the plan?" Rubin asked, placing the scope on the floor between his legs.

"It's a two-part move. One of us needs to get inside, while the other goes to the home address."

"David, I understand this is your job and your client, but things are becoming complicated.

Forcing this guy to test whatever is in your pocket and then taking his family hostage, do you really think that's necessary? This is not easy shit to get away with, especially without planning. This could bring down a lot of heat."

David tapped the steering wheel. "I know, brother, and I can't force you to stay. Do you want to bail?"

"That's not what I'm saying. I'm just concerned about where this will lead. Once he tests your vial, what happens next? What's the end game? Proper planning is essential; unplanned or unprepared actions lead to failure. With your background, you should understand that better than anyone."

"The agreement I have with the client is as follows: nothing more has been discussed. However, the scientist must carry out the test. We need to keep the family as collateral to ensure he completes the test and doesn't contact the police, either today or at any point in the future. After that, we're done. There are no further instructions."

"If I'm doing this, I'll go to the home, but I need to arm myself. If I'm heading into a well-off area, you can bet your ass there will be cameras everywhere. I need to change my appearance. I'm not taking any risks, so I have to go to my storage unit to gather the necessary items."

David sighed. Time was working against them, but he knew Rubin was right. Fastballs and thinking on your feet were never ideal. "How far is your storage unit from here?"

"At this time of evening, the roads should be clear. I keep my storage unit outside of London for a good reason. Fortunately for you, it's on this side of the city, about a twenty-minute drive. So, factoring in the drive there, getting my gear, driving back, and then heading to the address, it could take about an hour."

David kept tapping the steering wheel as he listened.

"Unless you want to take a risk, I suggest you wait until I'm in position before you move in. Otherwise, you'll lose the leverage you're after. You know just as well as I do that he'll want confirmation and proof of life; he'll need to see a visual of his family. I'm sure you can intimidate him to take the test, but chances are he'll report it to the police afterwards; they always do. The other option is more traditional and straightforward: just slot him. That way, we can avoid all this hassle after he's done what we need him to do. We'll destroy our phones afterwards."

David shook his head. "We can't take him out. First, the client hasn't instructed us to do that, and second, he's too close to the MP. It'll just open up a can of fubar." David took a deep breath. "Okay, I'll go in."

"Fine," Rubin replied. "That means you'll need to wait around here for an hour. My suggestion is to head out back like I did. Dressed like you are, you should be able to get closer now that it's dark. If he lowers the security shutters, you'll be in the blind."

"Agreed. I'll do that."

"Here, pass me your radio. They won't work over such long distances."

David handed over his radio.

"I'll take your car and move as quickly as I can, but I don't want to risk getting pulled over by going over the speed limit."

"Yes, I understand."

David undid his seatbelt, reached beneath the steering wheel, and opened a compartment he had cut into the dashboard. He retrieved his firearm and tucked it into his jacket.

"I'll tell you this: you'd better speak to your client and tell him to be on the ball. If that test is conducted before you're in there, that MP might be on her way back. If that happens and she shows up, you're on your own. How you handle that is not my concern. Additionally, this goes beyond our initial agreement. What was supposed to be a simple debugging task in a hotel room has now escalated into kidnapping. Your client had better have a safe full of cash because I need to be very well compensated for this. Do you understand?

David nodded and stepped out of the car. "The keys are in the ignition."

Rubin slid across the seat. "How old did you say the kids were again?"

"I didn't, but they are seven and four. Why do you ask?"

Rubin glanced at David. "No reason, just gathering information." He closed the door and drove away.

As David walked toward the observation point, he considered his options. If the MP returned and his client told him to put her down, it would create a serious problem. Targeting the scientist was one thing, but carrying out such an action against a member of parliament was a whole other level. Sooner or later, the law would catch up with them.

++++

Alix Gregory sighed as he glanced at his phone. Darius was calling. He closed his eyes and rubbed his forehead, wondering what he wanted this time. Putting down his briefing notes, he tried his best to ignore the call. Despite having attended the same college, Alix did not enjoy Darius's company; every conversation with him felt like an attempt to ask for something. However, since Darius was a significant donor to the party, the situation was complicated. Reluctantly, Alix answered the phone and adopted a pleasant tone. "Darius, it's always good to hear from you."

"Always good to speak with you, Prime Minister. I see your approval ratings are reasonably strong for this stage of your term."

"Well, we can only do our best," Alix replied, forcing a laugh as he waited to find out what Darius wanted.

"I know you're busy, but I wanted to let you know that we have a reception at the Lords this Saturday night."

Alix shook his head. Weekend receptions were rare, and most business was conducted during the week. "No, I wasn't aware. What's happening?"

"It's just a fundraiser. The board and I will be there, along with Lords Hawthorne and Gatesouth, as well as some of our top clients and salespeople. It's always a treat for them to be invited to the palace, as it makes them feel important. Of course, this is a significant benefit for us, as they tend to work harder once they return to work. As you know, product distribution has been stagnant for a while, which hasn't been helped by one of your backbenchers."

Alix rolled his eyes; he knew what was coming. He was all too familiar with how Helen Lord MP was attempting to undermine the cosmetic beauty business. Furthermore, the previous day, she had embarrassed him in the chamber during Prime Minister's Questions. He sensed that Darius was about to make his main point.

"What are you up to this weekend? I'd personally like to invite you to join us," Darius said.

Alix closed his eyes in frustration. After attending various engagements across the country and spending the entire week staying at Number 10, flitting between Parliament, he certainly didn't want to spend more time there over the weekend. "I'm going with my wife to Chequers in the morning after our briefings. We are long overdue for a weekend together."

"Weren't you there last weekend? I'm sure I read that somewhere."

Alix gritted his teeth. Every time Darius called, he had researched Alix's business activities in advance. When politicians asked questions, Alix was well-prepared by his team of advisors. He was also skilled in diplomacy, but that never seemed to work with his old college associate, who had financially supported his political campaign in the early days. "Well, yes, I was, but we weren't alone," he lied. "We had to entertain."

"Oh? I wasn't invited to that?"

"It was a political event rather than one for supporters."

"Well, my company is a significant donor to your party."

Alix bowed his head; Darius always had him at his mercy. His company had contributed a substantial amount over the years, all of which was declared, above board and in accordance with ethical guidelines. However, Darius had also provided private support for him on other issues. Occasionally, Darius would subtly remind him of this fact. "Yes, I know. Your donations and continued support are greatly appreciated. You are always welcome at Westminster and Number 10; you know that."

"Yes, I know that."

The tone of Darius's voice changed instantly from one of pleasantries to overt manipulation. Alix needed to find a way to escape this conversation. "I'm sure you'll all have a great time. I'd be happy to arrange for some bottles to be sent your way for the reception. By the way, I've recently started signing bottles of whisky. Apparently, they tend to do well in auctions and fundraisers, particularly among Americans. House of Commons whisky signed by the Prime Minister, if that interests you. As I mentioned, I'll be at Chequers; you can always stop by if you wish."

"Well, Prime Minister, on behalf of myself and the board, we appreciate your generosity," Darius replied, his tone condescending. "But that's very kind of you; however, even by your own admission, Chequers is not the most interesting of places."

Alix let out a forced laugh as he braced himself for the punchline.

"Oh, come on! Come and see all of us. I'll even invite a few members of the old gang from college, just a jolly boys' evening, if you will. You can shake a few hands and exchange a few smiles. No speech is required; your presence would mean a lot to us."

Alix rubbed his temple, struggling to find a way to exit the conversation. "Look, Darius, it may be difficult. I'm trying..."

"Do you know how much our market value has slumped in the UK and worldwide?" Darius interrupted.

Alix closed his eyes and took a deep breath to steady his voice. "I'm aware that your trade is suffering right now. Yes, of course. You have my sympathies."

"But do we, Prime Minister?"

"Well, of course you do. We are old friends, and..."

"And your MP is not helping matters."

Alix quickly glanced around, leaned forward on the desk, and lowered his voice. "She's not my bloody MP. Any ministerial ambitions she may have will be quashed."

"All the same, she is a governmental MP and therefore one of your own. Perhaps an appointment with the Chief Whip is in order after that debacle in the chamber yesterday?"

"Trust me, after the embarrassment she caused me, the wheels are in motion in that regard."

"Well, that's good to hear." There was a brief silence, and Darius felt satisfied that he had made his point. "Oh, come on, stop by, even if just for an hour. Come and meet the old boys and enjoy a little jolly with us. I'm sure we'll be happy to pay handsomely for some of those bottles of whisky you mentioned. I know the board that financially supports your party will be thrilled."

Alix rolled his eyes, "Look, I might be able to drop by. I'll need to clear it with the wife. You know how these things go; my plans change by the hour, and committing to anything is difficult."

"Trust me, old friend, we understand. But unless the skies start to fall, I hope you can make it. Guests will arrive at 7 p.m., and I don't think it will be a late evening. Besides, it would be great to have some one-on-one time with you again."

Alix swallowed, feeling uneasy about the situation. "I'll see what I can do," he replied.

"Of course. A formal invitation will be sent to you. Farewell for now, Prime Minister."

As Alix ended the call, he bowed his head in concern. Whenever Darius called, he always seemed to want something; he was both devious and intelligent. However, Alix couldn't ignore the facts, Darius's support for his political career was undeniable. Yet, that wasn't the primary concern; it was what Darius had covered up for him in college that truly worried him.

++++

Nestled in the undergrowth, David checked his watch. Twenty minutes had passed, and nothing noteworthy had occurred. There was nothing more he could do until Rubin returned from his lockup and began his way to the doctor's family home. He took his phone from his pocket, covered the illuminated screen with his hand, and called Darius. The call was answered almost immediately.

"Do you have an update?" Darius asked.

"Yes, I'm monitoring the subject as we speak. He is alone in the lab."

"Good. When are you going in?"

"My colleague had to collect some equipment we'll need. I know this call is encrypted, but I'll choose my words carefully. Once he's ready, he'll head to the subject's home address."

There was a brief pause. "Okay, are you sure that is entirely necessary?"

"Well, the subject may require some persuasion, and we might need leverage to assist us."

"I see."

"Look, I need to be clear with you. We are both taking exceptional risks here, and we value our freedom."

"And that is why I pay you well."

David closed his eyes and nodded. "Yes, that's not in question, but we need to think on our feet; matters could evolve quickly."

"I understand, but that's why you do what you do. You're professionals; it's in your nature to thrive under pressure."

David rolled his eyes. He knew that Darius cared little about their safety; his genuine concern was for the company and anything that might affect him or the board.

"I have cash here for your friend. I know that's how he prefers to be paid."

"That's the arrangement I've made with him, but I also need to share his views with you. Forcing entry into an industrial unit is one thing; entering someone's home and confronting a family is quite another."

There was silence on the other end of the phone. "What would you have me do, David? We are close to completion."

"I'm just presenting the facts. This is a tricky situation, and nothing can be taken for granted. Now, a family with young children is becoming involved, and we are unsure of the outcome."

"I understand, and I deeply appreciate your service. Does your colleague know who we are?"

David nodded slightly and smiled. This was the first time Darius had shown any concern for his own safety. He knew that Darius understood the nature of David's business, and if things went awry, it could have serious consequences for him. If Rubin were aware of all of the details, Darius wouldn't want the former Legionnaire coming after him. "No, your identity and that of the company are being withheld," David replied.

"I see. That's good to hear; our board values your discretion."

"When you receive the test results, what happens next?"

"As long as both of you ensure that the test is conducted with the strict understanding that the subject and their family will remain silent in the future, that's it. All we need is the vial you are carrying to be tested. Remove the one the woman from Westminster dropped off from the scene and dispose of it as you see fit. Once the test is completed, let me know the results, and I'll guide you from there. My phone will be on for you all evening. Do you have any further questions?"

"No, sir, not at this time."

"Good. I'll wait to hear from you then."

The light on David's phone screen dimmed. In the darkness, David rubbed his head as he watched the lone figure sitting at the computer. "Poor bugger," he murmured, fully aware that the stranger in front of him was about to face a terrifying night.

++++

Not fully prepared for the situation, Rubin pulled his cap down to cover his face as much as possible. He was aware of the locations of all the cameras, allowing him to avoid making eye contact with them. The car that David had lent him was parked around the corner in a dimly lit area. Rubin's storage unit was hidden in plain sight among over one hundred other units spread across five floors. Most of these units were likely filled with furniture and belongings of newly divorced couples trying to get back on their feet. From the outside, it was the perfect hiding place, visible to everyone yet remaining unobtrusive.

Finding available storage units in the southern region of the country with dependable security measures was a challenge. He discovered this particular storage complex while it was still under construction a few years ago; the paint was still relatively fresh, and the building was well-maintained. Industrial-strength lights illuminated the area around the facility throughout the night, and motion activated cameras monitored all activity within the inner perimeter. Given today's climate, it was much safer for him to store his equipment in a facility like this. In the past, he had used old farm outhouses for storage, but with rural crime on the rise, he could no longer afford the risk.

With his case of debugging equipment in hand, Rubin was ready with his key card as he slightly bowed his head and approached the entrance. He was aware that a camera was placed on the other side of the main entrance door. With calm determination, Rubin swiped his card through the scanner and entered his PIN code. A loud click signalled that he could enter as he pushed the door open. After ensuring it closed securely behind him, he headed directly for the stairway. Once he stepped through the door to the stairway, he looked up and tucked the key card back into his pocket. He sprinted up the steps to the second floor, knowing there were no cameras in the stairway. Upon reaching the top, he adjusted his cap and retrieved the key to his storage unit from his pocket. Given that cameras were installed at either end of the floor, he strolled casually, pretending to fidget with his key until he arrived at unit number 209. He looked around to make sure no one was watching before turning the key in the lock and feeling the mechanism click into place. Placing his case on the floor, he crouched down, pulled up the shutter, stepped inside, switched on the light, then stepped back outside to retrieve his case and closed the shutter behind him. To the casual observer, this unit appeared similar to others, filled with old furniture, mirrors, and random carrier bags containing clothes, nothing out of the ordinary. However, behind this façade lay a false wall that Rubin had constructed over several nights. It looked identical to the original wall, except the unit's overall length had been shortened by about three meters. The central brick in the fake wall was removable. As Rubin pulled it out, he gripped the sturdy handle he had installed tightly. Despite having small roller wheels embedded in the lower brickwork, it took significant effort to pull the heavy wall to one side. He removed his cap; the brisk jog up the stairs with his heavy case and the dragging of the artificial wall had elevated his pulse. Tossing his jacket aside, he plugged in a lamp and switched it on. He needed to think quickly as he surveyed his collection of work materials. In the car, he had camouflage clothing and a ghillie suit. It was essential for him to alter his appearance, including his clothing, to enter the lab technician's home confidently. Breaking in was not an option; that would create unnecessary chaos. He wanted to be welcomed inside. He rubbed his chin, contemplating his next steps. A cheap suit would likely suffice for his needs. He grabbed a duffel bag and stuffed it with plain black shoes, trousers, a shirt, a jacket, and a tie. From the side, he picked up a pair of glasses with fake lenses and tucked them into a pocket of the bag. Next on his list was an ID. Although he didn't have a valid police ID for the county of Kent, he did possess a counterfeit London Metropolitan Police warrant. He figured that being only about thirty miles from London, it might pass as legitimate. He planned to rehearse his story on the way there. His hair had receded years ago, so now he shaved it completely. He owned a collection of inexpensive wigs that looked passable until someone got too close. He placed a couple of these wigs into the duffel bag, along with a fake moustache that he tucked into his pocket.

Due to strict firearms regulations in the UK, he didn't keep many weapons in his unit. Smuggling them into the country had become more trouble than it was worth, and he could no longer trust street sellers. Whenever he used weapons here, he made sure to dispose of them as quickly as possible. He owned two clean shotguns that had never been used for any private sector work. He possessed an old sniper rifle, which was the only weapon that truly concerned him. If it were discovered, it would link him to a murder that had occurred just over a year ago. However, knowing that bringing rifles into the UK was more complicated than bringing in shorter weapons, he decided to keep it. He opened a metal drawer that had once held mechanics' tools. Inside, he found two handguns. While both had been used before, they had never been used in the UK, so he considered them to be clean weapons. In the country where they had been used, no one ever bothered with something like a forensic investigation. He picked up both handguns and ultimately chose a Smith & Wesson M&P because it came with the appropriate silencer. As he would be entering someone's home, he was aware that if he encountered any resistance in a densely populated area, he would need to act quickly and leave quietly. He opened another drawer, took the silencer from its sheath, and collected a couple of loaded clips, adding a box of extra rounds to his bag.

In the stillness of the room, he rubbed his forehead, making sure he had everything he needed. Satisfied, he picked up the duffel bag and walked toward the front of the unit, placing it next to his case. He then picked up the case, returned to the rear, and put it in the unit's hidden section. After switching off the light, he stepped back and began pushing the wall into place. He hoped no one else was in the building at this hour, as this process was far from quiet. As the wall settled, he wiped the sweat from his brow and replaced the central brick. He rearranged a few items to cover the wall as best he could, then grabbed his jacket and cap.

With the duffle bag slung over his shoulder, he locked the unit and estimated that he would reach the lab tech's house in about thirty minutes. Before leaving, he texted David to let him know he was on his way.

Chapter Sixteen

Helen glanced at the unappealing "all-you-can-eat" menu and quickly pushed it aside. Her stomach had been rumbling for the past hour, but with so much on her mind, she couldn't bring herself to eat. Sitting in the restaurant and bar area of her hotel, she picked up her phone and scanned the QR code on the table, hoping that a large glass of wine would help ease her tension. As she awaited the test results, she thought a drink might make the evening a little more bearable.

She checked her phone repeatedly, aware that Ryan was busy, and tried to avoid messaging him. Putting the phone down, she took a moment to survey her surroundings. The restaurant was reasonably busy, and the table she had chosen was tucked away in a corner. She wanted a quiet evening, free from interference from anyone else's conversations.

Earlier, Ben Tasker had messaged her, confirming that the police had taken away computers for examination, Alison's office had been sealed, and further forensic testing would be conducted. Now, it was up to Helen to take charge and continue the campaign.

Her hands shook slightly as she picked up her phone again. The lab results could be a catalyst for change. A quick check on social media revealed that her outburst during Prime Minister's Questions was no longer trending, and as the day wore on, only a handful of entries remained about Alison. Her friend had become yesterday's news. Still, she searched for any updates. The last entry from a news channel stated that Alison was still in critical condition.

"Hello. A large glass of white wine."

Helen smiled and nodded as the server placed the glass in front of her. "Thank you," she said.

"Would you like something to eat?" the server asked.

“I’m not sure. Is it okay if I sit here for a bit?”

“Yes, of course. This table is not reserved for the evening; however, the last food order is at 9 p.m.”

Helen smiled, “Thank you. I’ll keep that in mind.” As the server turned away, she felt relieved that she hadn’t been recognised. She thought to herself, ‘Imagine being famous.’ It must be challenging to maintain a private life when your name is constantly splashed across the media. Taking a large sip of the wine, she grimaced at its terrible taste, quickly realising why it was so cheap. What if Alix walked in right now? Just imagine the Prime Minister entering a place like this. There would be chaos, with everyone vying to get close to him, either to embrace him or voice their concerns. Her ambitions to rise from the backbenches were fading. If he did come in, he would likely either ignore her or approach her immediately to question her about her party loyalties. Considering it was Thursday evening, he was probably planning to head to Chequers to escape the pressures of being the country’s leader. Helen’s phone bleeped, causing her to spill wine on the table as she hurriedly reached for it. Her heart sank; the message wasn’t from the lab. As she read the text, she shook her head, realising the wording had been approved by higher-ups and carefully crafted in case it ended up in the hands of a journalist. It was from Sebastian Hetfield, the Chief Whip, demanding to see her first thing Monday morning. She put her phone down. That settled it: the Prime Minister definitely wouldn’t be talking to her if he showed up here. Her rebellious nature had attracted too much attention, and she knew it was only a matter of time before she would be summoned. However, by Monday morning, everything might change. With that in mind, she took a large sip of her wine, savouring the sense of satisfaction.

++++

David clasped his hands together and blew on them to warm his fingers. Crouched between the small trees, he felt the dampness settling in and was eager to move to get some circulation back into his body. Over the years, he had come to realise that he wasn't as capable as he once was. In his youth, he had been trained in the concept of mind over matter and had mastered it, but now, in his mid-forties, it was no longer as easy.

He had a clear view of the lab technician, who had barely shifted from his seat for quite some time. The vibration of his phone provided a welcome distraction. "What's your location?" he asked.

"About fifteen minutes out," Rubin replied.

David checked his watch. "That makes your ETA around twenty-five past eight. Can you confirm?"

Rubin glanced at the car's sat nav. "Roger that, but I'll need to do a quick reconnaissance to check for CCTV and those bloody doorbell cameras."

"Understood."

"I appreciate that we're communicating via these means, but can you confirm the next steps as best you can?" Rubin asked.

"I've spoken to the client. I'll need to go in. I'll need a visual confirmation for leverage once you've entered the property at your location."

"Understood. I'll focus on the adult."

"Can you let me know when you are in position?"

"Roger, will do."

"Okay, out." David put the phone in his pocket and rechecked his watch. He hoped that Rubin was truly reformed, as he claimed, and that he would remain calm and composed. David glanced at the lab technician and, satisfied that he wasn't being observed, stood up and moved towards the waterline. He stepped carefully down the bank and walked alongside the edge of the stream, mentally rehearsing what he would say to gain entry. As soon as Rubin was in position, he would go in, and barring any mishaps, it should be relatively straightforward.

++++

David received a text message from Rubin that said, "Can you talk?" He crouched beside the stream and called Rubin. "Yes, go ahead," David said.

"I've parked around the corner. As expected, this is a middle-class area, and a few properties have CCTV; some of the systems look modern."

"Is there anything at the subject's house?"

"Not that I could see, but it was a quick drive-by. I'll change and head over there if you want to go in."

"Roger that, I'm doing that now," David replied, putting the phone in his pocket and taking a deep breath. Anticipation surged within him as adrenaline flowed through his veins. He lost count of how many times he had carried out actions like this over the years, but it had been a while since he had done so on British soil.

++++

"Oh, for God's sake," Ryan exclaimed, accidentally knocking his mug and spilling coffee over the sides. He rubbed his eyes and glanced at the clock on the wall. Deciding to work for another two hours in the lab before heading home, he felt tired and increasingly careless.

Getting up, he headed to the kitchen for paper towels and caught sight of himself in the mirror. His eyes were bloodshot and discoloured, and he needed to return to work early in the morning. He was looking forward to a family trip to the Peak District in Derbyshire for some fresh air on Saturday and Sunday. The best part about this weekend was that he would have completed all his work, allowing him to put his phone away. He also planned to stop his office number from diverting to his personal phone. As he pulled at his eyelids in the mirror, he was startled by the sound of the buzzer at the front door. He tossed the paper towels aside. "Who on earth is at the door at this hour?" he muttered as he walked into the reception area and stood behind the main desk. Noticing a lone figure outside the front door, he pressed the intercom button, "Yes, what is it? We are closed."

"Good evening. My name is Stanley O'Dair, and I am a parliamentary researcher for Helen Lord."

Ryan shook his head, rolling his eyes in annoyance. He was tired and irritable. "So, how can I help you?"

"Ms Lord asked me to come by. Unfortunately, there has been an issue in her constituency, and she had to leave the area. She requested that I collect the results of the test you're conducting."

Ryan sighed and rubbed his forehead, feeling frustrated. He hadn't even started the test yet and was considering postponing it until the morning. Regretting his decision to take on the MP as a client, he said, "I'm sorry, but you've made a wasted trip. I haven't started the test yet, so you'll need to come back."

"Negative. I've come from Westminster and need to head back tonight. She asked me to deliver the results there."

'Negative... who talks like that?' Ryan thought to himself. It was just one vial; he couldn't understand why there was such urgency. "Look, it's late. Do you have some form of ID that you can show the camera?"

"Of course," the stranger replied.

Dressed somewhat oddly for a parliamentary researcher, he held an ID card up to the camera, but Ryan paid it little attention. "Look, I'm working on something. You're welcome to come in and have a coffee while you wait. I'll take care of it next."

"Thank you. I'm sure Ms Lord will appreciate it."

Ryan pressed the buzzer to let the man in. As the stranger pushed against the main door, he seemed more interested in surveying the building than in anything else. "I'm guessing this door locks behind me?"

It was an unusual comment, but the stranger was correct. "Yes, it does," Ryan replied.

"Good. Where do I follow you?"

Ryan sighed and gestured for the man to follow. "You can grab a coffee in there. Forgive me if I don't make it for you; feel free to help yourself. There's milk in the fridge if you want it."

David nodded and placed his fishing syndicate license back into his jacket, having carefully covered his name as he held the card up to the camera. He had taken a calculated risk, hoping the scientist wouldn't recognise what a parliamentary pass looked like. He followed the lab technician into the back area, which he had been monitoring for the last hour. After looking around to ensure no one else was present, he said, "You need to close those blinds."

Ryan returned from the kitchen with paper towels to clean up the coffee he had spilt. "I'm sorry, what did you say?" he asked as he dabbed at the puddle.

The man replied, "I said you need to close those blinds."

Ryan shrugged as he tossed the damp towels into the bin. "Why? There's nothing out there."

"Well, I've been watching you from out there for the last hour."

Ryan froze and shook his head. "You what?" he asked nervously.

"I said I've been watching you for the last hour. Did I say something that you don't understand?"

Worried, Ryan sensed the atmosphere was changing rapidly. The man spoke clearly, but his words were intimidating. "Why would you be out there? I don't understand."

David then took the Glock pistol from his pocket and placed it on the table beside him.

Ryan stumbled backwards in panic. "Who are you? What do you want?"

"All in good time. Now, if you wouldn't mind, please close the blinds."

Ryan suddenly felt a wave of panic wash over him as he shook, his mouth going dry. The exhaustion he had experienced just moments ago vanished in an instant. He rushed to the window and pressed the button to lower the security blinds. Turning to the stranger, he could feel his face flush as beads of sweat began to form on his forehead. "I've done what you asked. What do you want?"

David calmly raised his right arm and pointed at the computer in front of the visibly terrified man. "Please take a seat. We need to have a little chat."

Reluctantly, Ryan obeyed the instruction, his nervousness evident. David could tell this was a situation Ryan had never encountered before; it should be relatively straightforward.

"First, I should clarify that I'm a professional. Second, the weapon on the table is genuine. Third, I know you are alone in this building." David smiled, his demeanour unsettling. "That means you are all mine."

"Look, I don't know what you think I've done; I have a family," Ryan stammered, desperation creeping into his voice.

"Yes, I know," David replied, pulling a piece of paper from his pocket. "You are Dr Ryan Dobey. You live not far from here on Heronway Road, and you are married to Andrea. You have two daughters, Annabelle and Sophie, ages seven and four, respectively."

Ryan swallowed, shaking his head in disbelief.

"I wonder if you'll still be taking that break in Scotland?" David smiled coyly.

The man in the white coat trembled even more. "Was that you on the phone earlier?" he asked, clearly unsettled.

"Yes, my Scottish accent needs a lot of work," David wagged his finger playfully. "However, security lesson number one: never tell people what they don't need to know! It's not that difficult. You really should take your safety more seriously."

"What do you want?" Ryan demanded, his voice shaking.

"Your phone. Slide it across the table towards me, out of arm's reach," David instructed.

Ryan nodded repeatedly and pushed the device forward.

"Now, tell me about your security system and the cameras outside," David said calmly.

Ryan placed his hands over his chest in panic, his breathing becoming audible.

"You need to remain calm. Panicking leads to mistakes. Follow my instructions, and you may get through this. I'll ask again: tell me about your cameras."

Ryan wiped the sweat from his forehead and pushed his hair back. "Um, to be honest, that's not my area of expertise."

David raised his right hand. "Stay calm and think. Are the cameras connected to the internet, monitored or are they backed up somewhere on-site?"

Ryan shrugged. "We have a monitor in one of the side rooms where we play back recordings. It's an old system, backed up on disks, I believe."

David nodded. "Good. I'll address that issue later. Now, you had a visit from a member of parliament earlier. What is the status of her request?"

"The test? I haven't started it yet," Ryan admitted, worry evident in his voice.

David smiled. "That's good; everything is still in your favour." He took a box from his pocket and placed it on the table. "Where is the item she wanted tested?"

Ryan nodded towards another desk.

David immediately spotted a box with similar packaging.

"It should be in the fridge, but it hasn't been there for some time," Ryan said.

"So, just to confirm, you haven't tested it yet?"

Ryan shook his head vigorously in response.

"When did you last speak with her?"

"Um, when she dropped it off. She asked for the results to be given to her upon completion."

Just then, David's phone vibrated. The message informed him that Rubin was in position and about to go in. A slight grin appeared on David's face. "Excellent. Then we shall begin."

++++

Rubin brushed himself down as he approached Ryan's family home. Lowering his head to avoid any CCTV cameras, he stood at the foot of the driveway and noticed there was no doorbell camera outside the Dobey household. The street was quiet, and no one was around. He adjusted his fake moustache, straightened his wig and ill-fitting tie, and held the counterfeit metropolitan police identification in his hand.

The curtains were drawn, but the lights were on inside. While standing next to the front door, he could hear children playing inside. He took a tissue from his pocket, covered his index finger with it, and pressed the doorbell. After putting the tissue back in his pocket, he noticed a young child appear on the other side of the frosted glass.

"Mummy, someone is at the door!" the little girl shouted.

A door chain was pulled to secure the door before it was opened. A woman, probably in her mid-thirties, peered through the gap, looking him up and down. "Yes? Can I help you?" she asked.

"I'm sorry to disturb you, ma'am, but are you Andrea, the wife of Ryan Dobey?"

She immediately looked concerned as Rubin presented his ID for her to see. "I'm Sergeant Ellis, a detective with the Metropolitan Police," he said, quickly returning the ID to his pocket. "I was wondering if I could come inside; it's a private matter."

She placed a hand over her mouth in worry. "What's the matter? Is it something to do with Ryan?"

Rubin nodded. "It's probably best if we speak inside, ma'am."

"Oh yes, of course. I'm sorry," she replied. She closed the door, unlatched the chain, and then opened it again.

"Thank you, ma'am," Rubin said as he stepped into the Dobey household. He noticed the young girl he had seen through the door clinging to her mother's leg, while another daughter, a few years younger, appeared and waved at him. Rubin smiled and waved back.

"What's happened?" Andrea asked, her face as pale as a sheet.

"Shall we go inside?" Rubin suggested.

She nodded. "Yes, of course. The kids are about to go to bed. With Daddy not being home, they're acting up a little, I'm afraid.

Now, both of you, upstairs and get ready for bed. I'll be up in a little while; I need to talk to this gentleman."

"Oh, mum!" The older child protested, clearly unhappy about being told to go upstairs, as Andrea ushered Rubin into the living room. "Please, take a seat," she said.

"Thank you," Rubin replied, nodding as he sat down and took out his phone. He then messaged David and put his phone in his pocket. "Is anyone else here?"

"No. Just me and the girls, is Ryan okay? Has something happened? Is he in trouble?" she asked quickly, her voice laced with panic.

"No, he's fine. It's what he's about to do that we're more interested in."

++++

David read the message on his phone. Rubin was in, and for now, the lab technician was cooperating; he didn't want to alarm Ryan any further by mentioning that a mercenary was in his home. David stood up, picked up the small box containing the vial that the MP had dropped off, and placed it into his pocket before sitting back down. "How long will the test take?" he asked.

"It depends on what you are looking for," Ryan replied.

"What did the MP tell you about what's in my pocket?" David pressed.

Ryan's voice trembled as he struggled to maintain his composure. "Not much, just that it's a contaminated filler, as far as I know."

David frowned. "Contaminated with what?"

Ryan shook his head. "I'm not sure. Could you please explain what this is all about and what's happening?"

"All you need to know is that you will be testing the product in the box I've provided. Once you're finished, I will pass along your results, and I suspect that will conclude our business."

"Are you going to call Helen with the results?" Ryan asked.

David smiled, "No, I won't be doing that; someone else will take care of it. As long as you do what you're told, I'm sure everything will turn out just fine." He reached across the table and lightly tapped the Glock. "Now, if you could be so kind, let's get started."

Ryan swallowed, nodded repeatedly and picked up a pair of disposable gloves. "Would you mind if I get a cup of water?"

"Of course. Please make yourself comfortable; you need to be relaxed."

David closely observed Ryan's every move as he walked over to the chilled water dispenser. Ryan filled a cup, drank it immediately, then filled it again before returning to his workstation.

"Look, I should let you know that we have a variety of testing equipment here. The process will be quicker if you can provide some insight into what I'm looking for. Testing can last for hours or even days," Ryan explained.

"Well, let's hope for your sake that it doesn't take that long," David replied.

Ryan shook slightly and quickly looked away from the stranger's menacing eyes.

"Just run whatever tests you were planning for the MP using the product I've given you."

Ryan nodded quickly, sweat running down his temple.

"Tell me, what were you going to do for her, for the MP?" David asked.

"Well, considering what she paid and without getting too complicated, this is a standard experiment conducted over multiple scans. Ideally, there should have been more scans," Ryan explained.

"Go on," David prompted.

"We need to move to the machine in the next room, which will perform quality control checks. It's a quick experiment that utilises spectroscopy and NMR."

"What is NMR?" David asked.

Ryan hesitated for a moment, then replied, "Oh, um, nuclear magnetic resonance. NMR detects the magnetic properties of atomic nuclei in a magnetic field, and from that you infer chemical structure."

David nodded confidently, even though he didn't understand any of it.

"This test is a one-dimensional technique, given the timeline she requested. The process is non-invasive to the sample," Ryan explained quickly. "Essentially, I'm looking for detailed information about the molecular dynamics and interactions, absorbing electromagnetic radiation and…" He paused, noticing David rolling his eyes and glancing at the ceiling. Ryan coughed lightly, his body starting to shake again.

"Congratulations, Doctor Dobey, you certainly know your stuff and a lot of fancy words," David said, lowering his head to meet Ryan's eyes. "I just need to know how long it will take, even if it is a rough estimate?"

"Four scans: one hour and six minutes," Ryan replied.

David blinked in surprise. "That's a very specific time, Doctor."

"Well, specifics are my business."

David nodded. "Very well. Get to it then."

Ryan stood up and said, "I want to clarify that the time I quoted is only for the duration of the test. There is still preparatory work to be done, and I must emphasise from the beginning that I don't believe the findings will be conclusive. This should be considered merely a preliminary test; I wouldn't base any model or product on it. I need to make you aware of that."

David nodded, "Duly noted. I'll be sure to pass that information along."

"To whom?" Ryan asked.

David growled slightly under his breath as he stood up to retrieve his firearm. "That's not your concern. Now, get to work."

Ryan nodded quickly, picked up the box that David had handed him, and made his way to the lab next door.

David knew he had the doctor where he wanted him; the man looked terrified. With over an hour of waiting ahead, he glanced toward the kitchen. "Keep that door open," he instructed Ryan as he quickly leaned into the kitchen to switch on the kettle. As he entered the lab next door, he saw Ryan struggling to open the box of filler. Frustrated, Ryan put it down and scratched his head. "What do you do next?" David asked.

Ryan turned around quickly, trying to put on his latex gloves. "I, um, need a sample holder… um…"

David shook his head in irritation. Ryan was stuttering and panicking; his hands trembled as he opened the box containing the vial. "Be careful with that!" David cautioned. "Look, you need to calm down and take a deep breath."

The firmness in his captor's tone made Ryan feel even more uneasy. "It's easy for you to say; no one is pointing a gun at you!"

"I'm not pointing a gun at you, Ryan. Just be calm and take a deep breath."

"Okay, okay. I, um, need to prepare for the sample entry for the preparation chamber."

"Ryan, listen. You don't need to talk me through every phase. Just continue; let's get this done."

Ryan nodded repeatedly.

David could hear the kettle boiling. "Do you mind if I get a coffee?"

Ryan spun around. "Do I mind?" he asked, starting to laugh. "Is that a joke?"

David left the room and went into the kitchen, picked up the coffee holder, and nodded in pleasant surprise. "This is expensive coffee, Ryan. I guess you must be making a few quid in this business." He placed the coffee holder down when there was no response and headed back into the lab. "Do you want a coffee?"

"No, I bloody don't!"

"Suit yourself. Let me know when you are near completion."

✢✢✢✢

David glanced at his watch and, feeling increasingly impatient, took a deep breath. An hour and six minutes had passed. "Where are we, Ryan?" he asked.

"Nearly there. The machine is synced with the computer over there," Ryan replied, tilting his head towards the right side of the room.

David quickly retrieved his phone from his pocket and checked it because he hadn't heard anything further from Rubin. He could only hope that everything was stable at the other end.

"Okay, here we go. The results are coming through."

David stood up from his chair and put his phone away as Ryan removed his gloves and approached the computer. He dragged a chair over to the desk and sat down to read the screen.

A couple of minutes passed, but Ryan's body language grew increasingly uncomfortable. David noticed the lab technician shaking his head as he examined the results, his expression filled with concern as he rubbed his eyes.

"What's wrong? What's bothering you?" David asked.

"Um, this can't be right," Ryan responded.

"Why? What are you seeing?"

"It's just that the formula is a filler. The vial you gave me is 3 mm, and most subjects can safely take 0.5 mm at a time. Over time, they may take more. However, there's something else here, something that has no place in a cosmetic procedure." He rubbed his lips thoughtfully. "This cannot possibly be accurate."

"Such as?" David prompted.

Ryan turned to face David and took a deep breath. "This particular filler is designed for the lips, according to the box it came in, and I can see that it contains hyaluronic acid."

David shrugged, clearly not understanding the significance of what was being said.

"Hyaluronic acid retains moisture and is naturally produced in the skin. It has hydrating and volumising properties and can also reduce wrinkles. However, over time, the body metabolises hyaluronic acid, which is why subjects, or users, if you will, need to return for repeat treatments to replace what has been lost."

"And?"

"That's the beauty of it, if you like; there are many other fillers that contain calcium hydroxyapatite, poly-L-lactic acid, polymethyl methacrylate, and..." Ryan noticed the puzzled expression on David's face. "Anyway, the main component of this particular filler is hyaluronic acid, which is expected. I see nothing wrong with that. However, there is something else in the test results that concerns me, and I'm struggling to make sense of it."

"Go on," David urged.

"Well, the test I performed, using this technology and considering the cycles that have taken place, provides information about the presence of functional groups and stereochemistry. Essentially, it outlines any impurities or indicates whether the sample is contaminated," Ryan explained as he leaned back in his chair, deep in thought. "I did mention that this was a basic test; it was one-dimensional. I need more time to analyse it further."

"You don't have that," David pointed out quickly. "Tell me what you see."

"Unless the test is flawed or the sample is compromised, it seems there is an additional component present, as indicated by the aromatic peaks. To be honest, and as I mentioned, we would need more time for accurate analysis, possibly using 2D NMR, or gas chromatography..."

"You don't have it!"

Ryan scratched his head and raised his hands in frustration. "Well, okay, I'm suspecting that what I'm seeing is an opioid-like structure, possibly a derivative of diacetylmorphine."

David frowned. "Morphine?"

Ryan shrugged. "This isn't just a morphinan; this is a psychoactive compound."

David asked, "So, what does this mean?"

"As I said, this was a basic test, but to put it simply, it could be addictive if it enters the bloodstream," Ryan said as he leaned closer to the screen. "It originates from the dried latex of poppies. If this is true, it would mean there's a psychoactive agent hidden within the cosmetic filler, but that clearly cannot be accurate."

David stood behind Ryan and noticed him glance nervously at the handgun tucked into his belt. "Don't even think about it; you wouldn't be quick enough," he warned.

"No, no, I wasn't thinking that at all, I promise," Ryan stuttered, moving away from the screen and shifting his chair further back.

"So, Ryan, let me be clear: are you saying this could be addictive? If someone takes this, could they become an addict or something?"

Ryan scratched his head. "I'm saying that if the machine is calibrated correctly and the test is accurate, it could have opioid properties."

David looked at the screen, scanning the information but struggling to understand it.

"You know what an opioid is?"

David shot Ryan a brief scowl. "I'm not a complete fool. Yes, I know what it is and what it can do."

"Then you'll understand my concern. This is highly dangerous," Ryan replied, nervously rubbing his lips again. "The vial you asked me to test contains a byproduct that has a more common name."

"What is that?" David asked with curiosity.

"Look, I'm struggling with this. The dose is small, but the question is whether it's clinically possible to drip-feed this opioid into the brain as the hyaluronic acid metabolises. However, it seems that this sample you provided also contains diacetylmorphine."

David nodded nonchalantly, encouraging Ryan to continue.

"To put it simply, this is not unlike heroin," the scientist explained.

David stepped back a couple of paces, feeling just as bewildered as the anxious scientist. He moved toward the windows, needing to think as he watched Ryan's reflection in the glass. The MP wanted a vial tested, and according to Ryan, he had replaced it with one that might contain an opioid. Nothing about this situation made sense. He turned back to face the scientist, whose body was trembling with anxiety. "What do you want me to do?" he asked.

"I need you to remain silent. I have to make a phone call," David replied.

Chapter Seventeen

Given the circumstances, Andrea was coping remarkably well. Rubin had to supervise her as she put the children to bed. The eldest child asked if she was okay, and Andrea explained that Rubin was an old family friend and they would be talking downstairs.

They spent most of their time in silence in the front room. A couple of hours had passed, and Rubin knew that the test was ongoing. He sat on the sofa while the lab technician's wife occupied the chair opposite him. His gun lay beside him. Her eyes were red from crying, but she mainly remained quiet.

The walls were adorned with various pictures of the girls, alongside a few photos of Ryan, the scientist, smiling at the tops of mountains. He probably didn't have much to smile about now, and things were only going to get worse. To Rubin's knowledge, he had no idea that his wife and daughters had also been taken hostage.

Rubin told everyone in his network how much he had calmed down as he aged. He realised that communicating with his subjects and demonstrating who was in control was all that was needed. This marked a stark contrast to his past experiences of countering or working with warlords, arms dealers, and working covertly to fight cartels, work he no longer had any interest in. If he could earn as much from assignments like this as he did in his previous operational work, life would undoubtedly be easier. The lady sitting before him had her knees together, her hands resting on them. She couldn't look him in the eyes.

"Do you know how long this will take?" she asked.

Rubin shook his head. "I'll have a better idea once I hear from my associate. Your husband needs to run a test in his lab, and that's it. As soon as he's done, I'll be on my way, and your life will return to normal."

She nodded.

"Of course, that depends on your cooperation," he added.

"What do you mean?" she replied.

"Do you think I want to be here? Do you think I enjoy threatening you or your children? I'm not a monster. Those days are behind me. My path lies elsewhere now, with God."

Andrea looked surprised as tears streamed down her face again. "God! Do you think He'll forgive what you're doing? We are good people!"

"Irrelevant. Many good people die, and that's something I know all too well. You find yourself involved in something beyond your control, so you need to accept it."

Andrea wiped the tears from her eyes. "What do you mean by 'cooperation'?"

"Oh, that's quite simple, Andrea. You must never tell anyone." Rubin's smile was extremely intimidating. "I haven't upset or harmed your children; only you, and that's how I want to keep it."

Andrea shook her head repeatedly. "I'll never say anything..."

"Oh, you promise..." Rubin laughed. "They always say that, but rarely keep their word. Do you think I'm stupid?"

Panic set in as Andrea raised her hands. "No! No, I never said that. I promise..."

"Of course, you promise. But here I am, sitting in your living room with a handgun. We need to discuss the facts. Do I look like a loud-mouthed thug? Do I strike you as a wannabe tough guy who's been asked to do a favour by someone in a pub?"

"Well, no..."

"My colleague and I are professional private sector operators; we do what it takes. Do you understand? We are selected for our skills, and you won't find our services online or anywhere else. I have faith, but I live my life without mercy, and I won't hesitate. My conscience is clear in that regard. God has a plan for me."

Andrea nodded, feeling frightened.

"The people we work for are professionals, just like us. Keep in mind that I was here; my colleague knows I'm here, and the people we work for are also aware of it. We always know how to find you; there's nowhere you can hide. Never forget that we will never lose sight of you. Do you understand?"

She nodded again and replied, "Yes."

"Good. Now we wait to hear from my colleague, and hopefully, this will all be over for you very soon."

++++

David pressed Darius's number on his phone and waited as it rang. He pointed at Ryan, "You, go stand in the corner with your hands on your head."

Ryan quickly got to his feet. "I did what you asked. Can you let me go now? I can't help you any further!"

David replied, "You may still be of use." He gestured toward the corner of the room as the phone was answered.

"What have you established?" Darius asked.

David turned to check that Ryan was following his instructions. The terrified man in the lab coat stood trembling in the corner. David then gestured for Ryan to turn and face the windows. "The test has been completed, but the lab tech has some concerns," he reported. David could hear Darius taking a deep breath.

"How so?"

"Look, this is beyond my scope, but he claims the filler may contain a psychoactive agent. Does that make sense to you?"

"A psychoactive agent? What is he suggesting?" Darius pressed.

"He claims that some form of heroin derivative is present in the filler. Again, I must emphasise that this is beyond my area of expertise."

"Heroin! He's delusional; he's probably just nervous because of you."

"Do you want the test to be rerun? I must emphasise that time is of the essence." He turned his back on the technician and took a few steps away, lowering his voice to a whisper. "My colleague is at home; he's not yet aware of this."

"Give me a moment with this, David, will you? Hold on."

David pulled the phone away from his ear, surprised to find he had been put on hold. With the anxious technician in the corner of the room, he walked back to the workstation and looked at the screen again. The information he read, along with the scientific terminology, made him look away immediately; it was a language he didn't understand.

The call was taken off mute.

"Look, David, the MP wants the results, and as you mentioned, we have little time. Let her receive the results directly from him, but under no circumstances should she come to the lab to collect them. Have him inform her of the findings over the phone, and…"

"Sir, with all due respect, doesn't this concern you? He is convinced by what he has found."

"No, it must be a bad batch. We will proceed with the plan."

"Would you like to test the other vial, the one in my pocket?"

"No!" Darius responded immediately. "Please dispose of that in a safe place as soon as you can. Tell him to relay the results, ensure that the MP does not come to the lab, and call me with what she says; we need to know what her intentions are."

David nodded. "Yes, I'll do that right away."

"Thank you, David. We greatly appreciate your efforts, and you will be well rewarded."

After ending the call, David tucked his phone into his pocket. The conversation felt strange and concerning; something was unfolding. As the technician had explained in simple terms, David understood that what he had carried and presented must be illegal. He placed his hands on his hips and tapped his fingers, contemplating his next move. He realised he had nothing further to report to Rubin that would hold any significance. "Okay, Ryan, lower your hands and retake your seat," David said as he perched on the edge of a table, observing Ryan. The colour had drained from Ryan's face long ago; he sat in silence, clearly afraid of what was about to happen next.

"Okay, I need you to take a deep breath and get some water if you need it. Here's what you are going to do: You will call the MP and tell her exactly what you've discovered."

Ryan looked at David in shock. "You want me to tell her about the diacetylmorphine?"

David nodded.

Ryan nervously ran a hand through his hair. "You know this product is highly illegal," he said.

"That is not my concern," David replied. "My priority is my client, and this is what he wants. You will call the MP, explain your findings, and provide details if you wish. But understand this: I will be right here." He removed the firearm from his jacket and placed it on the table. "I will be listening to every word. If you say anything outside of what I'm telling you, your outcome will be permanent. Do you understand?"

Ryan nodded repeatedly and asked, "Can I have some water?"

"Of course. Just remember to stay calm. She mustn't come here. You'll share your findings with her over the phone, and that will be all. If she insists on coming, you need to come up with an excuse that she won't question; otherwise, there will be two body bags this evening, and you'll be leading her to her death. Am I clear? Have I said anything you don't understand?"

"No, I understand that part, but what if she wants the findings emailed to her?"

David paused, realising he hadn't considered that, and Darius hadn't mentioned it on the phone either. "You'll tell her that you'll send it tomorrow because a family emergency has come up, understand?"

Ryan stood up and pointed at the water dispenser.

"Yes, go ahead and take as much as you need."

Ryan filled his cup at the dispenser twice and downed the water.

David took Ryan's phone from his pocket and set it on the desk. He then nodded at Ryan. "Do as I say and make the call."

++++

"I need to check on my daughters."

Rubin sat with his hands on his knees, contemplating her request.

Andrea continued, "I need to make sure they are asleep."

"Why wouldn't they be, other than my being here? Is there anything unusual going on, something out of the ordinary?"

"I sometimes read to my youngest."

"It's a bit late in the evening for that." He could tell she wasn't being truthful and just wanted to see her children. However, her calm demeanour was remarkable. Rubin had encountered similar situations many times before: a fretting wife, a panicking husband, and screaming kids typically triggered his temper issues. Yet, her request seemed reasonable.

Rubin nodded, "I'll need to accompany you, and I'll ask you to leave your phone here."

Andrea swallowed and stood up.

"I'll follow you. They have been quiet so far." As she walked past him, he placed a hand on her shoulder, making her jump. "I never asked earlier, do you have nanny cameras or any devices in their rooms that record?" She shook her head, and he could feel her trembling. "Never lie to me; that would be very unwise," he warned as he removed his hand from her shoulder. He accompanied her upstairs. This time, without the need to oversee the children's bedtime routine, he observed the Dobey household with greater scrutiny. The house was immaculately clean, and as he passed by, he noticed numerous pictures of the children with Ryan and Andrea, depicting them as a close-knit, good-natured family. Judging by the home's interior design, they also appeared to be reasonably successful.

Upon reaching the landing, Andrea turned to face him, her

expression a blend of anxiety and intense protectiveness. "Please do not hurt my children; they are my world," she pleaded.

Rubin nodded. "That depends on you."

Andrea opened the first bedroom door and then the second. Both rooms were filled with toys. The eldest's room had a dollhouse and an old rocking horse, a piece rarely seen now and likely passed down through the family. As Andrea closed the second door, Rubin noted that both children were asleep. He felt a sense of satisfaction upon receiving a notification on his phone: "Call to subject underway. Stand by."

"It looks like your husband is complying," he said, locking eyes with Andrea. "Shall we have a cup of tea? Hopefully, this won't take too much longer."

++++

Ryan picked up his phone, his hands shaking uncontrollably.

"As soon as you dial, put the call on speaker. I want to hear every word," David instructed, grabbing a pen and paper from one of the desks. "I'll be writing down instructions for you. Any slip-ups will have severe consequences. You need to stay calm and talk to her as you normally would. Remember, she is not to come here." David nodded at Ryan. "You can go ahead now."

Ryan swallowed, his forehead perspiring as he unlocked his phone. His trembling hands forced him to place the phone on the table to access his call list. After selecting Helen's number, he pressed the call button and immediately activated the speaker. The call was answered after just one ring, and Helen sounded as if she were in a crowded place.

"Helen, it's..."

"I know, what have you found?" she interrupted.

Ryan could hear the noise of people around her.

"I'm just heading outside so I can hear you," she said.

Ryan heard the squeak of a door opening, followed by immediate silence.

"I'm outside. Please tell me everything," Helen said.

Ryan looked into David's eyes and took a deep breath. "Um, the test has been completed."

"Thank you for getting that done so quickly. What have you found?"

"Um… well, it's unusual," Ryan replied, unable to break his stare from David's eyes. "The findings indicate that it's a cosmetic filler, as we suspected. The major property in common terms is hyaluronic acid…"

"Well, that's standard. I know that based on my research."

"That's not all. There is also a byproduct."

"Such as? Go on!" Helen's excitement was palpable.

"It's difficult to pinpoint its exact use, but I found trace evidence of diacetylmorphine."

There was a brief pause. "I've heard of that. Is it…"

"Yes, it's a morphinan. It's a psychoactive compound, highly irregular, and it has no place in a product like this."

"You're saying you have a derivative of morphine right there in front of you!"

Ryan looked at David for guidance, and David nodded for him to proceed.

"Um… yes, we believe that's what we're seeing here, although I don't know the purpose of it."

"We? Has one of your assistants examined the findings as well?"

Ryan froze, and David rolled his eyes in annoyance, shaking his head.

"Um, no, just the colloquial 'we.' As I said, the purpose of this is unknown to me."

"Oh, come on, Ryan! You're a scientist; the purpose is abundantly clear, a psychoactive compound concealed so that innocent people would unknowingly take it!" Helen glanced around to ensure she wasn't being overheard.

Until that moment, Ryan had never considered why a derivative of heroin would be included in a cosmetic product, especially with a gun pointed at him. But now he understood what was happening and why an assassin was in his office. This was major pharma at work, with serious thought and research behind it. If this substance were introduced to the general population, it would lead to a catastrophe of industrial proportions.

Helen sputtered with excitement, "This is an exceptional finding! It validates our research and what happened to Alison."

Ryan's eyes widened in alarm. He had heard about the incident in London involving the woman from the television channel, and he suspected it was all connected as he looked at David.

"Right, I'm at a hotel just around the corner from you. I'll come immediately..."

"No! No, you can't. I'm sorry, but that's not possible right now..."

"What do you mean? This is evidence! We have Knightark Pharmaceutical cornered; don't you see?"

A handwritten note was passed to him. "Look, you can't right now," he said. Ryan reread the note, which said, "Think very carefully." "Um, yes, it's a family emergency, you see..."

"I can be there in ten minutes if I hurry..."

Ryan glanced at David, who shook his head calmly.

"Broken leg."

Helen sounded confused. "What? I don't understand..."

"Yes, one of my daughters fell out of bed and broke her leg."

David rolled his eyes, but it might work.

"Oh, that's terrible! Is there anything I can do to help?"

"Why? Are you a fucking doctor?"

David's eyes widened as he waved his hands up and down, trying to signal the lab technician to calm down. Ryan was beginning to lose control.

"I'm sorry, Helen. I need to leave; I'm sure you understand," he said.

"No, it's okay. I'm sorry to hear your news. Would you be able to email me the findings before you go?" Helen replied.

David shook his head. "I'm sorry, Helen, but I won't be able to complete the report at the moment..."

"Are you busy on Sunday?" she asked.

Ryan wiped his brow, his lips quivering and his hands shaking as David gestured for him to stay calm.

"So? Are you busy?" she pressed.

He looked at David, startled by the question, as David shook his head. "Erm... No... Why?" Ryan responded nervously.

"Right, okay. Here's what we're going to do: I have an arrangement with a very small camera crew, and now is the right time to act. With the evidence you have, we can't waste any more time!"

David's calm demeanour shifted as he observed both the phone and the scientist with suspicion.

"What do you mean, Helen?" Ryan asked, his confusion evident.

"Well, think about what this could do for your career! Imagine being the scientist who uncovers all of this! This is a global issue, don't you see?"

"Look, Helen, I need to get back home," Ryan replied, desperation creeping into his voice as he wished for the call to end.

"Yes, I understand. I apologise if I seem rude, but this is important. We are discussing an epidemic, a manufactured, lab-created addiction. You must recognise the significance of this!"

"Helen, I run a small lab. I'm not looking for fame or worldwide recognition; I want no part of this!"

"Nonsense. This is for the benefit of everyone."

A note was slipped to Ryan that read, "Hear her out."

Ryan rubbed his temples in frustration. "What do you want, Helen?"

"As I mentioned, the time is now! I need to make a couple of phone calls and arrange the location."

"Location for what, Helen? I don't understand."

"For a live YouTube broadcast."

Panic washed over Ryan as he glanced at David. David frowned, pressed a hand over his mouth in thought, and then quickly shook his head.

"I'm not doing that, Helen."

"Listen, you could potentially receive some sort of Nobel Peace Prize or gain industry recognition in your field. If you bring the results of tonight's test with you, I have more filler to test. We can test one live on air. It'll go viral worldwide, and we'll bring them to their knees."

Ryan shook his head, and silence fell between him and the assassin.

"Ryan, are you there?"

Ryan frowned as he read the note that had been passed to him. "Look, Helen, I have a family emergency. I'll think about it and call you back within the hour to confirm or decline my interest in participating in any of this."

"Okay, I understand that you have a lot on your mind right now. But think about what this could do for your business."

David was satisfied they had stalled the MP and bought a little time; he put a hand to his neck and made a cutting gesture.

"Helen, I need to go. I'll call you back," Ryan said, abruptly ending the call with the MP. He leaned back in his seat, a wave of panic washing over him as he looked at the menacing figure who had taken him hostage. "Are you serious? You really want to go through with this?"

"I'm not sure," the man replied. "There are other factors at play here. Get yourself some water; you did well. Then go stand in the corner. I need to make a call."

✢✢✢✢

Helen paced back and forth outside the hotel. She had them, she knew she did. Alison would be vindicated, and Knightark's connection to crime would soon be revealed. If the lawyers and police became involved, there was even a possibility of prosecutions, provided they could substantiate the allegations. Regardless, their plans would be thwarted.

Her relentless pacing caught the attention of a few diners inside the restaurant. Finally, she sat on one of the benches, grappling with the weight of her actions. This was sensational, a conspiracy that would likely become the subject of a documentary film, and she was in the perfect position to expose it. Taking a deep breath, she closed her eyes. With only two days to plan, there was much to organise. She had suggested Sunday to Ryan as the possible date for the broadcast, but his tone was not encouraging. Given what had happened to his daughter, his reaction was hardly surprising. His outburst was immediate, and she hadn't shown enough compassion for his situation. However, she was driven and focused on her own goals. She was acutely aware of the worldwide opioid crisis, and in this case, the substances would not be distributed as pain relief; instead, they would be taken by innocent individuals seeking to feel better about themselves. It was a paradox: people would pursue treatments to enhance their appearance or regain lost youth through fillers, yet the reality of those choices would be quite different.

She smiled, knowing she had a meeting with the Chief Whip on Monday. He wouldn't be so cocky this time, and she couldn't wait to turn the tables.

Chapter Eighteen

"Things have taken a surreal turn, Sir."

"What do you mean?" David could hear the surprise in Darius's voice.

David glanced behind him; Ryan was back in the corner with his hands on his head. "The results were communicated to the politician, and she was extremely excited about them. It was as if she had been expecting results like this. Does that make sense to you?"

Darius sat at his desk and put the phone on speaker. "Members of parliament are a strange breed, David, especially when they get a bee in their bonnet. What does she want to do with the results?"

"This is where I think you may have a serious problem. The results were read to her over the phone, so no evidence has been provided. She is taking the technician's findings at face value."

David lowered his voice. "She wants to run some sort of live test on YouTube this coming Sunday."

"What?" Darius laughed incredulously. "Are you serious? That's ridiculous!"

"I can only tell you what I heard. She wants the lab technician to rerun the test, live on camera."

"She wants to do the test from where you are now?"

"No. She hasn't confirmed the location yet. Apparently, she has a small camera crew or something. I've stalled her for now because I needed to talk to you first, but the lab technician will call her back within the hour to confirm or deny whether he will participate. He doesn't want to be involved, but I've told him the decision isn't his to make."

"I see."

"Sir?" David asked after a long pause.

"Did you say Sunday?"

"Yes. If you don't mind me saying, you don't sound alarmed by this. If the secondary test confirms what the first test showed and it's streamed live, that could pose a problem, right?"

"Yes, I suppose it would be a problem. David, can you take a photograph of the results the lab technician produced?"

"Yes, I can do that; it will be a photograph of his computer screen."

"And can you send it to me immediately?"

"Yes, that's not a problem. I'll send it as soon as this call is finished."

"Good. Here's what I want you to do. The MP's proposal is something we could not have foreseen. It's concerning, but we have little time. She won't be able to prove anything in the grand scheme of things."

"But aren't you alarmed by her publicly making these allegations?"

"It's just that, David, they are merely allegations and nothing more. Her tests won't prove anything; it will turn into a lawsuit frenzy. And if she's speaking on YouTube, she won't have parliamentary privilege to protect her. All things considered, let her go ahead."

David raised his eyebrows and quickly glanced behind him, confident that Ryan couldn't hear him. He was taken aback by Darius's unexpected remark, which heightened his concerns. "Sir, I must inform you that the lab technician does not want to be involved. I suspect he is beginning to put the pieces together. He has already told me he doesn't want to participate in the broadcast. Isn't that the better course of action?"

"David, Helen Lord is a meddler trying to play detective, and she isn't very good at it. She should focus on serving her constituents rather than engaging in matters beyond her expertise. Our great company has many moving parts and is well-resourced. Besides, we have friends in places that outrank her, so we needn't worry."

"What do you want to do about the lab technician?"

"It's now Thursday night, and you say she doesn't want to broadcast until Sunday. Do you think you can keep him under control?"

David rubbed his temples, feeling uneasy. The situation had become more complicated and time-consuming, requiring him to secure Rubin's services for an extended period.

"David?"

"Yes, yes, I think so."

"You think so, or do you know so?"

"I know so, sir, but that means keeping him on edge for a couple more days. It won't be easy, and it also means housing his family, if you understand what I mean."

"I know, and that's why I trust you."

David rolled his eyes; away from his expensive desk and lifestyle, Darius had no concept of how challenging these situations could be.

"Listen, David, we need to find a way to keep him under control. If you can obtain his phone numbers, we can monitor him from our end. My communications expert can track him if he decides to run. I assume your colleague is willing to cooperate for an extended period until this situation is resolved?"

"I'm not sure, sir. I need to check, but he usually prepares for situations like this. We know this line of work is often fluid. However, I must mention that my colleague is costly, and he will bring this up if I ask him to work continuously until Sunday."

Darius laughed, "You mercenaries, it's always about money! But don't worry about that. Just let me know where you'll be, and I'll arrange for a bag drop."

"I understand. I will discuss this with my colleague. If any issues arise, I will inform you."

"Make sure you have the necessary leverage to ensure the technician complies. Have him call the MP to confirm the broadcast. Please keep me updated on any changes or developments."

"Yes, sir."

"And David, remember nothing ever comes back to us. Once this is done, destroy everything, and I mean everything. Eliminate all traces and evidence; there must never be a shred of anything that could come back to us."

"Yes, sir, I understand."

"David, as always, we are grateful for your assistance."

"Yes, sir, thank you."

After the call ended, David turned to Ryan to discuss his next move.

Meanwhile, Darius looked at senior board member William De La Roche and asked, "So, how did I do?"

William nodded with a grin, sipping his Scotch. "Excellent."

++++

"Take a seat."

Ryan turned away from the wall and complied.

"Did you hear any part of my conversation?"

Ryan shook his head vigorously.

David offered a slight smile. "It's okay if you did, as this concerns you." He sat down opposite the lab technician. "I don't have good news for you."

Ryan swallowed, sighed, and then lowered his head.

"I could soften the truth, but you're a very intelligent man, far more so than I, considering your profession. So, I should tell you how it's going to be."

Ryan looked up with anxiety in his eyes. "What is it?"

"Well, we're going to be spending more time together."

Ryan let out a whimper as his head fell once more.

"If it's any consolation, I hadn't planned for this either. I was hoping to spend the weekend fishing, but that's now out of the question, along with any hill walking ambitions you and your family had."

He immediately looked up. "What about my family?"

David extended a hand. "Remember what I've told you throughout this process: you need to remain calm."

Ryan looked around frantically. "What do you want?" he shouted.

"Listen to me carefully. Don't shout, and don't anger me. Just understand that you are involved in something, just as I am. We come from different walks of life, but we are in this together," David said, his smile far from reassuring.

"I'll remain calm when I know what the hell is going on. I ran the test for you; now, what do you want?"

"Your test results are quite complex, to say the least. As far as I can tell, that's part of the issue, and you have to do the live broadcast that the MP wants."

"What! I'm not doing that! I lead a quiet life and want no part of it."

"But you have no choice, Ryan. It wasn't me who got you into this mess; it was Helen. You wouldn't find yourself in this situation if she hadn't contacted you."

Ryan scratched his head. "Look, I have a family, and..."

"Yes, we know that. My colleague is with them right now."

Ryan's expression turned rigid. "What?"

"Well, you didn't think I was the only one involved in all of this, did you?"

Ryan shook his head. "I just don't..."

"It was a rhetorical question. The test you will perform for the MP is scheduled for Sunday, so we have until then to get along. This includes me, you, my colleague, and your wife and two daughters."

Ryan jumped to his feet and charged at David. Anticipating the move, David quickly rose to meet him, easily parrying Ryan's attack and delivering a sharp palm strike to his face. Ryan stumbled back against his desk and fell to the floor, tears welling in his eyes as he rubbed his face.

"I don't want it to be like this, Ryan. It's unnecessary and exhausting. Now, sit back down and compose yourself; there is work to be done." David sat back down and took out his phone. "I think it's time for some visual confirmation. You need to be convinced."

David called Rubin and selected the camera function.

"What have you done?" Ryan screamed.

"I haven't done anything, but I should check. My friend can sometimes be a bit unpredictable; apparently, he's found God, who would have thought it?" David smiled as the call was answered. A picture of an empty sofa appeared on the screen. "It's okay; it's me calling. You can show yourself."

The camera turned around, and Rubin appeared on screen.

"How are things going over there?" David asked.

"Good, we're having a cup of tea," Rubin replied.

"Very civilised. That's more than I've been offered. Put the wife on screen. Ryan, you need to see this." David held the phone in front of Ryan's face. "You recognise your wife, of course."

"Darling, are you okay?" Ryan asked as Andrea appeared on screen. "This man is in my office, threatening me. Who is that with you?"

David quickly turned the phone around. "Alpha 2, we're experiencing some temperament issues on our end."

Ryan leaned forward, "Show me the phone!"

"Now then, Ryan, keep calm," David urged as he held the phone out.

"Are you okay? Where are the kids? Are the kids okay?" Ryan asked, his voice filled with concern.

"They're fine, darling. They're asleep upstairs. The man here hasn't harmed me. What happened to you? Your face looks red."

"This bastard hit me across the face."

"What have you gotten us all involved in now?" Andrea said.

Based on what he had heard so far, David sensed that the wife was far calmer than the husband.

Ryan held his hands toward the camera, tears streaming down his face. "I don't know, I don't know."

"Okay, that's enough." David pulled the phone away. "Alpha 2?" Rubin immediately appeared on the screen. "Change of plans, we are coming to you," Rubin frowned and immediately glanced behind at Ryan's wife.

Ryan buried his face in his hands as David took a few steps away from him. "It's complicated, but we need to spend the weekend with them," he said. Turning back to Ryan, he pointed and added, "You stay right there; don't move a muscle." Ryan looked up with a terrified expression, and David knew he would do anything he was asked.

Rubin stepped out of earshot of Ryan's wife. "What's going on? I didn't sign up for this."

"I understand. As I mentioned, it has become complicated. I'll explain when I see you. Is there anything I need to know about the area?" David asked.

"Nothing in particular. How are you going to get here?" Rubin replied.

"Hold on. Ryan, is that your car parked outside?"

Ryan nodded, looking unwell.

"We'll be coming in his car. Garage or the driveway?"

"Driveway. There's no doorbell camera or external CCTV."

Ryan covered his mouth with his hand and rushed to the toilet. David followed slowly behind to keep watch.

"How long are you going to be?" Rubin asked.

Hearing the lab tech retch over the toilet, David quickly evaluated the situation. "About an hour, I would guess. We'll be bringing equipment, and I need to sort out the CCTV system here." He shook his head, glancing at Ryan, who was doubled over the toilet, vomiting again. "We've also got some cleaning up to do."

David ended the call, quickly took a photograph of the lab results displayed on the screen, and sent it to Darius immediately. He put on a pair of latex gloves and entered the toilet, where he was met with an overpowering smell. The lab tech was in a bad state. "Clean yourself up," David said. "Then we need to deal with this mess, along with anything that I may have touched, and your CCTV. I also want to collect everything that came into contact with the contents of the vial. After that, you'll need to call the MP to confirm you'll do the test." He paused, glancing at the mess in the toilet, "Also, some air freshener wouldn't hurt."

++++

Andrea opened the front door.

"You took longer than I expected," Rubin commented as he stepped in behind her.

"Yes, there was some cleaning up to do," David replied, looking Andrea directly in the eyes. "Go to the car and help your husband unload. And remember, we will be watching you."

Ryan stepped forward to hug his wife.

"No!" David intervened. "Continue as if everything is normal, just in case the neighbours are watching. If we're seen, we'll be friends from out of town. Am I clear?"

Ryan nodded and walked toward the car. "Go help him then," Rubin added for Andrea's benefit.

David stepped into the house, leaving the door slightly ajar so he could keep an eye on Andrea and Ryan.

"What's going on, David? I thought we were done here."

"Me too, brother, me too," David replied, glancing through the gap in the door. The couple outside followed the instructions, but they looked nervous and uncomfortable as they unloaded their car. "Something unusual came up with the test results. To be honest, I'm not sure what we're involved in."

Rubin began pacing back and forth, pointing at David. "Great! You got me into this. First, it was a bug sweep. Now we've taken a family hostage. This is above and beyond, and you know it. This is serious shit now!"

David nodded and reopened the door to let the couple inside. "Take the gear to the kitchen," he instructed. "Is that everything?"

Ryan shook his head.

"Do not speak among yourselves until you're inside the house and the front door is secured. Understand?" They nodded in agreement as they made their way to the kitchen. Rubin watched them closely. "What is that? What are they carrying?"

"Lab equipment; there's going to be a second test," David replied.

The couple passed by, heading back to the car for more equipment.

"What happened with the first test?" Rubin asked.

"I'm not entirely sure; this is hardly my area of expertise. However, our new lab friend mentioned that some illegal drug was found in the cosmetic filler, perhaps a derivative of heroin or something similar."

"Really? How is that even possible?" Rubin asked, expressing his disbelief.

"I don't know, brother. Like I said, this isn't something I'm familiar with. When was the last time you had a cosmetic procedure?" David asked with a slight smile.

"Have you seen my scars? I've earned them, and I couldn't give a shit about how I look."

David smiled briefly. "You and I both. Look, I don't fully understand what's going on, but the MP wants to do a live broadcast on YouTube this Sunday."

Rubin shook his head in confusion. "A broadcast of what?"

"A second test."

Rubin scratched his head as they watched the couple unload lab equipment from their car's backseats. "You say this Sunday, but that's three days away!"

"I know; it looks like we're babysitting."

"For three bloody days! David, we'll never get away with this. This has escalated beyond a one-nighter. This isn't a simple action anymore."

"I understand. It's tricky. If you want to back out, I won't hold it against you; there's a high chance of compromise."

"Jesus!"

"I thought you didn't take the Lord's name in vain?"

"Oh, piss off."

David opened the door as more equipment was brought inside. "Is that everything?"

Ryan nodded.

"Okay, take it through. Is the car locked?"

Ryan shook his head.

"Drop the gear, then we'll lock the car. Remember to act normal, like nothing has happened."

The couple carried the last of the equipment into the kitchen.

"So, what do you want to do?" David asked.

Rubin considered his options. "You know, for me, this job is all about the money. But this, this is dangerous. We're on UK soil; this isn't like the old days. Trails will be left behind."

"So, what's your answer?" David asked.

Rubin raised his hands. "I'm not sure. I'll see how this plays out. I'll need to be compensated for my time."

David nodded in response. "I understand, brother. I've already made arrangements for that. I noticed you aren't wearing gloves. I have some in my bag if you need them. Make sure to wipe down anything you touched; we must leave no traces."

Rubin replied, "I need to get our bags from the car."

"Come to me," David instructed Ryan, holding out his hand. "Car keys."

Ryan handed them over, and from the gap in the door, David pressed the button to lock the car. "I'm assuming one of these is for the front door?"

"Yes, it's the one with the green sticker on top," Ryan replied.

David selected the key and locked the front door. "Okay, where are the spare keys for the doors and the car?"

Andrea and Ryan exchanged anxious glances.

"If you hide anything from us, things will get much worse," David warned, pointing at Andrea. "Go and get me the keys. Ryan, I want your phone."

Reluctantly, Ryan handed over his phone, glancing over his shoulder as Andrea retrieved the spare car key from a kitchen drawer and the house keys from a wall-mounted hook.

David nodded as she handed them to him. "Now you two can catch up, but do it carefully."

Ryan and Andrea immediately embraced each other. "Where are the children? Are they okay?" Tears streamed down Ryan's cheeks.

"They're upstairs, asleep," Andrea reassured him.

They continued to hold each other tightly while Rubin and David exchanged glances. David realised that if Rubin agreed to stay, it would mean a long few days ahead.

Chapter Nineteen

FRIDAY MORNING

Helen yawned and stretched her arms over her head. Deprived of sleep, she had spent most of the night planning her next strategic move. At least Ryan had called back and confirmed that he would undertake the test on Sunday. Although she attempted to rest at one point, the noise in the corridors outside her room kept her awake, as did her racing thoughts. After finishing her stretching, she tried to focus her mind. Once the test was successful, arrangements for media coverage would be made. Without a media agent, she would rely on her extensive journalistic contacts. Joanna, her trusted research assistant, would need to support her, but Joanna hadn't been included in her plans yet; she intended to call Joanna on Sunday afternoon after the vial test was completed successfully.

The somewhat dilapidated hotel offered only a limited selection of television channels, but fortunately, it included a news channel. She kept a close eye on it and on social media platforms. Despite her efforts, she couldn't find any updates about Alison, nor were there any political developments that might prompt the Prime Minister to leave the country on short notice. She wanted him to remain in the UK to fully grasp the gravity of what she uncovered.

Lying on her bed, she took her laptop out of its bag to review her notes. The register of members' interests indicated that Lord Hawthorne and Lord Gatesouth were financially benefiting from Knightark Pharmaceutical. This raised the question of whether others were receiving undisclosed cash payments for so-called "services." Although she had no concrete evidence, her suspicions were growing. According to the register, Lord Gatesouth received five thousand pounds per month but scandalously dedicated only four hours of his time to the company. Lord Hawthorne received the same monthly amount but declared six hours of consultancy services, resulting in exceptionally high hourly rates for both. Notably, neither of them had a medical background nor was involved in any related medical businesses. The only connection she could find was their academic history; they had both attended the same college as Darius Neith, the company's chief executive. Helen had not recognised this connection, but an online political website had. This prompted an inquiry when a shadow minister raised it in Parliament. However, the Parliamentary Commissioner for Standards dismissed it, likely because some evidence had already been presented. It was possible that the two Lords were engaged in work for the pharmaceutical company, whatever that entailed. In any case, the inquiry was dropped and has not been mentioned since.

She turned away from the screen to reflect. A great deal had changed over the past few decades. For some members of the House of Lords, particularly those with "old money," their sense of entitlement and hereditary positions raised questions about their relevance in the modern era. Having never been elected, this lifestyle of privilege was increasingly seen as inappropriate by many. Helen was aware of many career politicians who transitioned from the House of Commons to the House of Lords. At the same time, many continued their political work out of genuine concerns and beliefs. However, some were unsettled by public scrutiny of their external earnings. Public outrage occasionally surfaced when journalists examined political documents and financial records that had previously gone unnoticed, bringing those earnings into clearer view. This issue extended beyond the House of Lords; some members of her party in the House of Commons also received monthly payments for consultancy work. At some point, this would inevitably change, and an MP's salary would need to suffice. Despite receiving offers in the past, Helen took pride in refusing external work. She wanted to maintain a clean reputation, especially since she was already under public scrutiny due to her involvement with Alison and her campaign.

The television volume was muted, and the news channel displayed the time: 8:15 a.m. The room rate included breakfast, and she considered going downstairs, but, as the day before, her appetite was minimal.

++++

Standing in his front room, angry and tired, Ryan placed his hands on his hips. "Well, it's no bloody wonder they're calling me!" he glared at David. "What do you want me to say?" He had missed two calls from his office.

Rubin was upstairs, keeping an eye on Andrea and the children. A call had already been made to the school; the kids were unwell and wouldn't be attending.

"Calm down! Just message them back and say something urgent has come up, and you won't be in today," David instructed.

"And what about the missing equipment? It's not like that's going to go unnoticed!" Ryan snapped.

"Ryan, just tell them a new client has come up with something urgent. You can say you've had to create a makeshift lab. You're a smart guy; you'll figure something out."

"But we're on a deadline with our major client. It just doesn't sound believable."

David shrugged. "Tell them this is a bigger client and a major opportunity. Let's face it; by Sunday, you and the MP will be famous anyway."

"Look, I don't know…"

"Just do it! And another coffee wouldn't hurt," David said.

Ryan scratched his head and took a deep breath. With his hands shaking, he began to type a message on his phone.

David stood behind Ryan, watching intently. "Be careful what you write; I am watching you," he warned.

"Hello!"

A young girl entered the room. David knew her name was Annabelle, and she was a seven-year-old with a bright smile.

"Morning, Daddy! We aren't going to school today!" she declared, delighting in the news as she kicked the mattress on the floor in the front room.

"What's this doing down here, Daddy?" she asked, looking curiously at the mattress.

Ryan glanced at David and explained, "Oh, Mummy and I slept downstairs last night because we had guests."

Annabelle extended her hand toward David, speaking confidently for her age. "Hello, I'm Annabelle."

"Hello," he replied, shaking her hand.

"What's your name?" she asked, her curiosity evident.

Ryan looked up, not knowing the names of either of the house guests. David met Ryan's eyes as he shook his daughter's hand, and Ryan's face immediately turned pale.

"I have a nickname, you see. Do you know what that means?" David asked.

"Yes, I have friends at school with nicknames, but they're all silly!" she giggled.

David smiled. "My friends call me Alpha."

"The man upstairs is called that, too!" she added, still giggling as she left the room.

David then turned his attention back to Ryan. "Let me check that message before you send it. Hand me the phone; I want to read it myself."

David read Ryan's message to his work colleague, nodded in response, and sent it. "Good, I'll be keeping this." He settled back on the sofa, putting Ryan's phone into his pocket. "You have a lovely daughter, full of energy and full of life."

Ryan swallowed and placed his hands on his hips, unsure of what to do next.

"It's such a shame she's caught up in all this. Still, you don't need to worry; this will all be over soon if you do what you're told. Now, how about that coffee? You can tell me what your plans were for today and this weekend. Let's make sure we tie everything up."

++++

Dr John Farmer retrieved his daily newspaper from the mailbox next to the security gate. As he scanned the front page, he walked absentmindedly back to his front door. Dressed casually, he had some consultancy work scheduled for late morning, but little else planned for the day. The gardener was expected to arrive soon; the lawns needed mowing, and the flower beds required weeding after the intermittent rain over the past couple of weeks.

After kicking the front door closed, he entered the kitchen, tossed the newspaper onto the counter, and made himself a cup of coffee. Just as he picked up his mug, the buzzer sounded from the security gate, coinciding with a phone call. He quickly set the mug down, grabbed his phone, and noticed that the caller was Lisa. He recalled her mentioning there should be no contact until they met the following evening. "Hello?" he answered.

"John, it's Lisa," she said.

"Yes, just give me a moment. I need to let the gardener in." He quickly checked the camera on the intercom and pressed the button to open the security gate. "Hi, how are you doing?" he continued.

"Good, thank you. I just wanted to make a quick call to check if you're still attending tomorrow night."

"Yes, at 7 p.m. at the Lord's. I hadn't forgotten," he replied, surprised by the question.

"Great! It should be a wonderful evening. I'm really looking forward to all of us catching up socially, as it rarely happens."

John couldn't help but frown. This seemed quite odd; her tone was different from when they had spoken outside the pub. "Um, yes, I suppose," he said.

"Fantastic! It's been a long time since I've spoken to Lord Gatesouth or Lord Hawthorne. It will be nice to see them again."

"Yes, I know what you mean," he replied, though he didn't truly understand and didn't care about their highly paid consultants.

"Excellent. I'll meet you tomorrow night in front of St. Stephen's. The main entrance isn't far from there."

John already knew the way and nodded suspiciously. "Yes, that will be fine. I look forward to seeing you then."

"Great! Bye for now."

He looked at the phone with curiosity, unsure of what had just happened. A loud knock at the door startled him. He opened the door and greeted the gardener with a cheerful "Good morning."

++++

The phone was answered promptly with, "Office of Helen Lord MP."

"Tobias, it's Helen. Is Joanne there, please?"

"Yes, Helen. Please hold on for a moment."

Sitting on a train, Helen glanced at her watch; it was early afternoon. Before making any further plans, she needed to return to the Commons to check on her hidden cache in the restroom.

"Hi, Helen."

"Joanne, I'm heading back to the Palace. I just wanted to check that everything is okay."

"Yes, everything is fine. However, I received an email from the Chief Whip regarding you. He wants to see you on Monday..."

"Yes, I'm aware. I received a text from him."

"Nothing from journalists today, apart from one article published by the local paper. They've posted something on their website regarding the cancellation of your surgery appointments, and I suspect it will also appear in the print edition later. A constituent commented on the online article, expressing frustration over your cancellation, and this has sparked further negative commentary. The main concern seems to be that you're no longer taking local issues seriously. I'm sorry to say it's becoming quite heated, and the phrase 'death of beauty' is being thrown around."

Helen sighed and looked around the train carriage. Only a few passengers were present, and none were sitting nearby. "This was always going to happen, but as you know, I'm working on something, and hopefully, all will be revealed in a few days."

"Are you okay, Helen? You sound quite tense."

She glanced around again. "Yes, I'm fine, but thank you. Is there anything else?"

"Not really. I won't trouble you with anything more. Would you like me to draft a response to the article in the local paper?"

"No, that's not necessary at the moment."

"You mentioned you were coming back to the House. Is there anything you need? The building is as quiet as usual for this time on a Friday."

"No, that's fine. I just need to check on something. In fact, why don't you and Tobias take an early afternoon off?"

"Are you sure?"

Helen could tell that Joanne was pleased with her suggestion, so she quickly added, "Do you have any plans for this weekend?" If Helen were being honest, she wasn't really paying attention to Joanne's response; she just wanted to get into her office in peace. Giving the staff the rest of the day off seemed like the best course of action. "Well, that all sounds great," she continued. "Just one more thing: I may stay in town for the next two nights. Would you mind booking a room for me at the hotel across from the old Scotland Yard building, if they have availability? It might be difficult to do that so late in the day."

"Yes, I can try to arrange that for you."

"It's quite expensive there, so could you check if the Parliamentary rate is available? Some places still offer it."

"Of course, I'll call them now and send you a message."

"That's great, thank you, Joanne. Also, please make sure to lock my office when you leave, okay?"

"Of course, I always do."

"I know, it's just... never mind. Anyway, have a great weekend, and I'll see you on Monday."

"Thank you, Helen. You too! Bye for now."

Helen glanced around the carriage again and tucked her phone into her bag. The train should arrive at Charing Cross in about twenty minutes, give or take. A short tube ride would get her to Westminster.

++++

Rubin was asleep upstairs while David struggled to resist the urge to check the time; babysitting was painfully dull. Neither he nor Rubin had any desire to have children; it was a foreign subject to both of them. This meant they often had to engage in forced smiles, seemingly pointless conversations, and playful antics. Though neither of them enjoyed it, maintaining the facade was necessary to keep the children calm. To help make the time pass more easily, David and Rubin decided to take shifts for sleeping.

Ryan's message to the office had worked for the time being. A curious response had come back asking, "Who is this new client?" Ryan felt he had to reply; otherwise, it would raise suspicion. David advised him to say he would explain on Monday, once the "deal" had been confirmed. For now, Ryan's and Andrea's phones were safely in David's pocket, and they enjoyed a brief moment of peace. David had checked whether Annabelle had a phone; he knew many children had them these days. To ensure neither parent was lying, he even asked Annabelle directly. She claimed she didn't own one because she was too young.

The conversation among the adults was tense. Their polite exchanges felt more like formal acknowledgements, and even as they shared lunch, they kept a noticeable distance from one another. No one made any effort to bridge the gap. Earlier, when Rubin needed to use the toilet, he used a plastic bag in another room, tying it up along with the used toilet paper for later disposal. Despite wearing gloves, they scrubbed every item of cutlery, mug, and surface after use. The sofa David and Rubin had sat on was vacuumed, and its contents were bagged. A plastic sheet now covered the couch. The bed sheets would also need to be disposed of when they left.

During a conversation with Ryan, David learned some good news: the family's weekend plans included a trip to the Peak District National Park, nearly two hundred miles away. They hadn't booked any hotels because they intended to drive there and camp, which meant there would be no evidence of their trip or any missed reservations. While David didn't enjoy the situation, he realised it could have been much worse. The family had only informed a couple of friends about their getaway, and no one else. Their house was semi-detached, and they had a poor relationship with the neighbour on their right due to his complaints about their children being too noisy. Because of this, it was uncertain whether the neighbour would be home. As long as an unexpectedly curious neighbour didn't decide to stop by, things seemed relatively safe. Now, as a family, they sat together watching children's television.

Feeling a vibration in his left jacket pocket, David checked the message on his phone. It was from Darius. Darius had pinpointed their location; a member of his security team had tracked the family's phones. The message was clear: a security team member was en route to the house to drop off a bag and needed confirmation of the house number. There would be a knock on the door, the bag would be left, and no conversation would be necessary.

++++

Helen unlocked the door to her parliamentary office. Fortunately, there were few people in the central area of Portcullis House, and she hadn't encountered anyone on the main or second floor who wanted to stop and chat. After swiftly closing the door, she unlocked her personal office, placed her bag and laptop on a side table and closed the blinds. After wearing the same clothes for more than twenty-four hours, she needed to change. To accommodate the demands of politics, which often led to late nights or unexpected overnight stays, she always kept a change of clothes in the office. Quickly flipping through various blouses and dresses, she selected a plain-coloured dress from the hanging rail in the cupboard and began changing. In a hurry, she promptly placed her spare wash bag, handbag, and laptop into a medium-sized suitcase. She tossed her old clothes onto a chair, put on a jacket, and picked up the metal coat hanger that had held her dress. After hiding the hanger inside her jacket, she glanced in the mirror to ensure it was concealed. Satisfied, she put her phone inside her jacket, locked the door to her main office, and headed to the restroom.

Observing the camera at the end of the corridor, she hoped that overzealous police officers hadn't searched above the tiled ceiling of the single-occupancy toilet. After closing and locking the toilet door behind her, she hung her jacket on the hook on the back of the door. As she unwound the metal hanger, she kicked off her shoes and sighed at the toilet seat, which had been left up again. She lowered the lid and gently stepped on it. When she felt confident the lid could support her weight, she continued uncoiling the coat hanger, leaving the hook intact at one end. Standing on her tiptoes, she pushed up the ceiling tile and slid it across with ease. Peering through the gap, she found it too dark to see anything.

Placing the hanger in her mouth, she retrieved her phone from her dress pocket and turned on the torch mode. A massive sigh of relief escaped her when she spotted the envelope still in its place. After several attempts, she successfully hooked the envelope and pulled it toward her. Thankfully, the contents remained intact. Using the hanger, she pushed the envelope back into place and left the hanger within reach above another ceiling tile before replacing the tile she had removed.

Stepping down from the toilet, she looked at herself in the mirror.

There was no turning back now; it had to be done. Knightark Pharmaceutical would pay a heavy price for this.

++++

Rubin was still upstairs, and David didn't really care whether he was getting any sleep. In any case, his colleague was away from the family hell of watching children's television. If David drank any more coffee, he would be in constant need of the toilet, yet he struggled to stay awake amidst the overwhelming boredom. He rubbed his eyes, realising that he had lost his weekend fishing plans to this.

Three loud knocks on the front door abruptly interrupted the family viewing. David checked his phone, and a message confirmed that the delivery was outside.

"No one move; it's for me," he said, alarming the children with his tone.

"Can I go see who it is, Mummy?" Sophie asked.

Andrea shook her head. "Not this time, darling. As you heard, it's someone for Alpha."

"Aww, your name's funny!" Annabelle exclaimed, pointing at David. She quickly turned back to continue watching television.

David stood up and walked to the front room windows. The light outside was fading, but it was still bright enough to see through the net curtains. He had been too slow to get up and couldn't see anyone in the driveway or parked on the street. He had hidden the master set of keys in the hallway. Ensuring he wasn't seen, he retrieved the keys from behind the shoe rack, then unlocked and opened the front door. An unmarked cardboard box lay on the mat. After quickly glancing around, he picked it up, locked the door, replaced the keys and returned to the front room. "Andrea, could you fetch a knife for me to open this box?" he asked. She immediately glanced at Ryan.

"It's okay, Andrea; if you don't mind," David said as he settled back onto the plastic sheet on the sofa. He examined the box for any unusual markings or indentations. It looked clean, but he wanted to be cautious as he prepared to open it. David was surprised by the size of the knife Andrea had brought from the kitchen; it was a solid eight inches long, sturdy enough to be used for cutting meat. Standing a few feet in front of him, she held out the knife toward him.

"Sophie, be a good girl and pass me the knife Mummy is holding," David said gently.

"We teach our children not to play with knives," Andrea replied, concern evident in her voice.

David nodded. "Is that so? Well, I suppose a little oversight today couldn't hurt. Sophie, could you do that for me?"

The four-year-old smiled and stood up, heading toward the knife. "No!" Andrea exclaimed, quickly taking a couple of steps forward and dropping the knife at David's feet. "Please go sit back down and watch television, Sophie."

David observed Andrea as she returned to her seat on the opposite sofa, admiring her protective demeanour. He bent down to pick up the knife from the floor while Ryan and Andrea watched him cautiously. He began to cut open the box in several places; their expressions filled with concern.

Once David was sure the box was safe, he sliced through the middle section, disregarding the gaffer tape sealing the top and bottom. He pulled out an envelope, read the information printed on the front, and set it aside. The remaining contents of the box would satisfy Rubin: a bag containing a substantial amount of cash in mixed denominations of British pounds and euros. He decided not to count it in front of the family. The weight of the box alone indicated they were being very well compensated, and, considering their situation and where he was sitting, they certainly needed to be.

Chapter Twenty

SATURDAY MORNING

Helen reviewed her handwritten notes, mentally reciting the key points again and again. Tomorrow, when she spoke on camera, there would be no autocue; she needed to memorise the major points she had to address.

Sitting in a quiet corner of the hotel's breakfast room, she observed the waiting staff as they diligently attended to the various tourists. She was familiar with the hotel, having stayed there several times. Due to its proximity to Westminster, it attracted various parliamentary staff during the week. Joanne had made arrangements for her stay and secured a two-night reservation; the confirmation text informed her that discounted rates for parliamentary staff were no longer available. The previous evening, Helen had taken a bottle of wine to her room and worked into the early hours, typing and constantly refining her notes. The small production team had not been fully informed about the facts. She had confirmed their availability and booked them. However, they believed it was merely a YouTube political broadcast focused on the cosmetic beauty trade, rather than an investigation into the true extent of Knightark Pharmaceutical. She needed to call Ryan to confirm the location, but his last text message seemed unreliable. She was counting on him, and without his credentials and the evidence from the first vial test, her case wouldn't hold up. She needed a positive test to present live on air, and making accusations against a company that produced and distributed addictive beauty fillers was a serious matter. This company had financial resources and a board of directors that had presumably approved the product; all she had was a political party divided by her recent actions. If she got this wrong, the lawyers would come after her from every direction.

"Would you like another coffee?"

Helen smiled and nodded as she read the server's name badge. It was Chloe who refilled her cup. "Would you like some more toast?"

"No, thank you," Helen replied, smiling again. As soon as Chloe turned to serve someone else, Helen returned to her thoughts. She realised she hadn't visited Alison in the hospital, and her last text message to Mike, her husband, had not been read. Helen picked up her phone and called Ben Tasker. She hoped he might have some updates or know if the police had reported back to him after their search of the channel's headquarters.

"Ben, it's Helen Lord," she said when he answered.

There was a brief silence before he asked her to hold on. As she waited while sipping her coffee, he returned. "Helen, I had to step into another room. Why are you calling?"

Helen raised her eyebrows at his tone, which clearly indicated his displeasure at being called. "I just wanted to check in and see if there are any updates on Alison," she replied.

"It's nice to see that you're so concerned for me as well, Helen," he replied, his tone dripping with condescension. "Last night, I had to sit down with my wife and discuss in detail what you two have been up to. We feel nervous in our own home."

"Ben, I truly don't know what to say…" Helen began.

"Then why call? Do you have any answers? Are there updates that your political mind can unravel?" he shot back.

Helen slammed her coffee cup down, catching the attention of several tourists in the room. She took a deep breath and rubbed her eyes. "Ben, we couldn't have anticipated how this would turn out. We were trying to do something good here."

"You've already said that!" he replied, frustration evident in his tone.

"Listen, I'm going to do my best to put an end to all of this.

Can you give me any updates on Alison?" She could almost feel his anger coming through the phone.

"Look, this hasn't been made public yet, but… Helen… wait, hold on a moment."

Helen heard a female voice in the background asking, "Who is it?" followed by Ben saying, "I'm taking care of it…" His voice became muffled as he tried to cover the microphone. There was a brief pause before he continued, "Helen, my wife doesn't want me talking to you. Can you hear anything behind me right now?"

Helen subconsciously shook her head. "I can't. Why?"

"That's because you've scared us so much that we've sent the kids away to stay with friends, and we're considering doing the same."

"Ben, I'm sorry. I really don't know what…"

"To say. Yes, you've already said that as well. Let me get straight to the point: there have been no new updates from the police. Alison's office is sealed, staff members are being interviewed, and computers have been confiscated. We are struggling to keep our channel together! My staff are terrified, and your actions have stirred up trouble. You've poked a bear with a stick, and now he's angry, which is affecting all of us!"

Helen was at a loss for words.

Yes, the answer to your question is yes. Alison is more stable and has been moved out of the high-dependency unit. I believe she is currently in an induced coma, but her injuries are extensive.

There was internal bleeding, broken ribs, a broken arm, a punctured lung, a burst eardrum, and that's before we even consider the facial reconstruction she'll need if she survives," he explained with a sigh. "The police are still waiting to speak with her. Does that answer your question?"

"Yes, it does," Helen replied in a conciliatory tone.

"Whatever you are planning, I want no part of it. Do not call me again."

Helen pulled the phone away from her ear, realising that Ben had ended the call; his feelings on the matter were quite clear. With the phone still in hand, she bowed her head, considering all the lives affected even before the evidence was presented. She sipped her coffee, contemplating Ben's situation; targeting him wouldn't make sense. If there were to be another target, it was more likely to be her. However, nothing unusual had occurred to alarm her.

Lifting her head with resolve, she knew this needed to be addressed, and it hinged on one person. Given what Ben had said, it was only a matter of time before the police would be looking for her as well as the individuals responsible for Alison's condition. She called the lab technician; he had better not let her down because time was running out.

++++

It was the most surreal morning that David could remember in a long time. Saturday morning, children's television was on while Sophie and Annabelle played in the garden. They even sat together for breakfast. Participating in this family's suburban life was not as excruciating as he had initially thought; strangely, he was starting to adapt. Although he had not yet counted the money he received, a preliminary inspection indicated that the amount was significantly higher than he had expected. This suggested that further work may be necessary. For the time being, he had hidden the money underneath Sophie's bed, and her parents were none the wiser. The delivery box, along with the handwritten notes he had given to Ryan during his conversation with the MP, had been burned in the garden the previous evening. Both he and Rubin currently stored their waste in bags at the end of the garden, while their urine was collected in plastic bottles. David had informed Rubin about the delivery, and they planned to divide their respective shares before leaving. The envelope that accompanied the money was folded and placed in the back pocket of David's trousers.

While in possession of three phones, the one belonging to Ryan vibrated, and David could see that the MP was calling.

"Ryan, phone call!"

Rubin entered the front room, closely followed by Ryan.

"It's the MP. Alpha 2, can you watch the wife and kids while Ryan takes this call?"

The open-plan layout of the house allowed Rubin to keep an eye on Andrea and the children playing in the garden while also listening to the call.

David signalled for Ryan to take a seat. "I'm going to answer this call for you and put it on speaker. Be extremely careful with what you say," he warned.

Ryan swallowed, nodded, and took a deep breath as David answered the call and placed the phone in front of him.

"Ryan, it's Helen Lord," the voice on the other end said.

Ryan nodded, and David gestured for him to respond.

"Ryan..."

"Um, yes, I'm here. It's me," Ryan replied.

"Are you okay? You sound like something is on your mind," Helen asked.

David had prepared a pen and paper in case he needed to jot down notes for the lab technician with the stuttering voice.

"I'm fine, just, uh, playing with the kids."

"Great, yes. I apologise for disturbing you on a Saturday, but I just needed to confirm that you are still available for tomorrow."

David nodded.

"Yes, I'm fine. I'm looking forward to it."

Helen was a little taken aback. For a lab technician who sounded uneasy, his response was somewhat strange; nonetheless, she was pleased that he was still confirming. "That's good. I have the location we'll be using."

Ryan read the note that David had passed to him, which instructed him to remain calm.

"I'm at a hotel in central London. I'll text you the details. With the equipment you'll be bringing, I'm guessing you'll be travelling by car?"

Ryan looked David in the eyes. "Uh, yes. In fact, I already have the equipment prepared, although it's hardly going to be a sterile location unless you have one arranged." David nodded, pleased with Ryan's response.

"To be honest, I'm planning to use the hotel room I'm staying in. I need to arrange a later checkout on Sunday morning, but that should be fine."

"You say it's fine, Helen, but it's not ideal, far from lab conditions." Another note was passed to him.

"I'm afraid we'll have to stick to the timeframe, Ryan," she said.

The note warned him not to question any further. "Okay, we'll do that then."

"I've arranged for two people to join us. One will be in charge of sound, and the other will focus on filming. I have a YouTube channel that I rarely use, but I've checked and can still access it. As long as the broadcast quality is good, we are all set!"

Rubin turned around with a frown and locked eyes with David. The MP seemed almost excited about everything that was happening.

"Look, I'll text you the details now. By the way, I know I personally covered the cost of your first test. How much will you need for your trip to London for the second one?"

Ryan glanced at David, who shrugged and raised his hands, unsure of what to say.

"No charge," Ryan responded confidently. "It's a good cause, after all, and, as you mentioned, it's great exposure for my business."

David and Rubin nodded, satisfied with Ryan's response.

"That's appreciated, and it's true. Although it's not just good exposure, Ryan, it's great exposure!" David rolled his eyes.

"Okay then, Helen, I'll be on the lookout for your text."

"When you arrive, you can drop your gear at the front of the hotel. There's a car park around the corner, but I'm afraid it's at London prices."

Ryan nodded, "Don't worry, Helen, I'll take care of it."

"Amazing! I look forward to seeing you tomorrow morning. Will 11 a.m. be okay?"

David nodded; the sooner, the better, so he could escape from here.

"Yes, that will be, um, perfect."

"Great! Goodbye, see you in the morning."

"Bye, Helen."

David leaned over to check that the call had disconnected before picking up the phone and his handwritten notes.

"Very good. Tomorrow, this will all be over for you and us. Incredible though, isn't it?"

"What do you mean?" Ryan asked, rubbing a shaking hand over his forehead.

"When you spoke to her from the lab, you mentioned that one of your kids had a broken leg, yet she never once asked about her."

"I'd forgotten about that," Ryan replied. "May I rejoin my family?"

Rubin opened the doors to the back garden and gestured for Ryan to leave the room.

"No whispering," Rubin added as Ryan walked past him into the garden.

David joined Rubin at the back door. They watched as Ryan put an arm around his wife while they observed their children playing on a trampoline.

"You know, this is going to be a problem," Rubin said, turning to David. "We haven't discussed tomorrow yet."

"I know it poses certain risks."

"Oh, really? You think? A makeshift lab test in a hotel room? There will be cameras everywhere. License plate recognition systems will catch you as soon as you drive into the city."

"I drive into the city?"

"Let me be clear, David. I'm staying here with wifey and children. This is your op, your job, your client. I will not be accompanying the technician to the test. I believe I've made myself clear. If we both stay here, it poses a major security risk for both of us. If he talks, this place will be flooded with blue lights. I'm not going to have a firefight with the police on this street. Do you understand?"

David nodded, acknowledging that Rubin was right. They couldn't rely on trust with Ryan; even with his family as leverage, he might crack under pressure and reveal something.

Rubin continued, "The only advantage we have is that with a live broadcast, we will see events in real time. However, that doesn't account for how he gets to the location and back. So, what's your plan, David?"

"We need to create a threat assessment and an exit strategy in case we have to relocate the family. I don't want to be in the actual hotel room. Even with your disguises, I can't be close to the MP or the two civilians she has invited."

"No, you can't. If there's any compromise or suspicion, you'll need to take them all out, though. If that happens, it's game over, and I'll have to deal with the family," Rubin replied.

David looked firmly into Rubin's eyes. Rubin hadn't changed; whether he had found religion or not, it was merely a facade, a way to seek repentance for his past actions and what he was still capable of. "I'll think about it," David said.

"You do that," Rubin replied, as they focused on the garden, where the innocent family was caught up in all of this.

✢✢✢✢

SATURDAY EVENING

HOUSE OF LORDS RECEPTION, HOUSES OF PARLIAMENT, LONDON

In light of recent events, Dr John Farmer decided to drive and keep the evening alcohol-free. He planned to use the car park beneath the palace. For those with official accreditation to access Parliament, this car park was one of London's best-kept secrets: it was free to use and secure.

As he drove into Parliament Square, he noted that it was approaching

7 p.m. Entry into the building should be relatively swift; by this time, tourists would have left, and most staff and MPs would be away for the weekend. He made his way to the entrance he intended to use, located halfway along the length of the palace. The black gates were guarded by police officers, some of whom were armed while others were not. John signalled that he was pulling in, ready to present his invitation. Tourists lined the street, many taking photographs of the iconic clock tower, while others chatted with the police officers and carried souvenirs from the numerous shops and stalls.

As soon as the officers spotted John's Jaguar approaching, they cleared a path for him and beckoned him forward. John rolled down his window.

"Please switch off the engine, sir."

John complied as three police officers approached his car.

"What is your business on the estate, sir?" one of them asked.

"Good evening, officer," John replied, handing his invitation through the window to the officer who had spoken. "I'm here for the evening reception with Lord Hawthorne and Gatesouth."

The officer nodded and said, "May I see your identification, please?"

John was familiar with this process, having visited many times before. He handed over his passport and driving license to the officer.

"Guests are not usually allowed to use the underground car park," the officer remarked.

"I understand, officer. However, permission has been granted on this occasion because it is a weekend reception," John explained.

The officer nodded and instructed him, "Please roll up your window and leave the engine turned off."

John smiled and closed the window as the officer took his documents for verification beyond the gates. They would check both his invitation and identification. Although the officers were aware of the evening reception, they were correct that most guests typically entered the building through the main public entrance.

Tourists gathered around his car, with a couple even stopping to take pictures, showing their curiosity about who he was. John sat patiently, tapping the steering wheel for a few minutes.

When the officer returned, John rolled down the window to retrieve his documents. "Dr Farmer, your reception is in the Cholmondeley Room in the Lords. Have you been here before? Do you know where you're going?"

"Yes, officer, many times," John replied.

"Even so, without official accreditation, after you park, you will need to be escorted to the Lords, and a temporary identification will be issued for you," the officer explained.

John nodded as the gates were opened for him.

"Please follow the path around for a vehicle search before you park," the officer instructed, pointing in the direction John needed to go. "You may restart your car."

"Thank you, officer," John replied, edging his car forward as the police watched him enter the parliamentary estate.

He veered to the left, noticing the heavy gates close behind him in the rearview mirror. The cobbled road wound around and began to dip. He stopped at the barrier, where a sign instructed him to turn off the engine. Glancing at the clock, he realised he was late, he had agreed to meet Lisa at the main entrance at 7. Just then, his mobile vibrated; she had sent him a message. Two police officers approached his car with search mirrors and began checking its underside. While they worked, he quickly replied to Lisa, letting her know he had just arrived. One of the officers nodded at him as the red light next to the barrier changed to green. He restarted the engine, and as the barrier lifted, he drove into the underground car park. He observed that nearly all the parking spaces were empty as an officer waved to him, signalling where he should park.

After parking, John got out of the car and straightened his tie.

"May I check your invitation, please, sir?" the officer asked.

"Yes, of course," he replied, handing over the invitation.

"Have you visited the parliamentary estate before?"

"Yes, I've been many times. I know the way, but I understand that you'll need to accompany me." The police officer smiled and handed the invitation back. "Please follow me; we have some stairs to climb. Are you fit and able to do so?"

"Yes, that's fine, thank you."

"So, you're meeting with Lords Gatesouth and Hawthorne?"

"Yes, just an informal gathering."

"Well, I heard a rumour that the Prime Minister may drop by."

"Oh, really?" John was surprised that such sensitive information was being shared so casually.

"You must know some influential people," the officer remarked with a hint of humour.

David smiled briefly as they ascended a short stone staircase back to ground level.

"We'll cut through Westminster Hall and into Central Lobby. I've been informed that the Lords' chamber is open for you; some guests are already present. We'll need to stop on the way to obtain your temporary identification, and you will also need to undergo a search. I trust you have no objection to having your photograph taken for the identification?"

John smiled and shook his head.

"Good. Please follow me then."

++++

Rubin stood on the other side of the front door while Andrea greeted the delivery driver.

"Thank you! Please keep the change," she said.

"Most kind, thank you," he replied as she took the Chinese food from him.

"Come on, kids, dinner is here!" Andrea called as she closed the door.

Rubin nodded at her. "Well done."

"Considering you wouldn't let us go to the supermarket, this is the best we could do," she replied.

Rubin acknowledged her comment. "I don't usually eat this kind of food either; that's not what they serve where I live."

"And where is that, if I may ask?"

Rubin nodded and gestured for Andrea to head to the kitchen.

Ryan set the plates, knives, and forks on the dinner table.

David quickly removed the sharp knives and returned with more blunt replacements from the kitchen.

"Okay, let's see what we have," David said with enthusiasm. It had been a while since he had enjoyed what he would consider a decent meal.

"Just rice for me," Rubin quickly added.

After spending two nights with the family, both David and Rubin had adjusted to their situation. Conversation was sparse, but there was a general sense of etiquette among them. Ryan's shaking hands had calmed, and the pallor of his skin had returned to normal. Although Andrea and Ryan didn't like the situation, they had accepted their predicament, realising that worrying wouldn't change anything.

Annabelle was overjoyed with the food placed before her.

"Just try a small mouthful first, darling," Ryan suggested, "just in case it's spicy."

David instinctively seated Sophie at the table, as if he had done it a hundred times before. He quickly noticed Andrea's disgust at having touched her daughter.

The television had been turned off, and they all sat in silence as they began to eat.

"Okay, maybe just a little curry sauce," Rubin said as he leaned across the table and spooned some sauce from the container.

The silence in the room was overwhelming, punctuated only by the sound of metal cutlery clinking against china as they ate together.

"Alpha 1, Mummy said you are leaving tomorrow. Where are you going?" Annabelle asked.

"Annabelle, don't be rude. That's Alpha 1's business!" Andrea scolded.

David smiled at Annabelle. "Yes, I'm going to London with your dad."

"Aww, can't you stay longer?" she pleaded.

"No, Annabelle! He can't!" Andrea snapped sharply, her voice filled with frustration. Her sudden outburst surprised their eldest daughter. Annabelle looked upset, and no one wanted to deal with a crying fit.

"I need to return to work after spending time with your dad," David said, trying to keep his tone calm to reassure Annabelle and prevent her from crying. "And how is your Chinese, Sophie?"

Andrea slammed her knife and fork down on her dinner plate, clearly upset at the thought of their captors being near her children. "Will you please not?" she asked David, her voice strained with emotion.

"Darling, it'll be okay," Ryan said, gently taking Andrea's hand in an attempt to comfort her.

Rubin, unaffected by the upset at the dinner table, continued to eat his rice. The family's distress meant little to him. He was focused on tomorrow's departure and suspected that David's client would instruct him to execute them all before he left.

Chapter Twenty-One

"If you could please place the lanyard around your neck, Dr Farmer," the police officer instructed. "I appreciate that you are familiar with some parts of the building, but even with the company you are with this evening, you must always wear your ID. Your temporary pass does not grant you escorting rights, so you will need to be accompanied if you leave your designated area."

They paused outside the grand entrance to the Lord's chamber, where the intricately decorated doors stood wide open. "I can see that Lord Hawthorne is already inside; it looks like he is giving a tour. This is where I will leave you if you wish to go in."

"Of course, thank you for your time, Officer," John said, extending his hand. The officer shook his hand and kept a watchful eye on him until he was satisfied that John had made his way into the chamber. John spotted Lisa ahead and hurried toward her.

"Good evening," she said with a grin. "You're late."

"Parking and search procedures, you know how it is here," he replied.

"I don't, actually. At least, not when it comes to parking. I have little intention of navigating this evening sober." She leaned in toward John and whispered, "There are only so many bloody hands I want to shake. Evenings with the great and the good no longer excite me; in fact, I'm not sure they ever did."

John laughed. "My father used to love them." He noticed she was carrying two wrapped items under her arm. "What do you have there?"

"Pictures. For Lords Gatesouth and Hawthorne, just a friendly gift."

John was surprised by the gesture. "That's very kind of you! What are they of? The company logo? A syringe or something?"

She laughed. "Oh, you have a sense of humour. That's good to know; you need it in this bloody place." She looked him over from head to toe, taking in his tailored suit. "No, they're paintings of the palace. I thought they might like them, a peace offering or something, I guess."

"A peace offering? Have you upset them?"

"Not yet."

They both burst into laughter.

Their laughter caught the attention of Lord Hawthorne, who approached them directly. "Ah, yes, we've met before," he said, extending his hand. "You are both on the board, if I'm not mistaken."

Lisa shook his hand and introduced herself, "Yes, my Lord, I'm Lisa Wellings. I've been on the board for just over three years. Dr Farmer, how long have you been on the board?"

John also shook the Lord's hand and replied, "It's been eight years. My father was a senior board member until his passing."

Lord Hawthorne nodded, "Oh yes, a good man. I liked him very much. He was quite generous." John gave a slight smile; he did not doubt that his father had looked after Lord Hawthorne over the years.

"I was just explaining to the group over there that the Lord's ceiling is divided into eighteen compartments, each adorned with royal badges…" Lord Hawthorne paused, noticing that his guests seemed to lack the usual enthusiasm that most would show. He quickly smiled to lighten the mood. "You already know these things, don't you?" His guests nodded, albeit a bit awkwardly. "Alright, enough of the tour," he continued, noticing that Lisa was carrying a couple of wrapped items. "So, what do you have there? Is there a raffle happening or something?"

"Well, there is a fundraiser later, my Lord, but no, this is for you," Lisa replied as she handed him one of the wrapped gifts.

Lord Hawthorne looked genuinely delighted to receive a present; his face practically beamed with pleasure, as John quickly noticed.

"For me? Why on earth is that?" he asked.

"It's just a small token of appreciation from Dr Farmer and me, in recognition of the good work you do for the company," Lisa explained.

"Well, that is very kind of you, my dear," Lord Hawthorne replied.

Lisa tried not to roll her eyes at being called "dear" and instead smiled politely.

"Can I open it now?" he asked eagerly.

"Please do," she encouraged.

Lord Hawthorne tore into the wrapping paper enthusiastically.

John quickly glanced at the picture inside and had to look away to suppress his laughter.

"Well now," Lord Hawthorne said as he crumpled the wrapping paper into a ball and examined the picture. His expression revealed little about his thoughts.

John sniggered to himself, trying to maintain his composure. The image of the Palace of Westminster was a chaotic blend of clashing colours; a modern interpretation that could only be described as tacky. He turned to look Lisa in the eyes, uncertain of what game she was playing. The palace was adorned with historic images of Westminster, but this rendition crossed a line into crudeness. Lisa stood resolutely, clearly enjoying a joke at someone's expense.

"Well, this is thoroughly charming, Lisa. I'll be sure to display it in my office," he said.

"I'm sure everyone would be thrilled if you did, my Lord," she replied with a hint of sarcasm.

"Come now. I know you've been here before. Lord Gatesouth is taking the first-timers into the Royal Gallery," he leaned in closer to them. "It never fails to impress. I'm sure we'll keep your clients in good company this evening." He beamed with self-importance. "Champagne on the terrace, then, shall we?"

John exchanged a glance with Lisa, fully aware that their company would be footing the bill. "Well?"

Lisa nodded, "Yes, that would be lovely, my Lord."

✢✢✢✢

John handed Lisa a glass of champagne and glanced behind him to ensure that no one was listening before bursting into laughter.

Lisa accepted the glass with a smile. "What's so funny?" she asked.

"You! What were you thinking? That picture was truly terrible!"

"It was, wasn't it. I just wanted to see his reaction," she grinned. "Corrupt bastard."

John continued to laugh. "Well, cheers then!" They clinked their glasses together and took a seat outside on the terrace, which overlooked the River Thames. This view from the palace was John's favourite, and as the sun began to set, they sat in silence, watching thousands of people cross Westminster Bridge. Slowly turning, the London Eye, once thought to be a temporary structure, has now become an essential part of the London skyline, offering tourists an unforgettable view of one of the world's major capital cities.

Lisa stayed true to her word and quickly finished her champagne. She placed the glass on the table and crossed her legs. "So, have you given our earlier conversation any more thought?"

"Which conversation? I didn't understand your last call at all; it didn't sound like you."

"Oh, that," she smiled. "That was nothing. I suspect they are watching us in some way, so I'm just being cautious. No, I meant our previous conversation."

"I hope that's not the case! However, to answer your question, I honestly don't know what to do. Our vote was acknowledged but not officially recorded, so it doesn't count. They are pushing ahead with the new filler, and it can't be a coincidence that we're here tonight. You can bet that plans are being made here."

Lisa nodded, "I'm counting on it."

"What do you mean by that?"

Lisa tapped John on the arm and stood up.

"Lisa, why on earth is your glass empty?" Ronald Ward, one of the senior board members, appeared next to their table.

"Ronald," John said with a smile as he stood up to shake Ronald's hand.

"It's great to see you both. I wasn't sure if you would attend."

"Oh, nonsense! Ronald, I wouldn't miss it for the world," Lisa replied quickly.

John glanced at her. Her composure was perfect, and Ronald seemed oblivious to her patronising behaviour.

"Well, look, both of you, come and join me in the Lord's Bar. There are a few people you need to meet. They are great salespeople for us, and we are going to take good care of them tonight," Ronald said.

Lisa turned to John and nodded, "After you, then."

++++

Outside the House of Commons library, Darius Neith reviewed some of the Hansard briefing papers. These papers assisted members of parliament by documenting discussions held in Parliament, along with votes and ministerial statements. The parliamentary library served as an invaluable resource, with staff available to conduct research and support MPs. When representing a constituency or the nation, MPs are expected to have well-informed opinions on all subjects relevant to current politics and global events. Ideally, when questioned, an MP's response should be articulate, informed, and thoughtful, even if it conflicts with existing policies or differing viewpoints.

Darius turned the handle of the library door.

"It's locked at this hour, sir."

Darius glanced over his shoulder, released the handle, and nodded at the security officer. He found himself intrigued by the extensive knowledge a member of parliament was expected to possess, ranging from local issues, such as potholes in roads, to complex topics in global economics. Politics had never been his career choice, but for many, it was a passionate ambition. His friend, Alix Gregory, had pursued that path long ago. Through various debating groups he had attended during college and his focus on academia, it was clear that some people were truly suited for it. Darius looked at his watch;

it was approaching 7:30, and he assumed the other board members were already gathered downstairs. "Do you have any idea how long he's going to be?" he asked one of the three security officers standing nearby.

"No, sir. We only know that he is on his way," the officer replied.

Darius gestured to one of the officers. "Do you mind?" he asked, indicating that he wanted to walk down the corridor.

"Certainly," the security officer replied with a nod.

Parliament is a beautiful yet ageing building, and in certain areas, its age is evident. Various departments work around the clock to ensure that the building continues to function properly. Darius smiled when he spotted a mouse scurrying down the corridor. "I see you still have a mouse problem," he said.

"That's one thing that will never change here, sir," the officer replied with a hint of amusement.

Darius grinned at the security officer. He had often dined in the Churchill Room and other restaurants in the older sections of the building, where scuttling mice occasionally made an appearance. He had read that the building's proximity to the river and Westminster tube station contributed to the mouse issue, which was acknowledged but persistent. When the company had hosted clients at the palace in the past, they were often shocked to encounter such sights. Nevertheless, the mice seemed to be as predictable as the next scandal; both they and the palace appeared to thrive on it.

Two suited men caught his attention from the other end of the corridor. He could immediately tell by their stride that they were part of Alix's security detail. Although the Prime Minister usually travelled with a larger group of close protection officers, only two were visible at the moment. If there were others, they were likely downstairs with the cars. Nevertheless, seeing the two security officers confirmed that his phone call to Alix had been successful, and he was indeed here. Darius had managed to pull his old friend away from Chequers, and Alix would not be pleased about this unplanned visit to Parliament.

Darius spotted Alix approaching from the end of the corridor, flanked by two additional close protection officers. Alix walked briskly, no doubt eager to finish this meeting and leave.

"Ah, Prime Minister, it's so good to see you again," Darius said.

Alix briefly raised his hand in acknowledgement as he drew level with Darius. "I see you're still enjoying our library," he replied.

"I do; it's magnificent," Darius said as they shook hands.

"Not quite as impressive as the Vatican's library, but there you have it."

"I wouldn't know; I've never been there."

Alix smiled as he turned to his security detail. "It's an old college friend. I'll be fine."

Two of the close protection officers moved away, heading towards central lobby, while the other two who had accompanied Alix remained in place.

"That includes you too, please," Alix added.

"Sir, are you attending the event downstairs?" one officer asked.

Alix turned to Darius. "I don't know; am I?"

"It would be appreciated. We are raising money for charity, and your appearance would be most welcome," Darius replied.

Alix snorted. "Yes, well. Look, I'll call you if I decide to go downstairs. The palace is quiet at weekends; I'll be fine," he said to the remaining security officers.

"Yes, sir," they responded.

Once the officers were far enough away to speak privately, Alix expressed his frustration. "I don't appreciate being pulled away from a well-deserved weekend off."

Darius nodded in response. "I understand."

"Come on," Alix replied, gesturing down the corridor. "My office is this way. Let's find out why I'm really here."

++++

"So, where are we at?" Rubin asked.

David leaned closer, "What do you mean?"

"About your plan for tomorrow."

David tilted his head to the left a couple of times, signalling Rubin to step away from the others. Dinner had finished, and the family was now sitting on the couch, watching Saturday night television.

Standing by the garden doors, David lowered his voice. "We know that the MP is in room 216 on the second floor. I assume that since it's Sunday, other rooms will be available. I plan to call and try to book a room next door or as close as possible. It will need to be an early check-in."

"How are you going to pay for that? If you book online or over the phone, it will leave a trace."

"I'll use Ryan's credit card. I'll take it from him in a moment."

"Okay. But how are you going to get into the room?"

"We will arrive early, ahead of the meeting time. Ryan will check in, collect the key, and bring it out to me. I've reviewed the hotel floor plans, and I know that the elevators are located to the left of the reception area; there are three of them. I'll ask him to press the call button on all three elevators, so hopefully one will be at the ground floor when I arrive, allowing me to head straight up."

Rubin shook his head. "This plan has risk written all over it. What if he communicates with the reception in some way?"

"Let's not forget that we have his wife and children hostage. He has cooperated so far, and there's no indication that he would change that. You've seen how scared he is."

Rubin glanced over his shoulder, knowing that the lab technician would have a long day tomorrow. "It still won't work; he needs to be monitored, with every move observed."

"I know, and I've been thinking about that. You have your bag of tricks with you, right?"

"Yes, upstairs. Only the debugging kit was dropped at my lockup. What do you have in mind?"

"Put up a temporary camera outside the room I'll be using, so I can monitor the corridor, as well as have him wear a body camera. Do you have pinhole cameras with you?"

"I have one, and it could be rigged into one of his jackets."

"Do you have a decoy badge we can attach to the other lapel to draw attention away from where the camera is placed?"

"Yes, that's not a problem. I always carry something with me."

"As long as we can monitor his words and hand gestures, to be honest, I think it's the best we can do."

Rubin chewed on his lips, fully aware that he was just as much at risk as David. If Ryan made any slip-ups and revealed anything, it would quickly lead back to the home address. "I don't like this; I really don't like it at all."

"What's there to like? How else would you run this op? We've been given a location that is incredibly difficult to operate from. There will be eyes everywhere."

"And how are you going to get there?" Rubin asked.

"We'll take his car. Ryan can drive. Although my car's license plates are cloned, it would be just our luck if the owner of the original plates were involved in something as minor as non-payment of insurance or a speeding fine. I can't risk getting pulled over; at least Ryan's car is clean, as far as we know. I'll double-check that with him, though. I'll also need to borrow a couple of other things from you, such as a wig. I'll keep the visor down while we drive and will bow my head at every traffic light and interchange."

Rubin placed his hands on his hips. "It looks like you're going to be relying on me to get you out of this mess," he said.

"Look, this is the best plan I can come up with on such short notice. As long as I can get in and out quickly and he is being monitored, we should be fine."

"That's the problem, you said 'should.' Listen, if this goes wrong, I won't stick around. I won't be here when you come back."

"I understand, brother. But if this goes tit's up, we'll both find out quickly."

"I don't like being completely reliant on you," Rubin replied.

"Yes, I can watch the live broadcast, but I only have one laptop connected to the pinhole camera, and I'll need to give that to you."

"I also have a key fob camera that I can connect to one of the mobile phones. To anyone else, it will just look like a standard remote car key."

"Okay, that sounds good."

"You need to call or message me immediately if you feel compromised."

"I will, brother. You have my word."

"And if there is a compromise, what will you do then?"

"I won't have much choice but to force my way into the room."

"And then?" Rubin added.

"I'll have to put them all down."

"Yes, you will. But not with the weapon you have. We'll need to swap. You get his credit card, and I'll go upstairs to get my silencer."

++++

"Please take a seat," Alix said.

Darius scanned the dated room. "It's not Chequers, is it?"

Alix laughed. "No, but it does have its charm. It's an old building that wasn't designed with modern comforts in mind. Would you like a drink?"

Darius settled into the chair opposite the Prime Minister's desk. "Sure, what are you having?"

"I'll have a brandy. Do you still enjoy Scotch?" Alix asked.

"I do, thank you." Darius unbuttoned his suit jacket and rested his arms casually on the sides of the chair. "You have photographs and paintings of some of your predecessors here."

"Yes, I may not agree with all their politics, but they are historical figures who have served the public."

Darius smiled as a glass of Scotch was handed to him. "And is that how you see yourself? As a public servant and a figure in history?"

Alix smirked as he took a seat. "Not history just yet." He raised his glass. "Cheers."

"Cheers to you, old friend."

Alix nodded, picking up on the tone in Darius's words. He knew that Darius wanted something. "Look, I don't have much time. I've come to see you and to say hello to some of your guests."

Darius nodded, then downed the Scotch in one go, placing the glass on the desk before resuming his position, arms resting on either side of the seat.

"What do you want, Darius? Let's get straight to the point."

"I prefer not to discuss these matters over the phone, as you know."

Alix set his glass down on the desk. "And what matters are those?"

"Are you recording this conversation?"

"What!" Alix laughed. "What an incredible thing to say."

"Well, this is a private chat, old friend. These walls have ears. Your cabinet briefs members of the press as soon as they leave your meetings at Downing Street."

Alix dismissed the comment with a wave of his hand. "That's just a necessity of business. I used to do it myself before I became Prime Minister."

"Are we being recorded, then?" Darius asked.

Alix laughed and picked up his glass of brandy. "I certainly hope not, given what happens in this room!"

Darius nodded. "I suppose that means we'll have to trust each other, won't we?"

Alix leaned back in his chair with a sigh. "What's on your mind?"

Darius stood up and put his hands in his pockets. "As you know, these are challenging times. Our share price fell to an all-time low six months ago, and I've had to diversify the company, shall we say. I'm looking for reassurance, Alix, and my senior board is looking for it too."

Alix frowned. "Reassurance about what?" He shrugged.

Darius raised his hands as if he were drawing a picture. "I'm envisioning… an office visit."

"A what?"

"Yes, it just occurred to me that we don't have any recent pictures of us together, or of you with my senior board."

"I don't understand, Darius. I can't be seen as openly supporting private enterprise, especially not on the corporate scale you represent. You're neither a small nor a medium-sized business, and you don't have government contracts. It would be politically unwise; the press would criticise it because of our history together from college."

"Unwise, you say? We don't see it that way. We're thinking about support. Come and join us for a jolly, and let's take some photos. We have some lovely models you can be photographed with..."

"What?"

"Yes, not just women, before you jump to conclusions. Our products cater to everyone. We wouldn't want you to be labelled as sexist, after all."

Alix swallowed. "Listen, Darius, you know I can't do something like that."

"Of course you can! You are supporting innovation and pioneering science. I've seen your predecessors at factories, labs, and the like; this is no different. Your support helps us through this transition. Let's put the cosmetic beauty business back where it needs to be."

"Darius, look, we go back a long time, but I'm uncomfortable with this. Maybe the business secretary can do something..."

"My company has supported you throughout your entire career!" Darius quickly interjected. "We have financially backed you as you've risen from the backbenches. We need to make good on our investment."

"Christ, Darius, what the hell does that mean? Our association is very well known. Your financial support of me and the party is officially declared through all proper channels."

Darius nodded. "Quite." He stood before the desk, looking Alix directly in the eyes. "But what about what isn't disclosed?"

"Oh, for fucks sake!" Alix slammed his brandy glass against the table. "We cannot talk about these things here!"

"Why not? I thought you said it was safe to talk in here."

Alix rubbed his forehead. "Yes, but still…"

"And we need to make good on our investment!"

Alix took a deep breath and leaned back in his chair. "What exactly do you want?"

"Excellent! Straight to the point, that's what I like about you. Do you mind if I help myself to your Scotch?"

Alix shook his head and crossed his arms.

"So, old friend, we have an exciting new development in the pipeline, an adaptation of our core Hydra-Fillixir range of products. It's quite revolutionary, if I do say so myself." Darius selected a bottle from the tray on the side and returned to the desk.

"Well, that's good news, isn't it?" Alix asked.

"Yes, we are pleased with it, but our fortunes need to change as the cosmetic industry is currently in turmoil, and not just for us, I should add. None of us is helped by your meddling MP, and we will need to make some changes. The good news is that's where you come in."

Alix raised his hands. "Look, I'm handling that. She has a meeting with the Chief Whip on Monday."

Darius shrugged. "So?"

"What do you mean, 'so'? He'll bring her back in line! As far as I'm concerned, her parliamentary career is over!"

"She has support outside of this building."

"And she has enemies, don't forget that! If I were you, I would be more concerned about bloody car bombs in the capital. Someone targeted her associate, the woman from the TV channel. As far as I've been briefed, they were very close to one another."

"Yes, well, she's silent now, at least for the moment."

Alix uncrossed his arms and observed Darius's body language. "Oh, holy shit, don't tell me you had something to do with that!"

Darius erupted into laughter and poured himself a generous measure of Scotch. "We may be disappointed with your lack of support, but we are not murderous by nature."

"I wouldn't put anything past you."

Darius swallowed the Scotch in one gulp. "That hurts, especially considering how long we've known each other."

"I know what I see."

Darius stuffed his hands into his pockets and licked his lips. "Alright, here's what I need you to do. Your Chief Whip is very close to Lord Gatesouth. I need you to persuade him to pressure the Chief Whip; I want her out of here, gone."

"Darius, listen to what you're asking; she's a bloody Member of Parliament. It's not that simple. Yes, she's a maverick, but she was democratically elected. If she continues like this, she won't be re-elected at the next election..."

"That's two years away! She needs to be silenced, and I mean it."

"What the hell do you want me to do? No one will support her here. Her so-called bill will never pass; even the select committees won't entertain it. We can't just withdraw the whip from her; her campaign doesn't justify kicking her out of the party!"

"Well, maybe you need to remind our friend in the Lords that we also provide him with financial support."

"That's on public record, and..."

"Not all of it is."

"What do you mean?"

"He's paid much more than he declares."

"Christ, Darius, I really don't want to know."

"Well, now I'm telling you, so you do know!"

"Oh God!" Alix rubbed his eyes in frustration. "Why can't you talk to Gatesouth? He'll listen to you."

"Because you are the Prime Minister, and it would carry much more weight coming from you."

"He'll think you have something on me!"

Darius smirked. "Exactly."

Alix rose to his feet. "Oh, here it comes."

"We've never asked for anything from you before. We put you in your position, and now you need to deliver. Our shareholders expect returns, and you owe us a serious debt."

Alix scratched his head, clearly anxious.

"Don't take it personally, old friend. It's just business."

"You are no friend of mine, Darius."

"You were happy to accept our money, though. Let's not lose sight of that." Darius leaned over the desk. "We own you."

"How dare you! You are in my office. I'm the bloody Prime Minister of Great Britain!"

Darius smiled. "Yes, you are! But we do not forget."

Alix looked away. "Don't."

"It seems you do not forget either, old friend. Turmoil, if it ever gets out, could lead to unpleasantness that might bring down a government."

"You promised you wouldn't mention it again!"

"I had no intention of doing so, but you need to play ball, old boy. You're hardly the first person to sit in this office with a dilemma of conscience," Darius poured himself another large Scotch. "And you definitely won't be the last."

"You are ruthless and corrupt!"

"I'm ruthless and corrupt? It wasn't my drug party where a guest took a nosedive..."

"That's enough!"

"It wasn't me who asked for it to be covered up."

"I said that's enough!"

Darius swallowed his Scotch. "Well, it's always a pleasure to see you, old friend. I'm glad to see that you understand the way things are. I'm neglecting my guests and need to head downstairs. We will, of course, see you in a bit. I'm sure Lord Gatesouth will be thrilled to see you."

Chapter Twenty-Two

"Ah, Lord Gatesouth," Lisa greeted him.

The Lord extended his hand, although his body language suggested he didn't remember her.

"Lisa Wellings, board member of Knightark Pharmaceutical," she introduced herself.

"Oh yes, of course. Please forgive me. I've noticed that as I get older, my memory isn't as sharp as it used to be."

Lisa nodded. "Not at all. I believe you've met Dr John Farmer."

"Indeed. I was a good friend of your father. I have fond memories of him," the Lord responded.

John shook his hand and smiled.

"He was such a dedicated servant to your company, a true visionary."

John nodded. "Thank you, my Lord."

"So, what are your plans for this evening? I've been showing some of your clients around the Lord's Chamber and the gallery. For those who haven't visited before, it's always a wonderful spectacle."

"I'm sure they appreciated the tour and embraced the building enthusiastically," Lisa replied. "Oh, while I think of it, I have something for you."

Lord Gatesouth laughed. "That's completely unnecessary. I do what I can to help your company within the confines of the rules. This place is no longer what it once was, and many questions are being raised these days. I don't understand why we're not allowed to shout from the rooftops about British business, although, of course, you are global as well." He smiled. "It's frowned upon now. I give a nod to business, and I end up all over the press."

Lisa passed her glass to John. "Here, hold this for me." She then took the wrapped picture frame from under her arm and handed it over to Lord Gatesouth.

He set his glass down and took the gift with enthusiasm. "That's very kind. Shall I open it now?"

Lisa reclaimed her glass from John and nodded with a smile.

He tore open the wrapping and held the picture frame up to examine it. John looked away, trying not to laugh.

"Oh, well, this is an interesting take on the palace. I don't think I've seen an art piece quite like it," he said. He immediately placed it on the table and lifted his glass. "Well, cheers to both of you. It's so lovely to see you again." They clinked glasses together. "I shall hang it in my office."

Lisa smiled, fully aware that was never going to happen.

"So, I hear there's a new product coming soon, or perhaps a rebranding?"

"Yes, my Lord," John replied, taking a sip of champagne. "It's more of a rebranding, really. As you know, the cosmetic beauty business isn't what it used to be."

Lord Gatesouth sighed and glanced over his shoulder. "I understand, and I sympathise with your situation. We live in an age of litigation, where only the lawyers seem to benefit."

Lisa maintained her smile as she listened to the man who received payments from their company each month but contributed little in return.

"As I mentioned, this place, this Westminster bubble, is just not what it used to be," he continued. "Tell me, is there any way I can assist you? I'm sure your senior board members must have some ideas."

"Yes, my Lord. Darius Neath certainly has plenty of those."

He smiled at Lisa. Lord Gatesouth's public school education had served him well in the corporate world, and his status in the House of Lords further enhanced his advantages. While he might not be street-smart, he could certainly recognise a patronising comment when he heard one.

"Well, in that case, I should have a chat with Darius. I haven't seen him yet; is he here?"

"I haven't seen him, my Lord, but I don't believe he would miss this occasion." John nodded and raised his glass in a gesture of farewell. It was clear that the Lord was primarily present to ensure his revenue stream was secure, with the company's good standing being a secondary concern.

Lord Gatesouth raised his glass, "Well, I'd better go find him. Wishing you both a lovely evening," he said before turning away.

"My Lord," Lisa called after him, "don't forget your picture."

"Oh yes," he replied, raising a hand in acknowledgement. "I'm sorry about that. Remember what I said about my memory?" He grinned as he collected his gift. "I'm sure I'll run into you both later."

Lisa raised her glass, "I have no doubt." As soon as he moved away, she giggled and turned to John. "That picture is going straight into the bin."

✣✣✣✣

William De La Roche, a senior board member and Darius's trusted confidant, smiled as he walked briskly to the door to greet the head of the company.

With a simple nod of acknowledgement, Darius collected a glass of champagne from one of the servers and stepped into the room. As the Chief Executive Officer, his entrance was immediately noticed.

"How did it go with your old school chum?" William asked.

Darius gestured for William to move to the side of the room. "Where are our two Lords?" he inquired.

"They're around here somewhere; I saw them in the Royal Gallery not too long ago," William replied.

"Okay, good. How many people do we have here?" Darius asked.

"All the board members are present, along with around thirty to forty guests. Our main distributors are here, along with a select group of surgeons. One of them, over there, is Julian Darcy. He's becoming quite the media darling. He actively promotes our products and has made several appearances on television and social media. He is one of the few in the field championing the cosmetic beauty industry."

Darius nodded. "I'm not familiar with him. Is he on the payroll?"

William smirked. "No, and that's the beauty of it. He hasn't asked for anything."

"Really?" Darius frowned slightly as he surveyed the room. "It won't take long; they always ask eventually. Still, he could be useful."

"My thoughts exactly."

"The Prime Minister is on his way; at least, I'm guessing he is."

"Okay," William nodded. "Is that a positive sign?"

"Yes, my friend, I think so. He needed to be reminded of how things are."

"Let's hope he was listening."

"Trust me. He heard what I had to say."

"Good," William glanced around the room. "We may need him."

Darius gently waved at a couple who recognised him. "We'll see. People like that come and go, trying to make their mark on history before ending up in the waste bin."

William snorted with amusement. "And where is it now?"

"The product?" Darius nodded at another familiar face. "Not far; it should dock in the morning and will be taken to the bonded warehouse in Sussex."

"Good. Are you concerned about any delays at customs?"

Darius shook his head. "Not especially. The products are on pallets in cold storage, with about an even split between the new variant and the old. You know how customs are; the most important thing is to ensure the paperwork is correct. Our broker has taken care of that, since customs typically don't like inspecting cold storage under the best of circumstances. Even if they do inspect, what could they do? Test every single vial?" He took a sip of his champagne with a smile.

"True. Are the personnel in place at the warehouse?" William asked.

"Yes, the special projects company is handling that. Ronald will still oversee everything during the initial delivery."

"Good. He's the right man for the job. How long do you think the sorting will take?"

Darius nodded at someone else in the room and raised his glass. "A few hours, my friend, as it requires a great deal of concentration. I like to call it 'selective inventory.' I've seen a picture of one of the packaging samples. As I mentioned before, in the small print on every box, there is a line that ends with two full stops instead of one. It's so subtle that it will be overlooked by anyone else. For appearances' sake, that is the only distinguishing mark."

William grinned. "Brilliant. But forgive me for asking, I trust the special projects team is unaware of what is really in the boxes?"

Darius snorted, "Are you kidding? Absolutely not! They're just looking for a simple printing error. One thing you can count on with military men is that when you give them an order, they follow through diligently. I've instructed the team leader overseeing operations to pay them double time for their precision, as it's such a painstaking task. Once separated, the new product will be reloaded back into cold storage on the truck, and only then will the driver be given the location of the unregistered facility; it will never be discovered. I've arranged for a separate batch of the old product to be flown into a private airstrip in Kent. These will be added to the original product batch at the warehouse, so even if the police or customs officials show up, the numbers will match. The only part of the process I haven't decided yet is who among us will be at the hidden facility to receive the cargo. I intend to be there myself, but if I am unable to, one of the three of us will need to go. I trust I can depend on you if I need to call; I presume you'll be staying in town for a few more days?"

William nodded in agreement. "Absolutely, I'm not going anywhere. Too much has been invested in this, and I want to see it through to the end. Overall, this is good news."

Darius grimaced as he finished his glass. "This champagne is terrible."

"Yes, quite undrinkable. At least it was cheap."

They surveyed the room, filled with lively chatter, smiles, and laughter. Other board members moved about, and they quickly spotted John Farmer and Lisa Wellings, who were engaged in a friendly conversation. Lisa held a glass of champagne, while John appeared to be drinking orange juice.

Darius set his glass down and remarked, "Look at them all, like vultures at a free bar."

William smiled. "Yes, but they generate money for us. Darius, are you concerned about the exposure and all of this coming to light?"

"Are you?" Darius shrugged. "I've done everything I can, my friend. What can anyone really prove? We'll continuously rotate batches, and the secure cold storage facility will remain undetected. It's on private land, and only I know its location; I did this intentionally to protect all of you." Darius glanced around the room. "So what if someone has a reaction and tests positive for class A drugs? How could they possibly trace it back to us? We'll hold our ground; they have a drug problem. If it hits the fan, we can plant class A substances into their homes. And even then, if we face a serious issue, we'd cite contamination at the plant. We could sack a few people in Brazil and maybe imprison one or two of them. I have already arranged for the marketing team to develop a new gift card. If someone has a reaction, we will send them money through these gift cards. We will always know who they are and where they go. We will ensure they receive the original filler; their newfound addiction is their problem. We can maintain this cycle for years." Darius signalled for one of the servers to come over. "Take a look around you, my friend."

William glanced around the room.

"No, not here. Look around you, outside of this place," Darius said, acknowledging the waiter as he took another glass of champagne.

"When your driver takes you back to your hotel, pay attention to what you see."

"What do you mean?" William asked.

"Life on the street."

William laughed. "And what would you know about that?"

Darius smirked. "I'll tell you what I know, my friend. This country is heading for disaster. Look at the street corners and the roads you'll drive down later. The opioid crisis in your country was orchestrated brilliantly, concealed in plain sight. People on these streets fight tooth and nail for control, battling over territory for minuscule rewards. It has become part of our culture, like a plague. They fight and fight until someone else takes their place, and then it all repeats. It's a cycle of chaos, and I want no part of it. What we've created goes far beyond anything that has happened in your country." Darius paused to sip the cheap champagne. "Before that bloody TV program and all the lawsuits started, there was a cosmetic business on nearly every road across the country; it was as common as a charity or a vape shop. Yet battles are fought on street corners, all for control of their little drug empires. This is cunning, my friend. If you want to get away with crime, hide it in plain sight, and it will remain there for years. The cosmetic business will thrive again."

William and Darius locked eyes.

"We are geniuses, my friend, and nothing can stand in our way. Unlike the vultures in this room and those who kill each other every day out there, we will have total control. No street dealers, no gangsters, just the local cosmetic beauty clinic. Soon it will be all over the country, and beauty clinics will start to reopen again."

"And what about international distribution?"

"It's all in hand. The British will serve as our guinea pigs. We'll observe how the product performs and monitor any aftereffects. If everything goes well and the collateral damage remains within an acceptable range, we'll expand into the Far East and your country as well."

William lifted his glass. "And I'll drink to that!"

They clinked their glasses and took a sip.

Darius flinched. "Christ, I'm not drinking any more of this champagne. Let's head to the bar and find something more appropriate."

✢✢✢✢

Helen Lord glanced at her phone; it was nearly 8 PM. She had reviewed her handwritten notes multiple times, carefully rehearsing the content and what she would say during the morning broadcast. For the second time, she confirmed that the two owners of the small production company were aware of the location and would arrive on time. There was little more she could do. Now, everything depended on Ryan and his testing equipment; however, the test had to be conducted within the non-sterile constraints of her hotel room.

Standing by the bedroom window, she had a perfect view of the former Scotland Yard, the old headquarters of the Metropolitan Police. Outside, the scene was relatively tranquil. In the past, when the police were stationed in the building across the street, the area was a hive of activity. Journalists and camera crews would gather on the corners for hours, sometimes even days. Now, only a handful of tourists and occasional hotel guests passed by.

As she retrieved her coat from the bed, she estimated that it would take her twenty minutes to walk to the palace. She needed to collect the vials from Portcullis House.

✢✢✢✢

"Have you done your rounds?" Lord Gatesouth grunted.

"I've done my part. What about you?" Lord Hawthorne replied, swallowing the last of his champagne and nodding. "I'm finished with being called 'my Lord' for one evening."

Lord Gatesouth smiled. "I don't know; I rather enjoy it."

"Touché!" Lord Hawthorne responded, then noticed a picture

under Lord Gatesouth's arm. "Oh Christ, you didn't receive one of those dreadful things too, did you?"

"Well, I certainly didn't pay for it, if that's what you're implying!" Lord Gatesouth shook his head. "Have you ever seen anything quite so ghastly?"

"I know, it's terrible, isn't it?" Lord Hawthorne replied, glancing around to ensure that Lisa wasn't watching him. "She gave me mine," he said, nodding in her direction.

"Yes, same here. I need to return to my office quickly; I'm expecting an email. Do you want me to drop off your picture?"

"Yes, please do. Straight in the bin." Lord Hawthorne took his picture gift and handed it to Lord Gatesouth.

"Are you sure you don't want to keep it?" Lord Gatesouth smirked as he noticed the Prime Minister entering the room with a couple of bottles of whisky.

"Looks like your old friend has arrived," Lord Hawthorne remarked.

"So he has. Anyway, I'm heading to my office now. By the way, we have a private golf day at the club on Tuesday. You're welcome to join us."

"What, and get fleeced by you again? I can't compete with your handicap."

"Excellent! We'll play for money then," Lord Gatesouth said with a smile before heading towards his office.

William gently nudged Darius's arm, "He looks a little sheepish and isn't carrying his usual air of self-importance."

Darius turned from the bar and noticed the Prime Minister entering the room. "Well, at least he showed up," Darius remarked. "He must have something on his mind."

William smiled as he picked up his glass of Scotch from the bar. "Following your chat, he was hardly going to miss it. It looks like he's going to be signing bottles again."

Darius grunted, "It always raises a bit of money."

"Yes, I guess so. By the way, what charity is being supported this evening?"

Darius shrugged as he grabbed his glass from the bar. "I've no idea."

"Do you think he'll come over to us?" William asked.

"I wouldn't have thought so after our brief exchange. We'll keep an eye on him and make sure he works the room," Darius said, taking a sip of his drink. "I want to get value for money from him from now on."

Alix nodded as Lord Gatesouth passed by. As he watched him leave the room, he noticed Darius Neith and his American colleague standing at the bar. Alix had met the American a couple of times before; he recalled that his name was William.

When Alix glanced over at them, they both turned away.

"Ah, Prime Minister, I'm glad you could join us! What a joy! I had no idea you were coming," exclaimed Ronald Ward, a senior board member.

Alix set down the whisky bottles and offered his hand. "Please, call me Alix."

"Oh yes!" Ronald responded, shaking Alix's hand enthusiastically. "Let me introduce you to a few people. This evening, we have scientists, fundraisers, distributors, and surgeons in attendance. They will be thrilled to meet you."

Alix took a deep breath and shifted into political mode. He knew he was being watched and could feel the daggers of resentment from his old school 'friend' standing at the bar.

++++

After a brisk walk, Helen crossed the road from Broad Sanctuary into Parliament Square. She realised that her earlier estimates had been incorrect; the walk had taken longer than she had anticipated. From the corner of the square, she had a perfect view of the clock tower, which read 8:35 p.m. Surprisingly, a few officers were present near the public entrance to the palace. With events being quite rare at the weekend, it suggested that something was happening inside. As she walked around the square and approached the large black gates at the front of the building's perimeter, she noticed that tourists were enjoying their Saturday night, filling the square by the thousands. Helen smiled at the police officer in front of her, who recognised her and nodded in return. "Good evening, ma'am."

Helen took her access card from her handbag. "Good evening to you. Is something happening inside? There are police further down by the public entrance."

"Just a Lord's reception this evening, ma'am, with only around forty or fifty guests."

"Oh, I see." Glancing across New Palace Yard, she noticed two cars parked further ahead. Tucked away on the other side of one of the narrow archways, a couple of police close protection officers stood next to the vehicles. "Excuse me, is the Prime Minister here?"

"Yes, ma'am, he arrived a little while ago."

This puzzled her. "Shouldn't he be at Chequers or somewhere else?"

The police officer smiled. "I'm not privy to that information, ma'am."

Helen glanced at the cars again. "No, I guess you wouldn't be," she mumbled. "Excuse me, I'm sorry for all the questions. What is the event at the Lords, please?"

"As I mentioned, ma'am, it's just a small gathering."

"Yes, but who is it for?"

"Knightark Pharmaceutical."

Helen froze, a chill ran through her as she considered the possibility that they knew what she had discovered.

++++

Helen pressed her hand to her chest as she hurried across New Palace Yard. To her right, the Prime Minister's cars were parked down a narrow passageway. Her heart raced, and she felt flustered, descending into a panic. Knightark Pharmaceutical was in the building, and the Prime Minister was also present. She knew that the company's head had attended college with him; was this merely a coincidence? Regardless, the timing unnerved her, and she was now concerned that they might have discovered the hidden vials. As she quickened her pace and jogged to the escalator that would take her to the main floor of Portcullis House, she did not doubt the seriousness of her findings. Rubbing her temples, she took a deep breath. As she reached the main floor of Portcullis House, an eerie silence filled the space; you could hear a pin drop. The restaurants were closed, and the surrounding offices were locked. A few police officers were present, but no one else was in sight. She hurried to the elevator, feeling a wave of relief when one of the officers gave her a nod of acknowledgement, which boosted her confidence that they were not actively searching for her.

As the elevator ascended to the second floor, she was aware of the camera inside and did her best to maintain her composure. If her office hadn't been searched, she would take a moment inside there to gather her thoughts. Upon stepping out of the lift, she peered down the corridor. Throughout her time in Parliament, she could never recall feeling as nervous as she did on this occasion. The thought of what she suspected had happened to Alison lingered in her mind. As she passed the restroom, she noticed the door was unlocked and that she was alone on the floor.

Common sense suggested that if an investigation were underway, the police would be present or her office door would be sealed. Thankfully, the door appeared untouched as she pulled her keys from her bag and let herself in. After scanning her office, she immediately locked the door behind her and unlocked her private office. Nervously, she examined every corner of the room; at first glance, everything seemed normal as she secured herself inside. Although the temperature felt normal, she felt overheated and quickly removed her jacket, tossing it aside. She reached for the water bottle on her desk and drank it in one go. After dropping the empty bottle into the recycling bin, she took a moment to calm herself. Tomorrow was when everything would come to a head, and the people responsible were currently in the same building. She needed to retrieve the vials. As long as they were still hidden where she had stored them, it was just a matter of whether she dared to confront the drug dealers downstairs afterwards.

++++

Alix smiled and nodded as he accepted the audience's applause. His impromptu speech, which lasted about two minutes, pleased the attendees. He congratulated the pioneers of British business and expressed his gratitude for being invited to the event. Afterwards, he autographed the two bottles of House of Commons Scotch he had brought for the upcoming auction.

Lisa watched him mingle with the crowd and said with a smile, "He's a pro."

John responded with a grin, "You have to be when running the country."

"Not a job I'd be interested in," she laughed.

"Neither would I; I couldn't handle having my face in the papers every single day."

Lisa finished the rest of her drink and remarked, "Yes, quite. I did notice that he didn't mention our company in his speech; he just referred to British business in general."

"Yeah, I think there are rules about that now. I'm surprised he's here; he doesn't usually show up at our little gatherings."

"You should get a picture with him."

John laughed, "He's a politician, not a celebrity."

"That's not how they see it. Have you ever met a politician who doesn't enjoy being photographed?" John raised his eyebrows; Lisa had a point.

"Anyway, why don't you go get a picture with him?" She leaned into John's shoulder. "It's always good to have these things; you never know when those pictures might come in handy."

"What on earth do you mean?" John asked.

"Well, it's like they say: keep your enemies close. You know he attended college with Darius, right? It's been investigated by the Commissioner for Parliamentary Standards on several occasions, especially since Darius is known to be a significant financial donor. It always makes the press."

"And I bet the PM doesn't like this situation one bit. Just imagine: our company pays members of his party for consultancy, like Gatesouth and Hawthorne, and his obvious connections to Darius must weigh heavily on him. But I have to admit, I have no idea why he's here either."

"And my instincts are picking up on a problem," she said.

John grinned. "You're quite inquisitive. What makes you say that?"

"Well, you and I know about the new filler. Darius suggests it contains a compound that enlightens the user, whatever that means. Yet here we are, in this place of transparency that is also full of secrets, and the man running the country shows up at the weekend, no less. It just doesn't add up; something is going on. Oh, wait, look, he's coming our way."

"Well, whatever you're thinking, you've had a few glasses, and your voice is getting a bit louder," John whispered.

Lisa extended her hand. "Prime Minister, I'm so glad you could join our little gathering this evening."

"Please, call me Alix. I'm off duty," he replied, smiling as he shook her hand.

"I was just telling my colleague, Dr John Farmer, that I was surprised to see you here," she continued.

Alix turned to John and extended his hand. "Alix Gregory. I'd say I'm pleased to meet you, but your face looks familiar."

"Yes, Prime Minister. Lisa and I are board members," John responded.

"Oh yes, of course! And please, call me Alix," he said warmly.

Lisa seized the opportunity to ask, "So, what brings you here this evening?"

"It's quite simple. I stopped by my office and discovered that this event was happening. I went to college with your senior director, Darius Neeth, so I thought I'd drop in and say hello."

"Really? That's very kind of you. May I be so bold as to mention something? I noticed you had an uncomfortable moment in the chamber this week. I saw it on the news. It seems you have an MP who doesn't support this company, along with others in the cosmetics industry."

John winced in embarrassment and discreetly nudged Lisa's side. Despite being on first-name terms, the Prime Minister appeared unhappy to hear this viewpoint.

Alix forced a smile, looking directly into Lisa's eyes. He was not only taken aback by what she said but also wondered why he was being asked about this at a social gathering. Most people were usually pleased to see him in such settings.

"I apologise if my question makes you feel uncomfortable, Alix."

"Er, no, it doesn't. I'm just a little surprised to hear it, if indeed it was a question. But let me tell you something about politics: this place where we stand right now is the bastion of democracy, one of the most famous buildings in the world. Within these walls, we are allowed to express our views. If our views are suppressed, then where will we be? It is important to allow free speech, even when members of your party disagree with party policy, because it is those policies that guide us as we work to do what is right for the British people. I understand your point, and I hear it. However, I believe my words have addressed your concerns. We in government, as well as those in opposition, will always challenge each other, and that is what politics is about, even when we disagree."

John intervened, not wanting Lisa to press him further. "Fine words, Alix."

"Well, maybe not fine, but it's a Saturday evening, and it's been a long week." He smiled at them both.

"Oh, I forgot to mention. Dr Farmer would love a photograph with you, would that be possible, Alix?"

John instantly frowned. Whatever game Lisa was playing, or perhaps it was the alcohol, made him feel enormously uncomfortable. Embarrassed, John held up a hand. "That won't be necessary."

Alix laughed. "Nonsense, I'll hear no part of it."

"Great!" Lisa exclaimed as she took her phone from her clutch bag and motioned for John to move next to Alix. "Okay, all smiles then!"

John forced a smile as Alix, a professional at having his photograph taken, posed effortlessly while three images were taken.

Glancing to his left, Alix noticed Darius and the American watching him from the bar. Darius gave a nod and raised his glass to catch his attention.

Alix swallowed, saying, "Right, lovely to see you both. I see Lord Hawthorne is over there. I haven't seen him in ages; I should catch up." He shook hands with them both before adding, "I hope those pictures turned out okay."

"I'm sure they will be fine, Prime Minister," Lisa replied.

Alix smiled at Lisa, trying to gauge her tone. He then nodded to them and turned to head toward Lord Hawthorne.

John shot Lisa a glare. "Well, that was bloody uncomfortable."

Lisa smiled back. "Did you understand a word of that politician's answer he just gave me?"

John shook his head. "Not really."

"You said his words were fine!"

"I was trying to lower the tone. He doesn't want to be interrogated on a Saturday night.

Lisa nodded and paused to check her phone.

"What is it?" John asked.

Lisa shook her head and put her phone away. "Nothing, just checking on something. She picked up her empty glass. "I need a refill."

Chapter Twenty-Three

Helen peered through the blinds in her office, gaining a view of the main floor of Portcullis House. She noticed there were no gatherings of police officers or officials from the Serjeant-at-Arms department below. Her paranoia was creeping in, but she felt it was warranted. After making sure the blinds were closed, she removed her shoes and unlocked her office door. Licking her dry lips, she unlocked the main office door and peeked into the corridor; it was empty and silent. Leaving the office door ajar, she hurried to the restroom. As she pushed against the restroom door, she noticed her hands were shaking. The light flickered on as she locked the door behind her. Turning to face the mirror, she caught sight of her reflection; her skin looked pale and clammy. Frowning at having to put the toilet seat and lid down again, she stood barefoot on the toilet lid and rose onto her tiptoes and moved the ceiling tile aside. Taking her phone from her pocket, she turned on the torch setting. "Thank God!" she exclaimed, relieved to see the envelope still in place. Grabbing the metal coat hanger she had left in the ceiling void, she extended it to its full length and used the hook to drag the envelope within reach. Once she had a firm grip of the envelope, she pushed the bent coat hanger back into the ceiling void and carefully replaced the ceiling tile.

Now it was the moment of truth. Sitting on the toilet, she opened the large envelope and, to her relief, found the vials still inside. Leaning back against the toilet, she let out a massive sigh of relief.

++++

Alix approached a small group where Lord Hawthorne was speaking.

"Ah, good, everyone. I'm sure you know this is our Prime Minister, Alix Gregory," Lord Hawthorne said.

Alix nodded and shook hands with the four strangers. "Thank you for the introduction, my Lord."

"Why, Alix, that is very courteous of you," Lord Hawthorne said, nudging the guest on his right. "He doesn't usually address me as my Lord; it's usually just Charles."

The small group shared a collective laugh.

"There's a reason for that, Lord Hawthorne," Alix smirked. "That's because I'm in your part of the building. Come over to the Commons, and I will call you Charles!"

The laughter continued.

"Look, I'm sorry to interrupt your conversation, but may I have a word with you?" Alix said.

"But of course, PM," Lord Hawthorne replied, nudging the guest again. "So, what's gone wrong now?" Charles grinned. "Ladies and gentlemen, it was lovely to make your acquaintance."

Alix then guided the peer to the side of the room.

"I must say, I'm surprised to see you here, Alix. These buggers still keeping you on the payroll?" Charles smiled as he took a sip from his glass. "Is everything alright? You look a bit troubled."

"Yes, yes, I'm fine. Actually, I'm looking for Lord Gatesouth. I've scanned the room, but I can't seem to find him. Do you know where he is?"

"Owen? Yes, he's around here somewhere. He had to go back to his office, something about an email."

"I see," Alix replied, glancing at the bar where there were still eyes upon him.

"Do you want me to call him for you?"

"No, no, don't worry. I'll go down to his office."

"As you wish. Do you remember where it is?"

"Yes, Charles, I've been to his office before."

"Oh, by the way, he has a golf day scheduled for Tuesday if you're interested?"

Alix scoffed. "You must be joking. We're in the middle of an economic crisis. How would it look being photographed on a golf course with you two?"

"Ah, yes, I see, it's all about keeping up appearances. Never mind; we'll have you elevated to the Lords once your term is up. Easy money after that."

Alix laughed. "I'll keep that in mind, although I'm still too young!"

"You cheeky bugger! I'm definitely not going to bid on one of your autographed bottles of Scotch now!"

Alix smiled. "If I miss Owen and you see him, will you let him know I'm looking for him?"

Charles nodded. "But of course."

As Alix left the room, he caught Darius's eye and nodded.

Darius returned the nod and nudged William. "And there you have it, my friend; the puppet is going to work."

++++

If Alix were honest with himself, he should have called his close protection officers instead of walking around the building alone. After seeing Lord Gatesouth, he intended to return to his office and contact them from there. At weekends and at this time of evening, the Lords were even quieter than the Commons. As he ascended the staircase, he usually would have appreciated the peace of the old building if he hadn't so much on his mind; being alone felt like a luxury these days. Passing the smallest bar in the palace, he noticed it was closed, just like everything else. A few doors down, he spotted that Owen's office door was open. At least he could have a private conversation in there. After knocking a couple of times, Owen appeared at the door, surprise evident on his face.

"Alix! What on earth are you doing here? I thought you'd be at Chequers!"

"Yes, well, I've been hearing that all evening. I'll be heading back there shortly. Look, can I have a word?" Alix replied.

"Of course! Is something on your mind?"

"Regrettably so."

"Well, do come in, old boy. Care for a brandy?"

"Thank you. A large one is needed," he replied as he closed the door.

++++

Standing in New Palace Yard, Helen glanced up at the clock tower before quickly looking behind her. The Prime Minister's car and the chase vehicle were still in place. Clutching her bag tightly, she felt reassured knowing she had the vials. However, she was uncertain about her next move. Her nemesis was inside the building, more accurately, their representatives were. If there was an evening function at the palace, it was reasonable to assume that senior members of Knightark Pharmaceutical were also in attendance. The timing felt suspicious, but why was the Prime Minister in the building as well? Two close protection officers stood next to the vehicles, and she noticed a driver in the front car, his face illuminated by his phone. It couldn't hurt to ask a question, she thought.

As she approached, the officers fell silent. "Good evening. I'm Helen Lord, MP. May I ask how long the Prime Minister will be inside?"

"I know who you are, ma'am," one of the officers responded. "At the moment, we're not sure."

Helen nodded in acknowledgement. "May I ask why he is here? I'm not aware of any government business this evening." She understood that police officers might occasionally provide helpful information.

He replied promptly, "We are not privy to that information, ma'am."

"I see." It was evident they were unwilling to discuss the matter further. Sensing the atmosphere was slightly tense, she made her excuses and wished them a good night.

The opportunity was too great to pass up. Timing was everything, and her inquisitive nature compelled her to discover what was happening. As the clock chimed overhead, she made her way back to New Palace Yard, cutting across the cobblestones before pushing open the heavy doors to enter Westminster Hall. The close protection officers strode past her, moving quickly to the far end of the hall. This suggested that Alix wasn't far away, and she might finally get some answers. Quickening her pace, she passed the commemorative plaques on the floor and caught sight of the one dedicated to Winston Churchill, marking his lying in state in 1965. Glancing up, she saw the security officers already approaching the steps at the far end. Soon after, Alix appeared at the top of the steps and briefly addressed the two security men. He didn't notice her as he made his way down. Even at this time of year, she could feel the chill in Westminster Hall; it was always cold in summer and freezing in winter.

Alix made his way towards her, flanked by his security. She had not seen him since their clash in the chamber, and as soon as he looked up and met her eyes, he quickly glanced away in disgust, shaking his head.

"Good evening, Prime Minister. It's unusual for you to be here at the weekend," she said, tightening her grip on her bag, her hand trembling slightly. It was clear that he wasn't inclined to stop for a conversation, but he was likely just as curious about her presence.

"It's alright, officers," he said, gesturing for them to stop walking. "I had something to attend to, Helen. What brings you here?"

"I had something to attend to as well," she replied, gripping her bag so tightly that her knuckles turned white.

"Interesting," he responded curtly.

"Interesting indeed. Were you at the party in the Lords?" she asked.

He smiled and slipped his hands into his pockets. "I understand you have a meeting with the Chief Whip on Monday."

"Do I owe you thanks for that?"

"Oh, come now, Helen, you have your actions to thank for that.

Our party has held your constituency for some years. Don't blow it, will you?" He nodded to his security as they moved away from her.

She stood alone in the vast hall, which had been filled with tourists earlier in the day. A glance to her right revealed a police officer at the top of the steps, watching over her. Continuing her walk toward the steps, she casually glanced behind her. Alix also turned and made some remarks to his security while they held the doors open for him. His vehicle was already waiting outside. As she ascended the stairs, she reflected on the moment that had just transpired. It was evident that he had no liking for her at all. However, she had been democratically elected, and there was nothing he or the Chief Whip could do about it; this was about doing the right thing. Wasn't that what MPs were elected for? She considered this for a moment before dismissing the thought from her mind and saying good evening to the police officer.

Quickening her pace, she headed straight for central lobby. She would then turn right, head down the stairs, and along the corridor where most of the social rooms were situated. If this pharmaceutical celebration were not down that corridor, she would head straight to the Lords instead. She might as well introduce herself. What was the worst that could happen?

✣✣✣✣

Annabelle and Sophie had gone to bed, while Andrea and Ryan were cuddled up on the couch, watching television with a glass of wine.

Rubin nodded to David, inviting him to join him in the kitchen. "Do you want a glass?" he asked.

David shook his head. "I'll wait until after everything is done. For now, I want to keep my mind clear and my wits about me. Wine makes me sleepy."

"It used to have that effect on me, too," Rubin replied as he picked up the bottle to read the label.

"You don't drink anymore?" David asked.

Rubin shook his head. "I miss it sometimes, but that's when the problems start. It brings back too many memories; it's best for me to stay away from it. I made a vow to change my ways a while ago, focusing on my faith." He set the bottle down. "Do we have the jacket we're going to use?"

"Yes, I went through Ryan's wardrobe and found a suit jacket. I've left it in the hallway. Is the camera powered?"

"It is. I also checked the laptop, and both devices are functioning properly," Rubin nodded. "I'll need to show you how to use them in the morning. The corridor camera runs on three standard-sized batteries, ensuring it's independent of any external power source. My laptop is old and drains quickly; the pinhole program and app are installed on it, so plug the laptop in once you get inside. You can monitor the pinhole camera using the laptop, watch the corridor camera on your phone, and I will connect the fake car remote camera to Ryan's phone. I know it's not the most secure setup, but you may need to access the hotel's Wi-Fi for the corridor camera and the key camera if you're unable to create your own hotspot. My laptop has its own network, so you don't need to worry about that. Bring me his jacket in a bit, and I'll connect the pinhole camera and the decoy badge."

David nodded, "Will do. I've booked the hotel room; it's only two doors down from where the test will take place. I checked the email confirmation on his phone. How many clips do you have for your firearm?"

"Two, I have spare rounds if you need them. If you must breach the room, one clip should be all you need to finish them off."

David turned to check on Ryan and Andrea. "Let's hope it doesn't come to that."

"If it does, so be it, but it'll be a mess we could do without, and I'll be long gone before you get anywhere near here. However, if you do need to breach, ensure the cameras are switched off first. Do not kill them during a live broadcast; it will be bad enough as it is. Showing it to the whole world would bring heat down upon us from every authority and security agency."

"Like I said, as long as he does what he's told, it shouldn't come to that."

"And what about the money? I know it's upstairs. Should we carve it up when you get back?"

"That's what I was planning to do. I'll only be carrying a small amount with me. Unless you have other ideas and decide to take off with all of it before I get back!"

Rubin looked offended by the suggestion. "I wouldn't do that. Besides, I know you'd come after me."

"I would." They locked eyes.

"We have to trust each other, then," Rubin added. "But I warned you before: if this goes south, I'll be gone and gone quickly. I'll take care of the family and half of the available money. If I think you've been compromised or taken out, I'll be taking everything with me. You'll find me in Nepal if you manage to get through this and want to come look for me."

"I'll keep that in mind."

Rubin nodded as they continued to stare at each other. "You do that," he said.

After a brief pause, David continued, "I'm not going to discuss cameras or anything else with Ryan just yet. It will only make him more restless, and we need him to stay focused."

"Fair enough," Rubin said as he poked his head through the kitchen door. The couple were talking, but they immediately stopped when they noticed they were being watched.

"Are they okay?"

Rubin nodded and turned back. "As soon as you're back tomorrow, my part in this is done. I need to return to my storage unit, prepare the money for laundering, and then I'll head home. I was only supposed to be in the UK for a few days."

David went to the sink and poured himself a glass of water. "I understand."

"Do you have more work lined up after this?" Rubin asked.

David shook his head. "I hope not! I primarily work with this client and have a couple of others, but the work is intermittent. This current client is always involved in something. They have plenty of cash, but their business is struggling right now, so I understand. They are trying to get things back on track."

Rubin snorted in discontent. "Everything is a struggle in this country right now. I don't miss it."

"You prefer where you are?"

Rubin adjusted his position to keep an eye on Ryan and Andrea. "Yes, I feel more at peace; it's good for the soul." He turned his back on David as he watched the couple sitting together, holding hands and watching television. "Poor bastards getting caught up in all of this."

David kept a close watch on Rubin, the former Legionnaire. He knew that Rubin's statement was true. If Rubin left with all the money, David knew he would have to track him down, but Nepal was vast, and his colleague wouldn't leave behind any data trails that would be easy to follow. David took a sip of his water, bracing himself for the next day. He didn't care for Andrea or Ryan; they were just unfortunate souls caught in the wrong place at the wrong time. It was purely a business matter. However, knowing Darius's character, he suspected that Darius would instruct them to kill the family before they left, and he was well aware that Rubin would have no qualms about doing so.

++++

On the Commons side of the palace, Helen made her way toward the Lords, following the noise echoing from within. A wave of uncertainty washed over her as she contemplated whether to enter. Given her campaign with Alison, she risked being ejected from the private event, which would undoubtedly create a noteworthy stir. As she approached, clutching her handbag containing the fortunes of

Knightark Pharmaceutical, she drew on her nerves and a sense of empowerment. She possessed knowledge that they did not. Despite her apprehension about what might happen next, she remained resolute in executing her plan, and the test would proceed. Someone in a senior position within the company must have sanctioned this illegal and highly addictive filler; it had been created intentionally to generate profit and to promote addiction. The informant revealed the company's name but did not identify any of the individuals responsible. As a staff member, he likely did not have access to that information. However, someone on the board must have known who they were. She felt uncertain about her next steps and whether it was appropriate to raise such questions in this setting. Since becoming involved with Alison, she had conducted her research and familiarised herself with the names and photographs of the four senior board members, which were easily accessible on the company's website. There were also eight junior board members whose names she couldn't recall, but she might recognise their faces if she saw them.

Taking a deep breath, she noticed that the door was open, revealing about thirty to forty people inside, with no one checking invitations at the entrance.

"Excuse me, please."

Helen offered a brief smile as she stepped aside to let a woman exit the room. The restrooms were further down the corridor, and Helen kept an eye on her, wondering if she might turn around, but she didn't. The woman pushed open the restroom door and vanished from view. The woman hadn't recognised her, maybe she was being too paranoid and overreacting.

Suddenly, a loud cough startled her from behind. She turned to find Lord Gatesouth standing there. Though they had never spoken before, she recognised him from her research. He looked perplexed. "Do you have an invitation?" he asked. His voice was deep, and his tone was polite.

"Um, no. I was just passing through. I heard some noise and thought I'd see what was happening," Helen replied.

"Passing through? Your place is in the other house, not here in the Lord's," he responded.

"Oh, do you recognise me?"

"Oh yes, you're the one who has been upsetting the leader of this country, as well as members of our political party. I'm quite surprised to see you here at a gathering of people involved in the cosmetic pharmaceutical industry. I've heard you're strongly against it," he said with a patronising smile.

Helen swallowed, feeling immediately awkward. "I have my views on the subject, particularly regarding non-necessary surgery."

He stepped into her personal space. "They are much more than just views." He didn't blink as he stared into her eyes. "As I said, your place is in the Commons. Lord, isn't it? Quite ironic that your surname is that."

"And why would you say that?" Helen asked, maintaining her composure despite his efforts to intimidate her.

Taller than she was, he smirked and leaned in closer. She could smell the alcohol on his breath. "Because this is not the place for you, and it never will be."

They locked eyes as a well-dressed gentleman stepped through the door. "Ah, there you are, Lord Gatesouth. We were wondering where you had gone."

The Lord straightened his back but kept his eyes fixed on Helen.

"And who do you have here?" the gentleman asked, extending his hand. "Darius Neeth, CEO of Knightark Pharmaceutical."

Despite the pain this company was about to cause, he was charming, well-groomed, and well-mannered.

"This is Helen Lord, MP. She's in the wrong part of the building," Lord Gatesouth snorted.

"An MP, really? How fascinating," Darius replied with a smile. Helen tightened her grip on her handbag; she recognised him instantly.

"And she was just about to leave," Lord Gatesouth added.

Darius lowered his hand, noting that his handshake had not been reciprocated. "Nonsense, I won't hear of it. Please, do join us."

Lord Gatesouth frowned, diverted his stare from Helen, and turned to Darius with a look of surprise.

"So, will you join us?" Darius smiled. "Excuse me." Helen watched as he signalled to someone. A waiter appeared with a tray of glasses. "Here, take one of these." He handed her a glass of what Helen guessed was champagne and raised his arm to invite her into the room.

Lord Gatesouth turned to Helen as she lifted her glass with a smile. "Cheers, don't mind if I do," she said.

++++

"What are you doing? Do you know who she is?"

Darius smiled at Lord Gatesouth. "Of course. It's always wise to keep your enemies close. Let's see what she does, if anything at all."

"Sounds risky to me. You have clients here," Lord Gatesouth replied.

"What's the worst that can happen?" Darius said as they observed the member of parliament walking around the room. Her champagne glass was barely touched, and she seemed more interested in people watching while clutching her handbag.

Lord Gatesouth felt someone behind him. He turned to see the senior board member from the United States. "Oh, good evening, William."

"Good evening, Owen. What's she doing here?" William asked, glancing at the MP.

"It's anyone's guess. It was your senior director's idea to let her in."

"What! Darius, you didn't invite her, did you?" William's tone was incredulous.

Darius turned around with a grin. "Of course not. It's just good fortune. Before she leaves, I want to have a chat with her."

"Darius, are you sure? You know what her agenda is and the knowledge she claims to have about the new product."

"The knowledge she claims to have," Darius said, wagging a finger at William.

"What new product?" Owen Gatesouth asked.

"Just an innovation. My friend, we always try to stay ahead of the game."

"That's the way to run a successful business," Owen added.

Darius nodded. "Anyway, let's not stare at her. Care for a whisky, my Lord?"

Owen smiled. "Don't mind if I do, old boy."

Lisa Wellings had a sly smile on her face. "Well, I never! It can't be," she said.

John turned around with curiosity. "Why? What have you seen?"

"Not a what, a who. Isn't that the MP who's all over social media?"

"Over social media for what?" John asked.

"If I'm thinking of the right person, she's the anti-beauty MP. I read that she is friends with the woman who was the target of the explosion this week."

John followed the direction in which Lisa was looking. "Yes, I think it is her. I didn't expect her to be at this kind of gathering. What is she doing here?"

Lisa finished her drink. "Let's find out."

"Just be careful what you say," John quickly added.

Lisa set her glass on the table with a grin. "What do you mean, me?"

"I mean, you've had a few drinks, and she's an MP. You never know who she might talk to."

"Well, look, chances are she wasn't invited, so let's see what she's all about. She's probably gatecrashing anyway," Lisa said as she walked toward the MP.

John finished his orange juice and followed Lisa. It looked like the MP was scanning the room, taking stock of who was present.

✢✢✢✢

Helen stayed near the edges of the room, choosing not to approach anyone just yet. She wanted to observe who was present and hoped to find out if the Prime Minister had attended at some point. The man who had introduced himself was familiar to her; his polite invitation into the room surprised her. He must have known who she was. Lord Gatesouth had made his feelings quite clear; she wished she had recorded his aggressive remarks, in which he declared that she would never make it into the House of Lords, though she had never even considered that possibility. The old boys' club and its threats held little significance for her; they were relics of the past. Now, gathered at the bar, they studied her every move like an unwelcome insect. Lord Hawthorne had joined them; while she had met him before, and he had been pleasant in the past, they hadn't spoken recently. They turned away in an attempt to make their stares less obvious, but it was clear she was the subject of their conversation. As she took a sip of her champagne, she reflected on her surroundings and the company she was in. Her campaign must have gotten to them, and given the occasional scowl she received from the bar, she felt confident that she had made her presence known in the room. Her friend lay in the hospital, and she suspected that someone in the room was involved, although she couldn't prove it. The old saying came to mind: "It's not what you know, it's what you can prove." Tomorrow, she would discuss Alison during the broadcast. While she intended to make direct accusations about the company and their new filler, she couldn't outright name them for attempted murder. Her thoughts were interrupted when a couple approached: a well-dressed woman, likely in her early forties, and a gentleman of similar age. The woman smiled as she approached.

"I recognise you!" the stranger exclaimed.

"Really? What have I done now?" Helen smiled and took a sip from her glass.

"Yes, I'm sure it's you; you're an MP, aren't you?"

"You are correct. I'm Helen Lord."

"Yes, of course. I'm Lisa Wellings, and this is my colleague, Dr

John Farmer." They all nodded at each other, but there were no handshakes.

"So, why are you here? I thought you were all anti-us?"

"Us?"

"Yes, John and I are board members," Lisa explained.

She looked them up and down; their faces seemed vaguely familiar, but they were not senior board members. "I think I just met your senior figure. Darius Neeth introduced himself to me and invited me in."

"I'm surprised he did that, considering your stance. Am I correct in thinking you are behind the so-called 'Death of Beauty' campaign?" John said.

Helen rolled her eyes. "I never called it that, Dr Farmer. That was a tag created on social media. Journalists use that term in their reports because it generates stories."

John nodded. "That it does. All the same, you are most welcome here. I'm just a bit surprised to see you."

Helen glanced towards the bar; the men were no longer being discreet, as they all watched her in the company of two board members. She had their attention. "Well, Dr Farmer, I'm here purely by chance. I happened to be in the building and thought I'd drop in. And it wasn't me who started the campaign you mentioned; that was my dear friend, Alison Harwood. I trust you've heard of her? She was blown up this week; someone tried to kill her. I guess she knew too much."

At that moment, Lisa looked at John, and the atmosphere soured instantly. "I'm very sorry to hear about what happened to your friend. What do you mean when you say she knew too much?"

Helen tightened her grip on her handbag. The female board member who had asked the question seemed genuinely confused. "You really don't know?"

Lisa looked quite perplexed, while John shook his head.

"How's your share price? I read that it has tumbled over the last couple of years."

Lisa raised her arm for attention. "Would you like another drink?"

Helen shook her head. "I haven't finished this one yet."

Lisa collected a glass from the tray in front of her and nodded at the server with a smile. "It's not just about us, Helen. I'm sorry, may I call you Helen?"

"You may," Helen replied.

Lisa took a sip from her glass. "The entire cosmetic industry has declined over the past couple of years..."

"It seems you still have some money in the bank, enough to host a party like this. That, along with having members of the House of Lords on your payroll."

John looked away, coughing slightly under his breath. He glanced over and noticed they were attracting attention from the bar.

"Our consultants are widespread, not just within Parliament; we are a global company. To my knowledge, everything is declared and above board," Lisa replied.

"Is that right, Lisa? May I call you Lisa?" Helen inquired, noticing the prominent smile had quickly vanished from the junior board member's face. "It's good to have connections, I suppose. However, the level of consultancy that the two Lords, who are staring at us from the bar, can offer appears questionable, considering their backgrounds. If I'm not mistaken, they all attended the same college as Darius and our Prime Minister. I ran into the PM earlier. Did he stop by here as well?"

John tried to nudge Lisa, eager to move away from the conversation. Lisa glanced to her right, realising that the MP was correct; they were being watched. "I'm not involved in those matters, Helen."

"Lisa, you're a board member. That surprises me. Here's what I think: I believe you bought your way into this place to try to influence the government. I'm particularly interested to see how the police investigation unfolds and who might be implicated in planting explosive devices on the streets of London. I'm curious about that!" Helen drained her glass and set it aside.

John raised his hand to signal for calm. "Helen, what happened to your friend this week is truly awful. It was well known in the beauty industry that she strongly opposed cosmetic procedures. However, we are business people, and we, along with our competitors, would never wish harm on anyone."

Helen adjusted the strap of her handbag to secure it on her shoulder. "As a doctor, you can appreciate that injecting foreign substances into oneself purely for aesthetic reasons might have hidden consequences."

"Well, I hear your viewpoint, but cosmetic enhancements are still in their early stages in the grand scheme of things. Our products undergo scrutiny and must be approved for cosmetic use, but as I mentioned, it's early days. If future adjustments are necessary, then so be it."

"Adjustments that could potentially be addictive. What would you say to that?"

The conversation came to an abrupt halt.

Lisa swallowed, unsure of what to say. The MP seemed to know something, and, more importantly, she suggested a connection to the event that had occurred in London earlier that week.

Helen continued, "Your silence speaks volumes. I think I'll grab one more glass of this free champagne before I leave." She nodded at them. "It's interesting to have met you both," she said as she walked away toward the waiter carrying glasses around the room.

John nudged Lisa to get her attention. Her eyes remained fixed on the MP. "What do you make of that?"

Lisa shook her head. "I don't know," she replied, turning to look John in the eyes. "She mentioned addiction and attempted murder practically in the same sentence." They both turned to see Darius raise a glass in their direction with a smile.

++++

"I noticed you raised a glass to two of our junior board members, Darius, but what were they doing talking to her?" Ronald asked.

"My dear Ronald, we don't need to worry about such things," Darius replied with a sly smile. "I have everything under control." He leaned closer to his senior board member. "For now, just focus on tomorrow. The consignment will be arriving, so I'll liaise with the special projects team to ensure the right vials are separated. I'll confirm as soon as the other cargo is flown in."

"I understand, Darius, but I'm not comfortable with her being here," Ronald said.

"Okay, look. I'll have a word with her. Let's find out what's on her mind."

"Do you want me to come with you?"

"No, I'll talk to her alone. I want her to stay calm. Being surrounded by us will only make her nervous. I'll take her a glass and see what she has to say. If there are any problems, I'll have her removed."

Darius turned to the bar. "Anyone care for another drink, gentlemen?"

"Why not?" Lord Gatesouth replied. "Are you up for another one, Charles?"

Lord Hawthorne placed his glass on the bar. "I don't mind if I do."

"William, can you get the drinks in? Owen, do you have a moment?"

"For you, Darius. Of course."

"William, I'd like another Scotch, please." Darius placed his arm on Owen's shoulder and pulled him away from the others.

"Is something on your mind, old boy?"

"Just a little. Did Alix Gregory come to see you?"

"Oh yes, that." Owen nodded. "The troublesome MP, the one who is in this room now. I'll handle it."

"Owen, she's probing too much. You know how the new intake MPs are; they believe in justice and championing the will of the people. It's not like the old days. I want her gone, she continues to criticise our business, and I hate to say it, but people are listening to her."

"She hasn't directly named the company, has she?"

"No, not yet, but I have a feeling it's coming."

"If she does that, she'll find herself in legal hot water anyway. I don't know much about her, but she's no fool. When she was elected, she won by a majority vote; that much I do know."

"Look, I know she has a meeting with the Chief Whip on Monday morning. I'm also aware of the close relationship you have with him. Make it happen."

Lord Gatesouth sighed. "I'll gladly call him tomorrow, old boy, but to my knowledge, she hasn't broken any parliamentary protocols."

"Not yet," Darius replied, "but I have a feeling she's about to."

Owen had a mischievous smile on his face. "What do you know?"

Darius patted Owen on the shoulder. "I always know my enemies, my friend."

"Ha!" Owen laughed heartily, quickly turning around to check if anyone was eavesdropping. "I don't doubt that. You wouldn't be where you are without your cunning. Look, I'll call the Chief Whip in the morning. I'll make sure he's prepared, and if she steps out of line, she'll be out of here. I'm sorry, old boy, but that's the best I can do."

Darius nodded. "Thank you. That will be enough." He then steered Lord Gatesouth back toward the bar, where William handed him a Scotch. "Well, cheers, gentlemen." They all raised their glasses.

"Right, I'm going to have a word with the 'death of beauty' MP," Darius announced.

Lord Hawthorne nearly choked on his drink and sputtered, "Good luck with that!"

Darius grinned, turned away from them, and called the waiter over. After taking a sip from his Scotch, he thanked the waiter for the champagne and scanned the room. Not seeing her anywhere, he called the waiter back. "Excuse me, have you seen anyone leave the room?"

"I've seen a few people leave, sir, mainly heading to the restrooms outside. Did you have a specific person in mind?" the waiter replied.

"Yes, it must have been within the last couple of minutes. Her name is Helen Lord; she's an MP," Darius said.

"Oh yes, sir, I know who you mean. I just saw her leave."

Darius nodded. "Thank you." He quickened his pace, aware of what she was planning to do the next day. However, he was also eager to understand why she was there, which hadn't been part of his original plan. With glasses in hand, Darius hurried out of the room. He noticed other people in the corridor, but Helen was not among them. He quickly moved down the hallway and pushed open the door to Norman Porch. To his surprise, he found that the door to the Robing Room was unlocked. The light was on, but no one was inside. Exiting through the door at the other end of the Robing Room led him into the Royal Gallery, where he spotted Helen up ahead as she made her way toward the Prince's Chamber.

"Excuse me, sir, are you lost?" a security officer called out after him.

Darius glanced back and replied, "No, I'm fine, thank you. I need to speak with her." He quickened his pace in an attempt to catch up with the member of parliament.

"Sir, I need to see your security pass," the officer insisted from behind.

Darius chose to ignore him, but he could hear the echo of footsteps following him. "Sir, please stop where you are," the officer urged.

Darius picked up his pace. He had been in the Royal Gallery many times before and knew it was one of the largest rooms in the palace. If he didn't catch up with Helen at the far end of the gallery, he would have to give up the chase. Transitioning from a speed walk to a light jog, the security officer called out from behind, determined not to give up. Fortunately, Helen had stopped and was standing next to the Pugin table in the centre of the room in the Prince's Chamber.

"Ah, Helen! There you are! You disappeared quickly," Darius said as he approached, holding a couple of glasses.

"Sir, I must insist that you stop immediately!"

Darius turned to the officer. "I'm very sorry about that. One of our honoured guests left without finishing her drink."

Helen took a couple of steps towards him. "I'm not your honoured guest."

"Ma'am, would you like me to escort this gentleman from the premises?"

Darius looked the officer up and down.

"I do not recognise you, sir. I do not believe you are a passholder, unless you can produce one for me now."

"Well, can you?" Helen challenged. "You seem to have access to this place whenever you want."

Darius bent down, placed the glasses on the floor, and pulled a lanyard from his pocket. "I have one of these," he stated confidently.

"Sir, that pass is meant to be worn visibly on your person. It's also a temporary pass, so you are not allowed to walk around the palace unattended."

Helen smiled. "Well, this puts you in a tricky situation, and the armed police are not far away."

"I've brought you a drink."

"Ma'am, would you like the gentleman escorted from the premises?"

Helen assessed Darius from head to toe. He was determined, but it was clear he did not have access here. "No, he's with me."

"Are you sure, ma'am?"

Helen nodded.

"Please remember to display your temporary pass in the future," the security officer said.

Darius acknowledged him, "But of course." He bent down to pick up the glasses as the security officer left the room. "Now that I'm your guest, you're welcome to join me for a drink. It's not as full as it was; I think I spilt some while trying to catch up with you."

Helen took the glass from him. "I hope you didn't spill it on the carpets; they are very expensive."

Darius shrugged. "Just on the gallery floor, I think."

"Hmm," Helen said, taking a sip from the glass.

"What were you doing when I entered this room? You were standing next to the table."

"I usually do," Helen replied. "It's my favourite room in the palace. If members of the Lords aren't sitting at this historic table, I often stop here to take stock."

"It is a beautiful room," Darius remarked, studying the impressive marble statue of Queen Victoria sitting on a throne, flanked by two figures he did not recognise.

Helen observed him as he took in the individual paintings that adorned all four walls. "There are twenty-eight of them."

Darius looked away from the artworks. "I'm sorry?"

"Twenty-eight. That's how many pictures are in this room. Each one is uniquely beautiful, depicting people who played significant roles in history. And now, you find yourself in their presence." She flashed a brief, fake smile. "What do you want?"

Darius grinned. "Straight to the point."

"Of course," she replied, sipping her champagne. "Your charms won't work on me, and, frankly, this champagne is dreadful."

He laughed heartily. "I couldn't agree more; that's why I have Scotch."

"Touché. Now, what do you want?"

"I'm curious about why you showed up at our little party this evening."

"I just happened to be in the building and noticed something was going on."

"If that were the case, you would know it was us. Your very presence suggests you're up to something."

"And why would you think that?"

"Are you recording this conversation?"

Helen smiled as she sipped the terrible champagne. "No. Why are you?"

"No. I guess we'll have to trust each other, won't we?"

"I think you misunderstand me, Mr Neith. I don't trust you in the slightest, and no amount of cheap champagne or your expensive suit will change that."

He nodded. "Okay, you've made your point. But why did you show up?"

"Because I think you're a crook. You buy your way into places, thinking you're untouchable. You believe you have power over people when all you really are is a drug peddler."

"Wow! That's quite an accusation. I'm fairly certain parliamentary privilege does not extend to this room, beautiful or not."

"Well, you said you're not recording this, so it's your word against mine. What do you have to fear?"

Darius put a hand in his pocket and sipped his Scotch. "I have nothing to fear."

"Really? Let me tell you, knowledge is power."

Darius laughed out loud. "That's a statement without foundation, made by the very foolish." He took another sip from his glass. "Knowledge isn't power. Money is power, as money buys people with knowledge, and everyone has their price."

Helen rolled her eyes. "Proud of that statement, are you?"

"I quite like it. So, what is your price, Helen?"

"Oh, please. You and your elite crowd, with your inherited wealth, surround yourselves with people who have titles. Neither of the Lords at your party was ever democratically elected; they assumed their titles through their gentry status, which is why they are so arrogant."

"While that may be true, things aren't done here the way they used to be."

Helen nodded. "And that's called progress."

"That's one way to put it."

"And what would you call it?"

"Adaptation. Just like how I run my company. We must evolve in a declining market. You and your friend have caused us a great deal of damage."

"Really? Well, it was never personal; you and your company are just one of many." She stepped into his personal space, refusing to be intimidated by him. "But you made it personal, didn't you?"

Darius shrugged. "I'm sure I don't know what you're talking about."

"What happened to the informant?"

"Oh wow, you're being quite direct. As I mentioned, I'm not aware of what you're insinuating."

"My friend is in the hospital!"

Darius lifted his hands in a gesture for calm. "You're raising your voice," he said. "That security guard won't be far away; let's avoid shouting at each other. There's always someone listening around here. Besides, I read about what happened; it's quite concerning."

"Concerning!"

"Yes, no one wants to see those things happen on these streets."

"And the only connection she had was to your company."

Darius frowned. "You're out of line. She had many enemies."

"That she did. However, she didn't have any evidence against others who were trying to distribute heroin in this country. She only had evidence that your company is attempting to do so."

Darius smirked. "No one would believe something so outrageous and…"

"I noticed you didn't deny it," Helen interrupted.

The smile faded from Darius's face. He swallowed the last of his Scotch and looked Helen directly in the eyes. "So, what are you going to do about it?"

Helen handed him the half-full champagne glass and adjusted the strap of her handbag on her shoulder. "In time, you will find out, very soon, in fact. You sicken me. Profits before people, that sums you up. You're a verminous cretin."

Darius broke into a fit of laughter, "Come now, of all the things I've been called, that's probably the least offensive. I'm an innovator, Helen."

"You're a murderer in the making, and I'm not through with

you. You are enemy number one, and I'm going to nail you to the wall."

Darius scanned the artworks above him. "Well, at least it's not a beheading or being hung, drawn, and quartered."

"We'll see," Helen said as she stepped to her right. "Security!"

Darius looked down, smiling.

The security officer entered the chamber quickly. "Yes, ma'am?"

"Please escort Mr Neith to where he needs to be. I'm done with him."

"Yes, ma'am."

Darius felt a hand on his shoulder as he finished Helen's champagne.

"Come this way, sir," the officer instructed.

Darius glanced back as he was escorted into the Royal Gallery. Helen was glaring at him. "Thank you for the cheap drink," she said before disappearing from view.

Chapter Twenty-Four

SUNDAY MORNING

Rubin yawned and walked into the front room. The makeshift bed for Andrea and Ryan looked untouched. "Did you get any sleep?" he asked Ryan.

"Not really. You may have been here for a few nights, but knowing a gun barrel is never far away makes it hard to relax," Ryan replied.

Rubin shrugged. "Well, after today, if you do as you're told, your difficulties will be over." He nodded as David walked into the room carrying a couple of mugs of tea. Rubin took one of the mugs and glanced at its contents, clearly displeased.

"We're out of milk," David said.

"That's hardly a surprise," Ryan responded as he rose to his feet, stretching his arms overhead. "We've been housebound for the last few days, and you won't let us out, so we're running low on everything."

"And, as I mentioned, today your problems will be over," Rubin reiterated.

"Yes, Alpha 2," Ryan replied, his tone patronising.

Rubin raised his eyebrows. "As soon as your wife is out of the shower, it's your turn. You need to be fresh and focused today."

"Look," Ryan raised his hands in frustration, "I don't know what's going on here. How many times do I have to tell you this has nothing to do with me? You come in here and threaten my wife and children! What kind of men are you?"

Rubin sighed, eager for this assignment to be over. "It's just a job, don't take it personally."

"A man who threatens children? You're a fucking coward!"

Rubin spilt some tea from his mug as he pulled his jacket across, revealing his firearm.

"Oh yes, go ahead and shoot me. You won't get your bloody lab test done then, will you?"

"That's enough!" David stepped between them. "We need calm heads here."

"You think I'm an idiot? You're not going to let us go."

Rubin reclosed his jacket. "You have nothing to fear."

Ryan looked away, nodding repeatedly as tears began to well up in his eyes. "I don't understand how you live with yourselves. What have we done to you?"

"Ryan, you need to stay calm. In just a few more hours, this will all be over. We'll leave, and you can return to your life with your family."

Rubin looked away, tired of playing the babysitter. He knew David's words were nothing but a blatant lie.

"You won't," Ryan said. "I've seen films and read books. We've all seen your faces. If I say, 'I promise we won't tell anyone,' you're not going to believe that, even if we are being truthful."

"You'll just have to believe us," David added.

"Well, I might consider believing you, but I'm not leaving him, scarface over there alone with my family while I'm with you. What are you going to do to my children? What are you going to do to my wife? Are you going to wave your weapon around to feel powerful because of your underdeveloped endowments?"

Rubin's mug of tea fell from his hand as he threw back his jacket and reached for his handgun.

"Come here, you little shit!" he yelled, aiming the firearm at Ryan's head.

"That's enough!" David shouted, grappling with Rubin to ensure the weapon was pointed at the ceiling.

"What's going on!" The words were screamed at them from behind. They all froze in an instant. Andrea stood there in a dressing gown, her hair wrapped in a towel. Both children were at her side, looking highly distressed as Annabelle began to cry.

David glared at Rubin, urging him to stay calm as he instructed him to put the weapon away.

Ryan suddenly dove out from behind the two mercenaries and grabbed Annabelle, lifting her in an attempt to comfort her. "It's okay; we're just playing a game. Please don't cry," he said gently.

David continued to glare at Rubin. "Look, we're all exhausted, but we must remain calm," he insisted.

Rubin tucked the weapon back behind his jacket and took a deep breath as he eyed the lab tech.

"I'll do what you ask," Ryan said, taking Andrea's hand. They exchanged glances, silently agreeing, "We need to bring this to an end."

Rubin scowled as he looked the terrified man up and down. The man was justified in being scared, and his words were accurate. They would never let them go, and Rubin decided he would make sure of that personally.

++++

Reflecting on the previous evening and the day ahead, Helen had a restless night. Today was the day her name would make headlines, and it was also about vindicating Alison's campaign. Once the truth was exposed, the police would be forced to investigate Knightark Pharmaceutical. Helen hoped to deliver a significant blow against them, which could also assist the police in their efforts to find the perpetrators behind the assassination attempt. She recalled her encounter only a few hours earlier with Darius, the smug, privately educated and self-entitled man. No amount of tailor-made suits could save him now. Although her stomach was grumbling, she couldn't bring herself to eat breakfast. Instead, she asked for a fresh pot of coffee to be delivered to her room. As she glanced at her watch, she realised it was nearly 8 a.m. She needed to ensure the room was as clean as possible, without any signs that could be caught on film revealing her whereabouts.

The fridge, located beneath the kettle, held a selection of alcoholic drinks, fruit juices, and chocolates, none of which were complimentary. Today, however, there were also three vials placed next to the vodka miniatures. She picked one up, acutely aware of the power it represented. The vials had been out of cold storage for several days; she had read they should be kept in a cool environment. Rightly or wrongly, she had placed them in the fridge the night before. After examining the vial, she returned it to its place, closed the fridge door, and went to the bedside table for her phone. No messages were waiting for her. She rechecked her watch. Knowing that the lab technician would be driving from Kent, she estimated he could arrive in about forty minutes, barring any severe delays. However, she was aware that London traffic could be unpredictable. She guessed he would be leaving home between 9:00 and 9:30. The temptation to message him was strong, but it was still early. She decided to wait a little longer, and if she hadn't heard from him by then, she would follow up to ensure he was on his way.

++++

Alison Harwood had been moved out of the high-dependency unit. Although this update hadn't made the front pages, it was featured in several Sunday newspapers. Darius searched for more information on the police investigation. There were mentions of it, but no specific details were provided, and terrorist activity had not been ruled out. Due to a lack of leads, a press statement from Counter Terrorism Command indicated that the current terrorist threat level remains severe, with no changes expected. That was all Darius needed to know. He tossed the newspaper onto the pile on his breakfast table. Everything was in hand and going according to plan. He then picked up his phone and called William. An early riser, William would surely not miss the incredible breakfast at the hotel where he was staying.

The call was answered quickly. "Good morning."

"And how is your head today?" Darius asked.

A brief laugh came from the other end of the phone. "Nothing that one of your Brit breakfasts can't fix."

"I thought Americans hated British food?" Darius asked.

"Not this one. These breakfasts are one of the only reasons I come here," he laughed.

Darius could hear a lot of noise in the background; William must be in one of the restaurants. "Can you talk?" he inquired.

"Kinda. What's on your mind, Darius?"

"Everything is on track. Do you have any plans for today?"

"Not really. I was going to tune in to a certain YouTube channel later, but other than that… not much."

"Great! Do you want to come over to my place? I'll arrange for some drinks to be delivered, and I can also invite Hugh. Ronald has other business to attend to today."

"Sure, I don't see why not. It would be good to stay updated on everything firsthand."

"My thoughts exactly. The broadcast is at 11. Can you be here before then?"

"I don't see why not. I just need to arrange transportation."

"Okay, you know where to come. If there are any issues, I'll send a driver for you."

"Thank you, Darius. I'll be in touch. If all goes well, I should be with you in just over an hour. Oh, excuse me for a moment…"

Darius pulled the phone away from his ear with a frown.

"Could I order some more sausages, please?"

Darius rolled his eyes.

"I tell you, my friend, there are no sausages like these back home."

Darius nodded. "So, I'll see you in an hour then?"

"You will."

Darius hung up the phone and began tapping his fingers on the breakfast table. "Paul!"

His butler stepped into the room. "Yes, Sir?"

"I have a couple of guests coming over. Could you prepare the drawing room please? Also, put some bottles in the fridge and check that the ice machine is full."

"Yes, Sir. I will do that now."

"Thank you. Once you're done, you can take the rest of the day off."

"Sir?"

"I can manage perfectly well on my own. I'll leave some cash on the side for you. Enjoy your day off."

The butler smiled. "Thank you, Sir. That is most kind."

Darius nodded and smiled back at Paul. The butler had only been in his employ for about a year, and Darius wanted him out of the way for now. He texted Hugh to invite him over. Satisfied that everything was in place, he picked up one of the Sunday papers again.

✢✢✢✢

"It's a nice day. Would you both like to go play in the garden?" David asked. The two girls smiled and quickly ran to the back door. Andrea got up from the couch to let them out. "Join them if you'd like," he added. Without saying a word, Andrea stepped through the back door into the garden.

"I'm going for a shower," Rubin said as he disappeared from the room.

"Your friend is uncontrollable," Ryan remarked.

"He's fine. It's just been a long few days for all of us."

"Longer for us than for you," Ryan quipped.

David ignored Ryan's comment as he took Ryan's phone from his pocket. "There's been no communication from the MP so far; I suspect it's only a matter of time. She's dependent on you."

Ryan scratched his head in confusion. "I still don't understand what's going on. The test I conducted revealed serious irregularities. I don't know who your client is, and I don't want to. I also don't want to be involved in whatever we've somehow gotten ourselves into. However, you must see that this makes no sense. She wants to do a live broadcast, and I'll reveal the same information. If that's the case, it would be illegal. I'm completely confused, and if you're honest, so are you!"

"I follow orders, and you must do the same. There's nothing you can do to change that; you have to accept it."

"Oh, right. I just need to accept it. But what if the test shows something completely different? What happens then?"

"All I know is that this needs to be done."

Ryan shook his head. "I wonder what the price of your conscience is in all of this?"

"That needn't concern you."

"Well, when you're sipping cocktails on whatever beach you choose, I hope you can live with yourself for what you've done to us."

David heard movements upstairs and stood up. "Go join your family. We'll be moving soon."

As Ryan stood up, David placed a hand on his shoulder. "Don't try to run. Your neighbour's wall is too high, and the gate at the end of the garden is locked. Don't force my hand."

Ryan swallowed, nodded, and walked into the garden while David went upstairs. Rubin was standing on the landing, wrapped in a towel. David signalled for Rubin to join him in the back bedroom so they could keep an eye on the garden below. It was the first time David had seen Rubin without his shirt on; his torso was covered with numerous scars and poorly drawn tattoos. The ink patterns were unclear, as the ink had bled into his skin. "I've got to say, your tattoos are dog shit," David laughed.

"Listen to me, brother. These markings are earned."

David examined Rubin's back and arms. "They look a mess to me." He pulled the net curtain to the side to keep an eye on the family. Andrea noticed him immediately and looked away.

"You know nothing, and you have no right to comment on my symbology."

"Symbology? They look like line drawings done by a three-year-old; most of them have run," David laughed.

"My brothers in faith drew them for me at the temple. I had to earn them. They are traditional symbols carved into my skin. My markings are sacred."

David raised an eyebrow. "Whatever they are, they look like a bloody mess."

"Religion is not a beauty contest. These marks were etched into my body over several days as I sought peace."

"That doesn't sound peaceful to me."

"It's nothing compared to the pain I've caused others." David looked directly into Rubin's eyes, revealing, for the first time, a glimpse of remorse for his past actions. Rubin quickly averted his gaze and left the room to fetch his clothes.

David's attention was drawn to the girls who were giggling as they played on the trampoline. Ryan, the devoted father, turned to look directly at David.

Rubin returned to the room, dropped his towel, and began to change. "It's almost time for you to go," he said.

David nodded, keeping his attention on Ryan. "The car is loaded, and as long as nothing unexpected happens, we should arrive with plenty of time to spare."

"You need to communicate with me regularly. Any mistakes, and I'll have to take care of the family and leave."

Below, Ryan turned to take Andrea's hand.

"I understand. We need to exchange weapons now. Can you run one more test on the body camera?"

"I will, just before you leave. Now, listen carefully."

David turned away from the window.

"I'm putting a lot of trust in you. My life is in your hands. Don't fuck this up!"

"If things go south, you'll be the first to know. I need the bag with the static camera and your disguises." David felt a vibration in his pocket, pulled out Ryan's phone, and entered his PIN code. "It's the MP asking if we are on the way."

"How are you going to respond?"

David typed out a message and held the phone up for Rubin to read. "I'm telling her we are leaving now."

Rubin nodded, "Then go. I want this day to be over with."

++++

Helen took a deep breath of satisfaction as she read the text message. Ryan Dobey, the lab technician, was on his way. With the two people from production also confirming their arrival within the hour, everything was in place. She sat on the edge of the bed, knowing it was going to be a long hour's wait.

++++

"It's time." David stood at the back doors of the house and signalled for Rubin to come over. They exchanged weapons. "Do you have the silencer too?" Rubin nodded and handed it to him. "If everything falls apart, I'll contact you immediately."

"Make sure that you do," Rubin replied.

David watched as Ryan wrapped his arms around both of his daughters. "If you need to make a quick exit, take my car. And don't forget the piss bottles and shit bags in the garden."

"I won't forget," Rubin assured him.

"Bleach the shower and remove any towels we used."

"Will do."

"When you're clear, dispose of your phone and wipe all the data on it. I'll contact you through the usual portal if necessary."

"David, I didn't survive in this game for all these years without knowing what to do. However this plays out, good or bad, I'll be off-grid for a while. That is, of course, after you pay me."

David tapped his temple.

"What is it?"

"I've left something upstairs; get them from the garden."

"Pass me Ryan's phone. I want to run a final check on the key fob camera."

David handed Ryan's phone to Rubin and then sprinted up the stairs. He could hear Rubin calling the family in from the garden. Upon entering Annabelle's room, David knelt and reached under the bed. He retrieved an envelope, placed it in his pocket, and then grabbed a small bundle of euros before heading back downstairs.

At the bottom of the stairs, Rubin ushered him over and whispered in his ear, "Remember, you'll experience a brief blackout with the bodycam until the laptop is switched on. I've removed my password, and you'll see the file titled 'camera'; it's as simple as that. I've put the laptop in the backpack."

David nodded and picked up Rubin's backpack from the couch. He walked over to the hallway mirror. Applying the stick-on moustache was easy, but the male wig, which reached down to his shoulders, was uncomfortable and needed some adjustment. As he positioned the wig on his head, he noticed Rubin passing him a cap in the mirror. David then added a pair of fake glasses with neutral lenses. "God, I look ridiculous," he said.

"You look like a tree hugger," Rubin replied, "and don't use the Lord's name in vain."

David frowned at Rubin in the mirror. Laughter came from behind him, and Sophie pointed at him.

"You look silly!" Annabelle said, peeking out from behind her mother's legs.

"Alpha 1 is trying to disguise himself," Andrea said, her tone thick with disdain.

"He still looks silly," Annabelle repeated.

Rubin stepped closer to Ryan. "Have you said your goodbyes?"

Ryan nodded but then walked over to his wife and hugged her. "It'll be okay," he said, trying to comfort her. Andrea had been strong throughout this ordeal, but the embrace made her eyes fill with tears.

"Ryan, please. Come with me," David urged, gesturing toward the front door. "I'll keep in touch," he said to Rubin. "Here, take these." He handed Rubin Andrea's phone and the keys to his car. "I have my phone and Ryan's. Call me on his number only for emergencies or if you don't hear from me."

Rubin nodded. "Will do."

"Here, catch!" David said, throwing Ryan's car keys toward him.

Ryan's hands shook as he reached out to catch the keys.

"You're driving. Alpha 2, is the road clear outside?"

Rubin peered through a gap in the curtains and nodded.

David took one last look at his colleague and the family before ushering Ryan through the front door. Ryan pressed the remote to unlock the car doors, and they both climbed in.

"Lock us in, Ryan."

"The car automatically locks as we start to move."

Ryan's face was pale, his eyes red, and his hands continued to tremble.

"Listen to me," David said firmly. "You're no good to anyone in that state. You need to get a grip. In about an hour, this will all be over. Focus on that."

Ryan nodded repeatedly, brushing a tear from his eye.

Head towards London. Drive slightly over the speed limit, but never at or below it. Understand? We don't want to attract attention.

Ryan started the car as David pulled down the sunshade and glanced back. Leaving Rubin alone with the family concerned him. He was sceptical about Rubin's religious beliefs; something felt off, and he worried that Rubin might lose control.

David took a deep breath and gave Ryan's shoulder a tap. "Let's go."

++++

David glanced at the satnav on his phone; they were about twenty minutes from their destination. So far, they had been fortunate with traffic and should arrive on schedule. He hadn't exchanged a word with Ryan during the journey. For the first ten minutes, David kept a vigilant eye on the driver, but as the trip continued, Ryan seemed to compose himself and accept his situation. At every junction, crossroads, and set of traffic lights, David bowed his head. Cameras were everywhere in the city, and the risk of being caught was one he didn't enjoy taking. He looked over at Ryan, who had earlier gripped the steering wheel so tightly that his knuckles had turned white.

"You've changed," David remarked.

"What?" Ryan responded.

"You've adapted. It was courageous of you to stand up to Alpha 2 earlier. Quite commendable."

"Great, so now you hold me in awe, do you?"

"I wouldn't put it that way, but you did show courage." David looked out the window at the thousands of people going about their daily lives. At that moment, he wished he could be with them and anywhere but here.

"And what would you do if it were your family?" Ryan shot back. "You're nothing more than a pair of thugs. Point a gun at someone, and they'll do what you tell them."

"Well, that's just how the world works. You can't blame us for that."

"I can blame you for bringing that lunatic into my house!" Ryan retorted, his voice filled with anger.

He examined Ryan closely and noticed that his hands had started to shake again as he gripped the steering wheel tightly.

"You have no control over him."

"Alpha 2 works for me, and that's all you need to know."

"You say he works for you, but I don't see it that way. He's uncontrollable and unhinged."

"Alpha 2 has been through a lot in his life. A lab rat like you wouldn't understand. You've never been in the field; you've never had to survive in hostile environments where everything and everyone is against you. It's wrong for you to judge him, and who do you think you are to try?"

"I judge as I see, and since you don't know anything about me, it's you who is wrong to judge!" David smiled as he looked out the window. "Rubin and I have a job to do, and..." Suddenly, he froze and closed his eyes in anger for having mentioned Rubin's name.

Ryan, realising he wasn't meant to hear that name, began to panic. He lifted his hands off the steering wheel, "I never heard that! I never heard that!"

"Didn't you?" David grabbed Ryan's arm, "Tell me what his name is!"

"I didn't hear anything, I swear!" Ryan's panic intensified.

"Then what is it!" David yelled and grabbed the back of Ryan's neck.

"Um, it's..." Ryan stammered.

In that moment, David pulled his jacket aside, revealing his handgun.

"Alpha! It's Alpha, Alpha 2!" Ryan exclaimed desperately.

David buried his head in his hands, unable to believe his own stupidity. "God damn it!" he shouted, punching the car's dashboard. Taking a deep breath, he raised his hands in a calming gesture. "Just follow the road; we're not far from the hotel."

"I don't know what to say to you. I promise, I didn't hear his name."

"Then say nothing," David snapped, drawing a deep breath and pointing at Ryan's face. "Listen to me very carefully: you need to forget that name. I told you that you would make it through this. If he finds out you know his real name, that's it for you and your family. It only takes one press of this phone to make it happen!"

"Honestly, I heard nothing. Please believe me."

"You must never repeat it – never! Alpha 2 would have no hesitation in wiping you all out." David noticed how alarmed Ryan had become. "Listen, here's what's going to happen. When we arrive at the hotel, you will pull up to the entrance. Before you get out of the car, put on the jacket that's on the back seat. There's a camera hidden inside it; I will be watching your every move. You will head straight to the reception. If there is a concierge or doorman at the front, ignore them. You will carry your own bags, even if they insist on helping you. At reception, you'll check in using the reservation on your phone. I will give you your phone so you can confirm the booking. Do not attempt to call anyone or send messages; I will be watching you. Once you have your room key, you will see three elevators to your left. Press the buttons to call all three elevators at once. Hopefully, when I go in, I won't have to wait around in the lobby. I will head straight to the room. Do you understand?"

"Yes, but will I have the room key?"

"No, you won't. After you call the lifts, return to the car, hand me the key and your phone, and then unload your equipment. By the time you finish that, I'll already be in the room. The room is front-facing, and I'll be watching you from one of the windows above. You'll take the gear to reception, leave it there, and then return outside to move the car to the parking area located around the corner. Once you've done that, return, gather your gear, and go to the room."

"Your room?"

"Not my room, pay attention, the MP's room! I'll be watching you on-screen, and a secondary camera will monitor the corridor. My room is only two doors down from where you will conduct the test. If you communicate with the MP or the two people from production…"

"What are their names?"

"I don't know, and I don't care. Don't interrupt me; focus on what I'm saying. If I think you are trying to send hidden messages to anyone else, the room door will come off its hinges, and I'll kill all of you. Don't think for a second that I'm any softer than Alpha 2. But I'll tell you this: if things go wrong, he'll be the next person I speak to, and you know what that means."

Ryan took a deep breath and nodded.

"Oh, and this is for you as well," David said, pulling an envelope from his pocket and taking the jacket from the back seat. "I've placed the envelope in the jacket pocket. You need to read the instructions before entering the room, as they are written on the front. Do you understand?"

"Yes," Ryan swallowed nervously. "I think so."

"Also, you'll need to carry this," David continued. "I'm going to put it in the pocket along with the envelope."

Ryan glanced over, "What is it? A car key?"

"Sort of. It's a fake key, but it contains a hidden camera. You need to place this key on the table where you'll be working, but look, see this?" David held up the key fob.

"Yes," Ryan replied.

"This is the camera end. Position it on the table with the camera facing away from you. That way, I can see everything in the room and ensure you don't try to communicate without my noticing,"

Ryan took a deep breath.

"If you stay calm, you're going to get through this. If you don't, that hotel room will be the last thing you ever see."

Chapter Twenty-Five

"I feel privileged to have you open the front door for me, Darius," William said.

Darius smiled. "I gave Paul the day off. Come on in, my friend." He looked William up and down, noticing that he looked well-fed. "I see you had the extra sausages then."

William laughed as he stepped into Darius's house. "Is Hugh here?"

"Not yet, but he won't be far away." Darius closed the door and glanced at the security monitor mounted on the wall. "Please, come through. Would you like something to drink?"

William shook his head. "It's a bit too early for me. So, where are we at?" He followed Darius into the drawing room, where a large wall-mounted television displayed the YouTube home page, with the volume muted.

"Please, take a seat. According to the trackers, the consignment arrived in the UK about an hour ago, and we're just waiting to hear about customs clearance."

"Good. What about the MP?"

"I received a message from our asset a few minutes ago; they should be arriving at the hotel any time now."

"What do you think will happen with the live broadcast?"

"To be honest, my friend, I'm not sure. We'll have to adapt to the events as they unfold."

William sat down, took a deep breath, crossed his legs, and looked at the TV screen. "I'm confident we can manage that."

"Of course we can." The intercom on the main desk buzzed. "Good, Hugh has just arrived. As you can see, my friend, everything is going according to plan."

++++

David sent update messages to Darius and Rubin, informing them that the hotel was only a couple of roads away. "How are you feeling?" he asked.

Ryan found the question difficult to comprehend. He was still getting used to seeing David with a moustache and long hair. "Is that a serious question? I'm bloody terrified!"

"Okay, let's set that aside since we're about to arrive. Do you know exactly what you need to do?"

Ryan nodded. "I think so, yes. It's just..."

"Just what?"

"I'm worried something will go wrong."

"It will only go wrong if you let it," David reassured him. "It's the next left, and turning left again will take us right in front of the hotel."

Ryan switched on the car's indicator as David took Ryan's phone out of his pocket. Ryan took the left turn but nearly drove past the hotel, slamming on the brakes as they were jolted forward.

"Jesus! Take it easy."

"I'm sorry, alright? I'm just nervous. I didn't see the hotel's turn until it was too late."

"We're not supposed to draw attention. Stay focused!"

The car slowly approached the hotel's front.

"How close do you want me to get?"

"What? Get as close as anyone else would. You're just dropping off baggage; stop panicking."

"There's a doorman ahead," Ryan pointed out.

"Remember what I said: politely say no and head to the reception."

Ryan parked the car.

David stared at Ryan. "Well, are you just going to sit there?"

"Erm, right, yes. Should I switch off the engine?"

David handed him the phone. "No, leave it running, just in case it doesn't start again."

"This car has always started."

"Don't tempt fate. Now, open your phone's email app and you'll find the booking confirmation for the room. Move quickly; get out of the car, the doorman is approaching, and I don't want him to see me too closely." He handed the jacket to Ryan. "Put this on. I will be watching."

Ryan nodded, his nerves evident as he stepped out of the car, awkwardly putting on the jacket.

David raised a hand to his face and rubbed his temporary moustache; this pretend grooming provided some facial cover. He kept a close eye on Ryan as he engaged in a brief conversation with the doorman. Whatever Ryan said must have been satisfactory; the doorman paid David no attention and started heading back to the front of the hotel. Ryan then ascended the short flight of steps and disappeared from view. David took a deep breath and patted himself down to ensure the firearm was precisely where he needed it. This was the grey period, and he hoped Ryan hadn't figured things out. The jacket camera would be on, but until the program on the laptop was opened, David couldn't hear or see anything. He checked that his gloves were in one of the jacket pockets. In this heat, wearing gloves may attract unnecessary attention, so he would put them on when he got into the elevator. Although there was likely a camera in the elevator, he assumed that security didn't monitor it closely unless necessary. From his position, he couldn't see the reception area; everything seemed to depend on fear and whether Ryan would follow instructions. David tapped his fingers on his thighs as he waited. Outside, there were no obvious security guards; only one doorman was present. He kept his head lowered behind the sun visor, knowing that if anything went wrong, he would immediately read it in the doorman's actions. For now, the doorman nodded and smiled at guests as they entered and exited the hotel. "Come on, come on," David mouthed silently, feeling that too much time had passed. His finger-tapping quickened as he began to consider that he might have to go inside.

David's fingers stopped tapping when he saw Ryan finally appear at the top of the steps. He watched closely to ensure that Ryan didn't say anything to the doorman as he approached the car. Ryan got in and handed David the hotel key.

"What took you so long? You were ages!"

Irritated, Ryan frowned and replied, "There was a queue. I thought you said you could see everything."

"Don't be cocky. Give me the phone."

Ryan let out a brief sigh before passing the phone back to David.

"Right, I'm going to grab my backpack. You unload the gear and take it into reception, then move the car before a parking warden notices it," David instructed, pointing at Ryan. "You remember where the car park is?"

"Yes, I've saved it in my memory," Ryan confirmed.

"Good. Don't mess this up!" David said as he exited the car, opened the rear door, and grabbed the backpack. Slinging it over his shoulder, he leaned back inside the vehicle and added, "And don't forget to read the envelope."

"Why is there a poppy badge on this jacket?" Ryan asked.

"What?"

"Well, it's not that time of year, is it?"

"Listen to me dickface. Service people should be supported all year round, not just once a year."

"It's just that it might attract attention."

David narrowed his eyes. "That's the point; it's a decoy."

"I don't understand."

"Oh, for God's sake. It's a decoy! The enamel badge is bright red, right?"

Ryan nodded.

"So, human eyes will be drawn to the badge, not to the hidden camera on the other lapel. Do you get it? Now stop stalling and do your job!"

Ryan swallowed nervously as David closed the car door and walked toward the hotel steps. David nodded slightly at the doorman but avoided making direct eye contact. With the room's passkey in hand, he bypassed the reception desk and headed straight for the elevators. As he approached, he noticed a couple entering one of the lifts and slowed down, not wanting to join them. When their lift door closed, the next lift to the right was already open. So far, the lab technician had carried out his instructions. With his head bowed, David stepped into the elevator, stretched the cuff of his jacket over his index finger to avoid leaving a fingerprint, and pressed the button for the second floor. As the lift ascended, he placed his backpack on the floor, put on his gloves, and waited for his floor to arrive. The elevator's automatic voice announced, "Second floor." When the doors opened, a woman stood waiting to enter. She smiled and asked, "Am I getting in, or are you coming out?"

David's heart skipped a beat when he realised it was Helen Lord, the MP. He pushed past her and immediately turned left, quickly heading down the corridor. Behind his fake glasses, David squeezed his eyes shut in annoyance; what the hell was she doing there? He reached the room as quickly as possible, hearing the lift doors close just behind him. He tapped the keycard over the sensor, glanced over his shoulder, and let himself into the room.

Helen frowned at the rudeness of the man who had pushed past her; he didn't turn around or apologise for making contact with her. As she stepped into the lift, she shook her head at the behaviour of some people. She noticed that he was wearing gloves. Gloves at this time of year? It was unusual. Perhaps he had a skin condition, she thought, brushing down her blouse as she pressed the button for the ground floor. When the lift doors opened, she quickly made her way to the front of the hotel. She was pleased to see Ryan unloading his equipment. Acknowledging the doorman, she moved briskly down the steps. "Ryan, I'm so glad you could make it! You're early!"

He froze the moment he saw her, looking deathly pale.

"Are you okay? You look as white as a sheet."

"Um, yes," he replied.

Helen noticed that he kept glancing up at the hotel's façade.

"What's the matter?" she asked, moving closer to follow his line of sight. He seemed to be studying the rooms above. Helen spotted a curtain twitch, but nothing else of note.

"Oh, it's nothing. I've just never been here before. It's an impressive building," he replied.

"It is. My room is just above," she said. "I saw you unloading and thought I'd come down to give you a hand."

Ryan's eyes immediately widened, and his pulse quickened. He stopped unloading the equipment and began to tremble. He knew that if she had seen Alpha 1 with him, it could spell disaster, and he could burst down here and lose control at any moment.

"Ryan, are you sure you're okay?" she asked, noticing him glance up at the building again.

"Um, yes, I'm fine. Thank you. If you could help me take my gear to reception, that would be appreciated," he stammered.

Helen nodded, sensing that something wasn't right with him, but it didn't matter; he was here, and that was what mattered most. "What are you going to do with your car? I don't think you can leave it out front."

"There's a car park around the side. As soon as I unload my gear, I'll move it."

Helen nodded sceptically. "Okay." Although she didn't know him well, he seemed frightened about something.

"Would you like help with that, ma'am?" the doorman asked as he approached her.

"Yes, possibly. Let me check. Ryan, how much more stuff do you have?"

Ryan unloaded a couple of cases from the car's boot. "That's about it."

"Let me go get a trolley for you. What room are you in, ma'am? I'll take everything up for you."

"Thank you. That's very helpful. I'm in room 216."

"Not a problem. I'll be back in just a moment."

Helen smiled at the doorman as he walked back up the steps. "That will save a bit of legwork. I'll go with him; don't forget, Ryan, room 216. I'll meet you up there."

Ryan nodded. "I'll go park the car."

As Ryan got into the car, Helen noticed him looking up again. She waited at the base of the steps and watched as he drove off. His behaviour was unsettling, and he didn't look well. Helen walked to where he had parked and glanced up at the rooms above. There was nothing out of the ordinary, but she could tell something was troubling him.

++++

David closed the hotel room door, quickly dropped his backpack and key card onto the bed, and went straight to the window. Pulling the curtains slightly to the side, he had a perfect view of Ryan unloading the car below. With little time to prepare, David knew he needed to act quickly. Remembering he had held the plastic room key card just before putting on his gloves, he quickly grabbed it from the bed, rubbed it briskly against his clothing to remove any fingerprints, and placed it on the sideboard next to the door. He then took Rubin's firearm from underneath his jacket and walked back to the window. The MP was now outside the building, talking to Ryan as he unloaded the car. Even from here, David could see how uncomfortable Ryan looked, constantly glancing up at the windows. David attached the silencer to the gun, set it aside, and quickly retrieved the laptop from his backpack. As the computer powered on, he navigated the desktop and selected the "camera" file. After one more click, an image appeared on the screen. The body-worn camera provided him with a clear view of the MP in conversation, and soon the doorman joined them. Turning up the volume, he heard the doorman offer to assist with their bags. However, something immediately caught his attention. The MP turned around and appeared to be looking up at the bedroom windows at the front of the hotel. She was also asking Ryan questions about his health. Their lives depended on Ryan staying composed. If the MP suspected that someone had got to him, David would have no choice but to intervene. Keeping an eye on the screen, David entered the passcode on Ryan's phone and opened the app that Rubin had installed. The camera and microphone were both operational, but the phone screen remained dark, displaying no images. He could only hear occasional indistinct words and sounds, as if the microphone was being rubbed against something. The camera concealed in the key fob was still in Ryan's jacket pocket, but at least it was functioning. He lowered the volume on the audio and plugged the phone's charger into the wall. For now, he would use Ryan's data; if any data warnings appeared, he would switch to the hotel's Wi-Fi.

From the body-worn camera footage, David could see that Ryan had returned to the car. He needed to set up the last camera, as the MP would be back in the corridor within minutes. A glance through the peephole in the door revealed that no one was standing directly outside. The small wireless dome camera that Rubin had given him had self-adhesive strips on its underside, allowing him to attach it quickly to the wall on the other side of the door. Although he hadn't seen it, he assumed there was a hotel camera monitoring the corridor, so he would do this as quickly as possible. David snatched the door open and glanced outside; the corridor was empty. He quickly affixed the camera to the side wall and closed the door again. Grabbing the power lead for his phone, he connected it and opened the camera app, gaining a visual feed of the corridor. After confirming that all three cameras were functioning, he felt satisfied. He then took off his glasses, the fake moustache, and removed the uncomfortable wig and cap. Setting the makeshift disguises beside the keycard, he ran his fingers through his hair as he dragged a chair in front of his new operations centre. He made sure the firearm was within reach and took a deep breath. Ryan was in the car, and all David could see was the dashboard. It was a tense moment; Ryan could easily make a run for it and drive away. David understood this, knowing he might consider the same option if he were in Ryan's position, but the difference was that Ryan had a family to worry about. David tapped his gloved fingers on the desk, his eyes focused on the images from the pinhole camera. It was now a waiting game; if Ryan were going to make a move, it would happen soon. For the first time, the operation was out of David's control and, for a brief moment, it was now in Ryan's hands.

++++

"I wish you hadn't signed us up for this!"

"She's already paid; what can I say?"

Yvette crossed her arms, clearly displeased. As the sound technician for today's broadcast, she felt frustrated. "It's Sunday morning! I had to cut last night short because of you, and I was having a good time."

"I figured you'd been out; you're in a bad mood, are you hungover?"

Yvette looked out of the taxi window and shook her head.

"We're almost at the hotel. Are you staying long?" the taxi driver asked.

"Oh, no. We're just a small camera crew working for a couple of hours," Matt replied. He was in charge of filming the party political broadcast.

"I see camera crews all the time in this city. You don't seem to have much equipment with you," the driver observed.

"It's all compact these days, not like it was years ago," Matt answered.

"Oh, right. Are you filming anyone famous?"

"She'd like to think she is," Yvette snarled as she continued to watch the passersby.

The taxi driver raised his eyebrows, signalling that their brief conversation was coming to an end.

"Interviewing an MP on a Sunday? How tedious," she remarked.

"Wow, this is exceptional whinging, even for you!"

Yvette flashed a patronising smile at her co-worker.

"It shouldn't take too long. She's interviewing a scientist, and we'll be done in an hour. It's a live broadcast, so no editing, it's a breeze."

Despite Matt's reassurances, Yvette remained displeased to be there, and nothing would change her mind.

"Right. Here we are," the taxi driver announced as he pulled up in front of the hotel. "Do you need a hand with your things?"

"No, we're fine, thank you," Matt replied, taking a couple of notes out of his jeans pocket. "Here you go; keep the change."

"Thank you very much! I see the doorman is on his way over," their driver laughed. "He always is. He's been here for years, always looking for tips."

"Well, we won't need him, and I've just given my tip for the day," Matt replied.

The driver laughed as Matt stepped out of the black taxi. "Here, pass me the tripod, will you?" Yvette handed it over, along with a couple of collapsible lighting stands. Matt then grabbed his camera bag.

"Do you need a hand, sir?" the doorman asked.

Matt smiled and replied, "No, we only have a few things. Thank you."

Yvette exited the cab, carrying a bag of remote microphones over her shoulder.

"Well, have fun, you two!" the taxi driver said, casting a sideways glance at Matt and rolling his eyes, implying that Matt might have a challenging day with Yvette.

Matt smiled as the doorman closed the taxi door behind them. "Do you know where you're going, sir?" the doorman asked.

"Yes, to the second floor," Matt responded.

"Very well. The elevators and stairs are to the left of the reception area. You won't miss them."

Matt nodded in thanks to the doorman, noticing that he lingered a bit longer than necessary. However, as he had already mentioned to the taxi driver, he had given his tip for the day.

Yvette caught up with him as they walked up the stairs into the hotel. "An hour at most. You'll see," he said to the disgruntled sound engineer.

++++

David stood at the bedroom window, hidden behind a curtain, with his firearm tightly gripped in his right hand. He had noticed a taxi pull up outside, from which a man and a woman emerged. The man was carrying a tripod and other equipment, likely indicating they were the camera crew the member of parliament had been expecting. With no way to contact Ryan, David felt uneasy. He maintained a careful watch at the front while also monitoring the laptop from behind the curtains. The lab technician had been sitting in the car for some time, and from the pinhole camera's view, David could see that the car had stopped moving. He was reasonably sure he was at the car park, but the length of the delay suggested that Ryan was weighing his options. "Come on, man, don't mess this up," David murmured to himself. He was in a dilemma; if Ryan didn't move soon, David would have to leave the hotel and confront him in public in the car park. If Ryan decided to drive away or make a run for it, David would be forced to call Rubin; if he did that, the family would be killed, Rubin would disappear, and to complicate matters, David had no means of transportation. Throughout his years working in the private sector, this was one moment where he had little control. "Come on, Ryan!" he muttered as he rubbed his lips. David returned to the cameras and set the gun down. He knew Ryan couldn't contact anyone and had made no attempt to disconnect the camera he was wearing. David glanced at the wig, knowing that if Ryan didn't act quickly, the operation would end before it even began. He began tapping his gloved fingers on the desk, hitting the surface harder with each tap. "Come on!" he urged. Suddenly, he stopped as Ryan moved and stepped out of the car. Ryan's action of locking the car door after exiting revealed something about his psychological state; he appeared to be in control. "So, where are you heading, lab rat?" David sighed with relief as he watched Ryan struggling to pay the parking meter with coins. After placing the payment receipt on the car's dashboard and relocking the vehicle, Ryan soon emerged at the top of the road, facing the hotel.

He was doing as instructed. David nodded, satisfied that everything was proceeding as planned. He glanced at Ryan's phone as it rang, noticing the MP trying to reach him. There was no turning back now.

Chapter Twenty-Six

The dresser in the hotel room would have to suffice as Ryan's makeshift laboratory table. The doorman helped Helen move it to the centre of the room. After tipping him for his assistance, he did not ask any questions and neatly arranged Ryan's equipment and bags on the bed. For the moment, that was the least of her concerns. Given that the car park was just around the corner, Ryan had been gone unusually long. As she stood by the window, feeling restless, she kept checking her watch. Perhaps the car park was full; she hadn't considered that possibility. It would be best to check. Helen picked up her phone and called him, but the call went unanswered. Running a hand through her hair, she felt her pulse quicken. Ryan had appeared unwell when he arrived, so her concerns seemed justified. He had shown up early and brought his equipment, so it would be strange for him to back out now. "Yes!" she exclaimed with relief as she saw him appear at the top of the hotel driveway.

There was a knock at the door, and a glance at her watch revealed it was nearly 11 a.m. She opened the door with a beaming smile as her production team arrived. "Hello! It's great to meet you finally," she said, noticing the equipment they were carrying as she welcomed Yvette and Matt into the room.

"And you, Miss Lord," he replied.

"Oh, please, call me Helen. So, you must be Matt, and I'm guessing this is Yvette?"

They confirmed who they were. Matt smiled warmly, while Yvette seemed somewhat disinterested.

"So, where would you like us?" Matt asked.

"I'll be with Dr Ryan Dobey, and you'll be filming both of us. Unfortunately, we have to work with this as a table. Can you set up around it?"

"That's a very dark dresser, Helen," Yvette replied with a shrug. "We'll try to lighten it as best as we can."

"Ryan has just arrived and will be setting up shortly. I'm not sure if he'll drape a white protective cloth over it, but I think that would help."

"It would," Yvette agreed as she took a couple of radiomics from her bag.

"Yvette, could you set up the lights while I assemble the camera?"

She nodded as Matt positioned the camera tripod.

"Are you shooting with just one camera?"

"Yes, Helen. Since it's a live broadcast, this approach will be easier. If you're interested in working with us again in the future, we can explore multiple camera options and cover various angles; all of that can be incorporated during the editing process. You mentioned it was just an interview."

"Well, it's a bit more than that, to be honest. Ryan will be conducting a test."

"A test? What kind of test?" Yvette asked.

"Based on our discussions, you're aware of my stance in the media. I'm striving to change the laws surrounding the use of cosmetic surgery. Many people are unaware of what substances are being injected into them, and that's the focus of today's filming. If we execute this correctly, it could reach millions of viewers."

Yvette looked at Matt in surprise. "I thought it was some sort of party political broadcast?"

Helen laughed. "Hardly, Yvette. Quite the opposite."

"I'm confused, Helen. What exactly are we filming today?" Yvette inquired.

Helen nodded. "I intended to brief you before we started filming, but the doctor…" She was interrupted by a knock at the door. "Ah, that must be him now. Ryan is running a test on a vial of cosmetic filler, which I believe is illegal."

Matt immediately paused setting up the camera. "Illegal in what way?"

Helen smiled. "You'll find out!"

"Look, I'm sorry, Helen, but our name will be attached to this project, and we are just a small production company. Can you tell me what makes this illegal?"

"Oh, just the minor detail that heroin is involved," she replied, turning her back to them as she opened the door. Matt immediately exchanged concerned glances with Yvette.

"Ah, good. Come in, Ryan," Helen said. She noticed Ryan folding a white envelope and quickly tucking it into his jacket pocket as he stepped into the room. His skin looked incredibly pale. "This is Yvette and Matt; they will be handling the filming."

"Pleased to meet you," Matt said as he stepped forward to shake hands with the doctor. However, he quickly withdrew his hand and wiped it on his trouser leg, realising how clammy the doctor's hands felt. The doctor skipped any pleasantries and didn't say a word, making his way directly to the equipment on the bed.

Helen closed the door behind them. "Ryan, will this dresser work? If so, do you have a cloth to cover it?"

Ryan nodded in response.

His behaviour was quite unusual, unlike the first time she had met him. Helen felt it was necessary to check on him. "Is there anything I can do to help?"

Ryan shook his head and began unpacking his bags. Not wanting to alarm the others, Helen whispered to him, "Are you sure you're okay? You don't seem like yourself."

He nodded, "I'm fine, Helen, honestly. Let's get this done."

She looked at him suspiciously. "Okay, if you're sure."

"So, to confirm, Ryan is going to test the contents of a vial. Will you be interviewing him or doing something else?" Matt asked.

"And how long do you think this will take?" Yvette quickly added.

Matt frowned at Yvette; she was not being discreet about her displeasure at being there.

"Actually, that's a good question, Yvette. Ryan, how long do you think the test will take?"

"About an hour, Helen, give or take. It's just a basic test, not what I would classify as exacting science," Ryan replied.

"Oh, I didn't realise it would take that long, especially since we know what we're looking for," Helen remarked, noting that she may have seen Yvette rolling her eyes. "Um, Matt, I'm guessing you don't want to film me for an hour, right?"

"Probably wise not to; it won't be engaging unless Ryan explains every part of the process. You'll lose viewers. That reminds me, I'll need access to your YouTube account."

"Not a problem. How do you want to do that?" Helen asked.

"The camera is synced to my laptop. We'll run it through there after I've got Wi-Fi. Ryan, would you like to talk about the process during the broadcast?" Matt inquired.

Ryan looked shocked as he placed a set of car keys on the dresser. "I'd rather not!"

His facial expression showed that he genuinely meant what he was saying. Regardless of what was on his mind, Helen didn't want to push him further. "Okay, everyone, I plan to read some handwritten notes first, and then we'll review Ryan's test results and go from there."

"Are you really sure about this, Helen? Heroin in a beauty product sounds like something out of science fiction," Yvette remarked.

'Well, she's blunt,' Helen thought, but she kept her opinions about Yvette to herself. "On the contrary, this is a scientific fact, secretly manufactured in a lab. Did you say you have a white cloth, Ryan?"

He nodded and tossed a cloth to her. He noticed Helen picking up the keys from the dresser. "Be careful with those!" he snapped.

Helen froze in shock, holding the keys and wondering why Ryan had reacted so aggressively. "I'm sorry, Ryan. They're just keys. I meant no harm."

He took the keys from her and helped her cover the dresser. Helen noticed that once he was satisfied with the cloth, he placed the keys back on top of it. "Are you sure you're alright, Ryan?" she asked.

He nodded and rubbed his forehead, which was lightly beaded with perspiration. "I'm fine, honestly. Please stop asking."

"Okay," Helen replied, holding her hands up. She noticed that Matt and Yvette were whispering to each other.

"Listen, she's a paying client," Matt said, glancing over his shoulder to make sure they weren't being overheard. "You're being a bit snappy."

Yvette bit her lip and shrugged. "Aren't you at least slightly concerned about this? Heroin, lab testing... I thought we were working on a political piece."

"And so did I," Matt quickly replied. "However, we should adapt. It sounds crazy, but as I think about it, it could attract a lot of viewers, which would be beneficial for us."

Yvette nodded. "Maybe. But what if she starts making accusations and naming names? It could lead to lawsuits."

"Perhaps, but that won't be our problem. It's her channel, and she'll be the one making those claims."

"I just don't want it to come back on us." Yvette stopped speaking as Helen watched them.

"Would anyone like a coffee?" the MP asked with a smile.

++++

Two rooms away, David sat focused on his laptop screen, shaking his head and rubbing his chin as he listened to the conversation between Ryan and the MP. "Calm down," he muttered under his breath. So far, Ryan had followed instructions and read the envelope David had given him before entering the hotel room. He had also remembered to place the hidden camera in the car key to capture what was happening behind him. However, the lab technician was anything but calm; the MP's persistent questioning about Ryan's well-being was concerning. David rubbed his eyes, realising that

Ryan was under immense strain. There was a genuine risk that he might crack under the pressure. David placed his hands on either side of the laptop and tapped his fingers on the table while keeping Rubin's gun close by. Things could escalate quickly. As expected, two civilians were responsible for filming the broadcast. They appeared worried about something; David noticed them engaged in hushed conversations that Rubin's microphones could not capture. The corridor had seen little activity, with only the occasional resident returning to their room. Ryan was currently setting up his equipment and had informed the MP that the test would take approximately an hour. David glanced at his watch. He needed to update the others, although he wasn't confident that everything would hold together.

++++

"Ah, good. Our asset is in position," Darius said as he set his phone down.

"Did he say anything else?" Hugh asked.

"Yes. The test may take an hour, so they won't start the broadcast until it's nearly complete."

Hugh nodded. "Anything from Ronald?"

Darius shook his head. "Not for a while. Only when he mentioned he was making his way to the warehouse."

"So, no word about customs yet?" William enquired.

"Nothing, my friend." Darius nodded at the senior board member. "These matters always take time. But for now, everything is on schedule."

"I'm worried about the outcomes. This test was never part of the plan," Hugh admitted.

Darius acknowledged Hugh's concern with a smile. "Something was always going to happen. Although I must admit, we couldn't have anticipated a leak from the facility. Treachery weaves its way throughout society."

"And what if someone else leaks something?" Hugh asked, his brow furrowing.

Darius grinned at William. "I have plans in place for that, and it has been addressed."

Hugh glanced at William, who looked at the floor with a smirk. "Oh, okay. I won't ask."

"Trust me, Hugh," Darius said, nodding reassuringly. "It's all under control."

✢✢✢✢

Given everything that had happened over the past few days, Helen was eager to get started. She paced back and forth in the room while Ryan assembled his testing equipment. Twenty minutes had already passed. Matt sat patiently in the corner, closely monitoring his laptop, while Yvette sat with her arms crossed, appearing somewhat bored.

Noticing Ryan put his hands in his pockets while he assessed his setup, Helen seized the opportunity to push forward. "Are you ready?" she asked.

Ryan's shrug didn't inspire much confidence. "It's as good as it can be, but as I mentioned before, it's hardly an ideal environment, and we are using my portable spectrometer."

"Don't worry, Ryan, I have every confidence in you. Are you going to change? That jacket doesn't seem appropriate for a test." She noticed Ryan tense up instantly.

"Um, no, I'll keep this on," he replied.

"Sorry, I don't mean to question your professional judgment, but I expected to see a lab coat."

"Um, well, no, sorry, I forgot it. Besides, this keeps me warm," his smile was far from convincing.

"Right. Okay. Sorry, are you cold? I've noticed you perspiring from time to time. I can check if the heating works if you'd like. I haven't tried it at this time of year."

"No! Honestly, Helen, I'm fine." Ryan raised his hands in an attempt to reassure her and wiped some sweat from his brow. "Look, as I mentioned, this is not ideal. I'm not sure what this is going to prove," he replied.

"We'll see!" Helen said, her excitement evident as she opened the fridge door and took out one of the vials. Ryan took a deep breath and put on a pair of latex gloves. He took the vial from her. "This is vindication," she added.

Ryan swallowed as he took the vial and nodded in response.

"Would either of you like another coffee? It might be a little while before we start filming," Helen offered.

Matt glanced up from his laptop, satisfied with the camera position. "Yes, please, Helen. Yvette, could you move the light on the right hand side a bit further to the right?"

Yvette got up. "Yes, I'd like another coffee too, Helen," she replied while adjusting the light. "Let me know when you're happy with it, Matt."

"A little further, please, and just slightly closer to Ryan," Matt instructed. On his laptop screen, he noticed how bloodshot Ryan's eyes were, and he could see the lab technician's hands shaking slightly. Ryan seemed preoccupied, and it was affecting his demeanour. Matt had overheard the MP repeatedly asking the lab technician if he was alright, but that wasn't his concern; he was there to film and had been paid for it. "That'll do, Yvette. Thank you, we'll connect the radio mics when the test is nearly complete," he said. The on-screen image was as good as it was going to get. Now, all they had to do was wait before filming began.

++++

Over an hour had passed when Ryan stopped to take a deep breath. "I'm only a few minutes away from completion," he said.

With a coffee in hand, Helen moved to Ryan's side. "Great news, it's taken longer than I hoped."

"These machines take time to warm up, and if I'm honest, they should have had more time."

"Do you have any preliminary findings?" she asked.

Ryan shook his head as he studied his laptop. "I'm keeping an eye on the software, but not yet. I should have a structural answer soon. It shouldn't take much longer."

"Alright, Helen. Are you ready to start?" Matt asked. I've logged into your YouTube account, and we can go live as soon as you're prepared. Yvette, can you attach the radio mics, please?"

Helen set her mug down and picked up her notes while Yvette attached a radio mic to her. Taking a deep breath, she nodded at Matt. "Just give me a moment," she said as she pulled a chair over to the dresser and sat next to Ryan.

She glanced to her left and noticed that Ryan looked incredibly uncomfortable. "Are you ready?" she asked as Yvette attached a radio mic to Ryan's lapel.

Ryan took a moment to glance at Matt and Yvette. "I want to be filmed as little as possible. If you can manage the broadcast without filming me, I'm fine with that."

"You're joking, right?" Helen laughed. "This will be the making of you!"

++++

Darius read David's message on his phone: "Gentlemen, we are about to go live." He stood up from his seat behind the desk, grabbed the television remote, and joined William and Hugh. The three of them turned towards the wall-mounted television as Darius unmuted the volume. "Would either of you like a drink?" he asked. This could be very interesting."

++++

Rubin and Andrea were sitting in the front room, waiting for Helen's broadcast to start on YouTube.

Rubin put his phone down after reading a message from David:

"Send the kids to play upstairs. We are about to go live. Now we'll find out what your husband is made of."

He noticed Andrea swallow nervously as she sat in fear. "Both of you, please go play upstairs," she insisted.

"Aww, Mum, it's nice outside," Annabelle complained.

"Annabelle, please do as I ask and take your sister with you."

Andrea glanced at her captor and the scars on his face, fearful for her family and what might happen next.

++++

Helen placed a glass of water beside her, took a deep breath, and nodded at Matt.

Matt completed his final checks on the laptop. "Camera is ready. Okay, we're going live in 3, 2, 1," he said, pointing at Helen.

Helen looked up from her notes. "My name is Helen Lord, MP. As many of you are aware, this week we witnessed an attack on the streets of our capital. My friend, Alison Harwood, left her home to go to work and became the victim of an attempted assassination, resulting in life-changing injuries. She has now been transferred from critical care; however, her recovery is expected to take a significant amount of time. Alison was appointed to Channel 8 television, where she oversaw programming in the aftermath of the now-cancelled series The Beauty Beach. The winner of The Beauty Beach was Megan Lauders, who received extensive cosmetic surgery as her prize. The surgery she underwent had disastrous consequences, leading to life-changing implications for her. After a lengthy legal battle, she successfully sued Channel 8 television and the production company responsible for the show. The production company went bankrupt, while Channel 8 barely managed to survive. Although the exact amount awarded in the lawsuit settlement remains undisclosed, it is rumoured to be in the millions of pounds. This landmark case changed television and ignited a debate on cosmetic surgery. Consequently, similar lawsuits emerged globally, empowering individuals of all genders to utilise this legal precedent to protect their rights. Many individuals who experienced negative aftereffects from unnecessary surgeries have discovered they had valid legal cases, and numerous plaintiffs have succeeded in their lawsuits. With each successful case, the influence of those in the cosmetic surgery industry has diminished. Throughout this period, Alison has played a crucial role in keeping the conversation alive. To this day, a significant percentage of people remain unaware of what is being put into their bodies. Yet many do so, often due to societal pressures and the influence of social media. Cosmetic surgery has been practised for many years, and many argue that it is still in its infancy, with numerous studies yet to provide a comprehensive understanding of its lasting effects." Helen paused to sip a glass of water. "Today, I am joined by Dr Ryan Dobey, the principal laboratory technician from Geographica Pathology Services. He is currently conducting tests on a vial that was sent to me. The contents of this vial, as these tests will demonstrate, will reveal the disturbing practices of a corrupt pharmaceutical company facing declining profits. What you will see on screen today has the potential to trigger a new drug epidemic unlike anything we have ever experienced before. It could lead to addiction among people from all walks of life." Helen paused and glanced at her notes. "A few months ago, Alison was approached by an anonymous source who claimed to work in a laboratory in Brazil in Central America. This lab synthesised a new beauty filler. The development process took months, and human testing resulted in fatalities, disfigurement, and addiction. The company behind this exploited vulnerable individuals, many without families, the poor, and the helpless, people who could easily disappear and wouldn't be missed. They treated these lives as collateral damage in their reckless pursuit of profit." Helen paused to sip her water, noticing the alarmed expressions exchanged between Yvette and Matt. "Alison brought her findings to me and communicated with the source, who bravely decided to blow the whistle on what was happening. Worryingly, the whistleblower disappeared a little while ago, and neither Alison nor I know their whereabouts. We believe the pharmaceutical company became aware of the whistleblower. Although I cannot provide further details, I am genuinely concerned for their safety. So, why are we here today? Why am I broadcasting to you live? The reason is that the whistleblower managed to send me samples of the vials. They did this because they shared Alison's beliefs, and we needed to publicly disclose what had been engineered and what was about to unfold. My collaboration with Alison has been widely publicised. We have faced online backlash, and both of us have endured abuse, which at times has been deeply personal and intense. Despite that, we pressed on, driven by the truth. Today, I am going to prove what is really going on." She glanced to her left and asked, "Ryan, how are we doing?"

"A couple more minutes, I would think."

"Good. Dr Dobey performed a test just two nights ago that proved a rogue and illegal contaminant had been created. The contents of the vial are packaged and ready for distribution." Helen was momentarily distracted as she noticed Ryan take an envelope from his pocket. "This will not stop. It will not end, and I'm telling you this today so you are aware of what has been happening. This will not be covered up. You need to know so that you can make informed decisions for the future."

Helen took a deep breath. "The whistleblower in Brazil was a senior technician. The board of the pharmaceutical company approved the creation of the Brazilian lab, which was established solely to promote addiction."

Ryan coughed slightly under his breath, "Ready."

"And now, we are about to prove this. This so-called beauty filler has been designed to continuously release a powerful and illegal drug into the brain, allowing you to unknowingly receive a Class A narcotic substance injected directly into your face. That drug is an opioid containing diacetylmorphine, commonly known as heroin, and I am officially naming Knightark Pharmaceutical as the company responsible for creating this product."

++++

Hugh jumped to his feet, his hands pressed against his face in shock. "What the fuck! She just named us, Darius!"

William also stood up from his chair, looking at Darius with concern.

Darius, however, remained seated. "Gentlemen, please stay calm. Let's see how this plays out."

++++

Yvette covered her mouth in shock. "Jesus Christ, Matt! She just named a company!"

Matt placed his hand on Yvette's shoulder and whispered, "I know. I know, but what can we do? We can't cut her off!" They both looked at the MP, concerned about what would happen next.

"Dr Dobey has now completed his evaluation. He has been testing a well-known product manufactured by the previously named pharmaceutical company, called Hydra-Fillixir. This scientifically modified version of their Hydra-Fillixir brand is part of their core range of fillers available worldwide. Although it appears similar to their other products, this variant contains diacetylmorphine," Helen announced as she watched him read the screen. "What have we discovered, Doctor?"

Ryan swallowed. "Um, well, I'm not sure what you were expecting."

Helen turned to acknowledge the camera. "You know what we are looking for, Ryan."

"Well, yes, I know what you think you're looking for, but the properties of the vial you gave me appear to be consistent with what I would expect to find in a cosmetic beauty filler."

Helen froze. "What!"

"Yes, look at my screen; it clearly shows that it contains hyaluronic acid, which helps retain moisture and elasticity in the skin."

Helen snatched at the screen in disbelief. "And what else?"

"I don't see anything in this test that is illegal. There's no indication of any illegal properties. I configured the system for this test to look specifically for what you suspected. You mentioned diacetylmorphine, but I assure you it's not present here."

Helen's hands began to shake. "You can't be serious! You tested this two nights ago! Where are the results from that night?"

Ryan opened the envelope and handed it to Helen. She immediately began to shake her head in panic. "But this! This isn't the same as it was the other night; this isn't what you told me!"

"Yes, it is. I may have made a mistake," he replied.

"But..."

"I'm telling you, there is nothing illegal about the vial you gave me."

Helen covered her mouth with her hand, realising the gravity of what she had just done. "Oh my God!"

Ryan stood up and began to walk away as the MP pointed at him. "They've got to you! What do they have on you?"

Ryan shook his head. "I don't know what you're talking about!"

In a panic, Helen dropped the printout and pointed at Matt. "Turn off that camera now!"

✢✢✢✢

Darius leaned back in his seat, laughing. "I can't believe she fell for it; she played right into my hands."

Hugh shook his head in disbelief. "What exactly did I just witness? She mentioned heroin during a live broadcast!"

"Yes, she did. But did she find any?" Darius replied with a smirk.

William paced the room, laughing to himself. "Come on, how did you pull it off?"

"Pretty simple, my friend. We knew about the informant," Darius explained, glancing at both men for confirmation. "So, I arranged for four vials of our core filler to be sent to the member of parliament. I made sure they were shipped from the lab in Brazil, and as far as she was concerned, they came from the informant."

William continued to laugh. "Brilliant!"

"And that is where our asset came into play. He ensured the new product was tested and that the findings were communicated to the MP over the phone. However, there was no credible evidence to support those findings; it was merely hearsay. It was a calculated risk, gentlemen. Nevertheless, between the MP and Alison Harwood, they had enough information to proceed with some form of broadcast. Now, where is their credibility? I can hardly believe she fell for it." Darius stood up. "And that, gentlemen, is how you carry out an assassination live on air. Let them assassinate themselves."

"But she named us, Darius?"

"She did, Hugh. She named us and accused us of being involved with Class A drugs. She made this accusation on a public platform without a shred of evidence to support it. Our lawyers are going to destroy her. There is no coming back from this for her."

"You didn't need to press Lord Gatesouth after all," William remarked.

"Oh, I don't know. It doesn't hurt to rattle our well-placed advisors. Besides, I couldn't have fully known how this was going to play out," Darius said, beaming with pride in his brilliance. "She'll be all over the news this evening and in the papers tomorrow. And let's not forget her meeting with the Chief Whip in the morning, I'd love to be a fly on that wall! Gentlemen, she is gone. The death of beauty is over, and I think a toast is in order." Darius moved to the side of the room, where Paul, his butler, had prepared a bottle of champagne in an ice bucket for them.

"So, what became of the informant? You never did say," Hugh asked.

Darius lifted the bottle from the ice bucket. "Do you really want to know, Hugh?"

"When you put it that way, I'm not so sure!"

Darius began twisting the muselet holding the cork in place. "You can say what you like about the cartels, but they are masters of disposal." He removed the muselet, pulled the cork from the bottle, and grabbed three glasses. "It can't be done in this country, my friend, but in South America, it is possible. I dare say that William knows what a sky burial is."

William snorted, "Yeah, I know."

"Well, I don't," Hugh admitted.

Darius nodded at William. "Do you want to tell him while I pour our glasses?"

William replied, "Sure, it's a tried and tested technique. You take the informer, the enemy, or whoever, to the middle of nowhere. Shoot them in the head, then remove all their clothes and lay them face down. Next, you take a machete and make criss-cross cuts down their back, on their backside, and along the back of their legs. And then you wait."

"Blimey, I wish I had never asked," Hugh said, taking the glass that was handed to him. "Wait, wait for what?"

"Vultures," William explained. "They feed in such a frenzy that nothing is spared, absolutely everything. It's perfect; there's no real trace evidence left. That's why it's called a sky burial. Afterwards, they shit the remains all over the land." William nodded as Darius passed him a glass.

"Far more effective than any pig farm," Darius added, setting the champagne bottle aside. "That's where betrayal gets you. All you need are vultures to do your dirty work. Fortunately, the only vultures we have to deal with in this country are already on our payroll."

They all laughed as Darius set down his glass, hearing his phone vibrate from behind him. He picked it up and read the message. "Well, well. It's Ronald. He's heard from the driver that our consignment has cleared customs," Darius said, smiling with satisfaction.

"How many have gotten through?" Hugh asked.

"As long as there are no breakages, the estimate is around nine thousand vials," Darius replied.

"Amazing," William said, raising his glass.

"Quite unprecedented," Hugh added as he lifted his glass.

"Gentlemen," Darius raised his glass, "to us and our successes. We are now officially in the opioid business."

Chapter Twenty-Seven

Despite the broadcast ending, David remained vigilant, closely monitoring the four individuals in the hotel room, aware that the tension among them could escalate at any moment.

In the garden of Ryan's family home, Rubin paced anxiously, deeply concerned about the situation. David was trying to reassure him during their phone conversation.

"Yes, I know. I'm monitoring everything; it's under control," David said.

"Listen! We watched the broadcast. The MP clearly asked if someone had got to him. That could lead back here!" Rubin paused his pacing, noticing Andrea in the front room. The worry in her eyes made him uneasy; he needed to prevent her from making a rash decision.

"Alpha 2, there's currently no indication of that," David replied. "I'm watching all of them on camera. It seems the camera crew is about to leave."

"Are you sure it's wise to let them go?"

"What? You can't be serious. They know nothing about what's going on. I'm not clipping them based on a maybe and having this whole place go off.".

"They pose a security risk."

"Not that I can see. They're just doing their job."

"Something feels off here."

David sat down, watching the laptop. "What do you mean?"

"The test from two nights ago. What was that all about? The live test I watched appeared to yield normal results. I don't know anything about cosmetics, but something definitely feels off."

"Look, don't worry about that. I'll be speaking with the client later. If I hear anything suspicious, even the slightest concern, you'll be the first to know."

"This is making me nervous. I have zero control over this operation."

"Trust me. Just keep an eye on the subjects. We'll be heading back to you soon. I'll message when on route." David could hear Rubin take a deep breath on the other end. He couldn't predict what his colleague would do next. "Did you receive my last message?"

"Yes. If there are any changes and I'm not satisfied, I'm out of here."

"Roger that. I'll be in touch, one way or another."

"Alright." Rubin hung up.

David hadn't been entirely truthful. He hadn't heard anything to suggest a compromise, but serious drama was unfolding just two doors away.

++++

Ryan hurriedly packed away his equipment, eager to leave the room as soon as possible. The MP's statement, "They've got to you," had been aired live, and in doing so, she had put both him and his family at risk.

Helen sat with her eyes closed, rubbing her temples. "What have I done?" she murmured.

"I'm not an expert, Helen, but I think you just accused a company of illegal drug manufacturing without a shred of evidence," Yvette said as she hurried to pack their production equipment. She quickly took the radio mics from the shaking hands of Helen and Ryan.

"Helen, I cut the broadcast as soon as you asked," Matt added. "But your YouTube account is… well, how can I put it? It's gone viral, completely off the scale." He was monitoring Helen's page. "It's being shared everywhere."

Feeling overwhelmed, Helen buried her head in her hands. "Can we delete it?" she asked.

Matt started folding up the tripod, having already put his camera away. "Well, yes, of course. But I'm afraid it's too late now. It will be everywhere, there will be screenshots, and others will film it with their phones, and so on. Oh, wait…" Helen looked up and saw him scrolling on his laptop. He let out a heavy sigh. "It's already been picked up by one of the national newspapers. A journalist has written an article about it. 'Maverick MP Loses The Plot In Bizarre Science Experiment,' is the title."

"Oh God," she said, leaning back in her chair and running a hand through her hair. "Just delete it."

Matt sighed. "If you're sure, but I have to warn you, you can't stop this from spreading."

"I know. Just do it anyway," Helen replied.

"I hate to say it, but the comments are… well, they're not very flattering. Last chance."

Helen nodded. "Please, just delete the bloody thing!"

Matt deleted the video, logged out of Helen's account, and closed his laptop. He noticed that Yvette was anxious to leave. "Um, Helen, we really need to go. I'm worried that this hotel might not be pleased about the broadcast being made from here. If the news channel is on downstairs, and this gets mentioned, and if the doorman sees it, he could make the connection. I don't want to be around if that happens, accusations of human trials and heroin and all that."

Helen leaned forward in her chair, resting her head in her hands. "Okay, that's understandable."

Matt slung his camera bag over his shoulder and picked up the lighting stands. Feeling quite awkward, he nodded at Ryan. "Well, we'll be off then." He glanced at Yvette and tilted his head towards the door. Without hesitation, Yvette left without saying a word. "Well then, good luck to you," Matt added as he closed the door behind him.

Yvette was already at the elevator and hurriedly pressed the down button. "I'll say this," she remarked as the doors opened and Matt joined her, "that was no ordinary political broadcast. She's not getting my vote." They stepped into the elevator and quickly descended to the exit.

++++

As David watched the corridor camera, he saw the camera crew departing the hotel room. The woman exited first, closely followed by the man. They moved quickly toward the elevator, exchanging a few brief words as they waited for it to arrive. Once they were inside the lift, David turned his attention to the windows. Below, he observed them leaving the hotel and hurrying to the end of the road. The man, whom David recognised as Matt, hailed a taxi from the street corner. Unlike what Rubin might have done, allowing them to leave was the wise decision.

As he returned to his seat, David reflected on Rubin's additional concerns. The point raised by Rubin was significant: the member of parliament's comment about Ryan being "got to" could potentially raise questions. However, it seemed unlikely that the police would follow up on such an offhand remark. There was a greater chance that Ryan's friends or neighbours might see the broadcast and come to check on the family's safety, but even that seemed unlikely. For now, they would monitor events as they unfolded. The key fob camera had been knocked to the side, displaying a side wall, but was still transmitting audio. The footage from the body-worn camera showed Ryan hastily packing his equipment. All Ryan needed to do was maintain his composure, and this situation would soon be resolved.

++++

"You and I need to have a serious conversation," Helen said.

"I don't know what you mean, Helen," Ryan replied, trying to sound calm.

"Oh, stop being so ridiculous, Ryan! Look at you, you can't wait to get away from here."

Ryan felt his heart racing, and he knew he was sweating. "Of course I want to get away! You accused a company of wrongdoing while I was sitting right next to you. I don't want to be implicated or associated with this!"

"Wrongdoing? Are you serious? How can you say that?" Helen

began pacing the room, her hands on her hips. "Look at you! You're shaking, you've been off all day, and you're as pale as a ghost. Something has happened to you!"

Ryan quickly zipped up one of his bags. "Honestly, I don't know what you're talking about. I just ate something last night that didn't agree with me, that's all."

Helen was furious as she pointed at Ryan. "That's not all! Where are the original test results? What you presented here is not what you told me on the phone!"

Ryan sighed. "I told you, Helen, I could have been mistaken."

"That's utter bullshit, and you know it. People in your profession don't make mistakes. Now, tell me what's going on."

"Helen, it's nothing. Please, I ran the test for you, and that's what you asked me to do."

Helen stepped into his personal space, noting the fear in his eyes. "What have they done to you? What do they have on you?"

++++

Two rooms away, David hurriedly put on the wig and moustache while keeping a watchful eye on the laptop screen. The situation was escalating quickly. He peered through the spyhole in the door, then opened the door swiftly to remove the corridor camera. As the door closed behind him, he quickly turned off the camera using the phone app and put it into the backpack. Standing over the laptop, he picked up the firearm. Ryan had to be exceptionally careful with his words, or the hotel door would come off its hinges.

++++

Ryan picked up the car fob from the dresser and placed it in his jacket pocket. He didn't bother folding the white sheet; instead, he crumpled it quickly.

"Ryan, look. Please tell me what's wrong," Helen pleaded.

With his back turned to her, he hurriedly stuffed the sheet into one of his bags. "I've told you enough times today, nothing is wrong."

"You know I'm in a lot of trouble because of this."

"That's your doing, Helen! I never wanted to be involved in the first place. I lead a quiet life and have no desire to be in the news like you."

"There will be fallout from this, and according to Matt, it has already started."

Ryan spun around quickly. "So? That has nothing to do with me."

"But it does, doesn't it?" Helen replied.

He turned his back on her, quickly grabbing his bags.

"There could be legal ramifications. If you are withholding evidence..."

"Evidence of what?" Spittle flew from his mouth in anger. "I don't work for you. You can't make me do what you want. Are you going to detain me here, or should I call security?"

Helen studied him as he repeatedly avoided looking her in the eyes. He was right; Ryan was not her prisoner. "No, that won't be necessary," she replied.

"Then can I go?" he asked.

Helen shrugged. "As you rightly pointed out, you don't work for me. You can leave whenever you'd like."

He nodded. "Then I'll do just that." Laden with his bags, he puffed as he made his way toward the door, then paused. "I don't suppose you could open the door for me, could you?"

Helen stood right beside him, and as he avoided her eyes again, she opened the door. No words were exchanged as she watched him walk toward the elevators. He quickly glanced back, panic evident on his face.

Helen slammed the door, knowing her career was in tatters.

✢✢✢✢

David let out a massive sigh of relief and set the firearm back on the table. That was close. Although Ryan hadn't maintained his composure, he hadn't revealed anything. The MP would never know how close she had come.

David deleted the apps on both phones and disconnected the body-worn camera from the laptop. He quickly checked his reflection in the mirror; his makeshift disguise would have to suffice. Sitting at the dresser, he carefully dabbed at his moustache while unplugging the laptop. As he folded the power cord, he noticed several files on Rubin's desktop. One of them was labelled 'G.' Curiosity got the better of him, and he decided to open the file. It was substantial in size, and Rubin's old laptop took a few seconds to access the folder. Inside were several videos and hundreds of graphic images. David froze in horror as the disturbing images flooded his mind, falling back into his seat in shock. His breathing intensified as he raised his hands to his head in disbelief, resting his elbows on the dresser. "Oh God," he mumbled in anger. Glancing at the ceiling, he realised he had seen enough and slammed the laptop shut. Shaking his head in disgust and placing his hands on the dresser, he knew he needed to compose himself and focus on the task at hand. Ryan was probably already out of the building, and he needed to reach him immediately.

Throwing the laptop and power cord into the backpack, he grabbed the hotel key from the side and put on his glasses and cap. He would have to deal with what he had seen later.

++++

CHEQUERS – OFFICIAL COUNTRY HOME OF THE PRIME MINISTER, AYLESBURY, BUCKINGHAMSHIRE, ENGLAND

Alix glanced up from his notes. "Come in," he said.

His wife, Eleanor, stood at the door.

"Darling, you don't have to knock," he smiled.

"I know you don't like to be disturbed at this time on a Sunday," she replied.

"Oh, please," he said, putting down his briefing notes. He had been studying the questions that would be asked at the upcoming Prime Minister's Questions on Wednesday. "I wish they'd scrap this ridiculous televised debacle."

Eleanor smiled while holding her phone.

"Dave from Chertsey is asking for Viagra on the NHS for his erectile dysfunction!" Alix mocked.

"Wait, that's not a serious question, is it?"

Alix stared at his wife, and they both broke into fits of laughter.

"Have you not checked your phone?" she asked.

Alix, half-reading his notes, shook his head. "No. I switched it off."

"What about the landline?"

Alix shrugged. "I pulled it out of the wall. What's wrong?"

"Seb just called me. He said he couldn't get through to you."

"Sebastian, the Chief Whip?"

Eleanor nodded.

"He knows not to call unless it's really urgent."

"He says it is, and he wants to speak to you immediately."

Alix looked surprised. "Did he say what it's about?"

Eleanor shook her head. "No, just that it's important."

Alix leaned across the table, picked up his phone, and switched it on. "If it's Seb, I'm guessing it has to be an internal issue, something related to the party."

"That's what I thought," Eleanor replied.

"What the…? My phone is going crazy!" Alix exclaimed in shock as his device flooded with incoming messages. "There's a message from Gatesouth and others about Helen."

"Which Helen?"

"I'll tell you which Helen: that bloody woman who challenged me in the chamber this week."

Eleanor approached his desk. "Oh yes, the one who blindsided you, the 'Death of Beauty' MP."

Alix shook his head as he tried to decipher the messages. "I don't understand what's going on. I'd better call Seb."

"Do you want me to leave the room?"

"No, darling, it's probably just party politics. Although I have no idea why I'm being disturbed by it." He called the Chief Whip and put the phone on speaker. "Do you want a drink?" he gestured to his wife.

She shook her head as Sebastian answered the call. "Seb, what's going on? Eleanor said you called."

"Alix, something has happened. You need to be aware of it immediately. Haven't you seen the news?"

"No. Why? I've been going through my briefing notes." Alix said as he switched on the TV, muted the sound, and immediately selected a news channel.

"Alix, I've never seen anything like this before. In a nutshell, Helen Lord conducted a live broadcast on YouTube in which she accused Knightark Pharmaceutical of being involved in the drugs trade."

Alix was taken aback, locking eyes with Eleanor. "What! Darius's company?"

"Yes. She conducted some half-assed lab test…"

"Wait, how does she know how to do something like that?"

"Sorry, no, actually, she didn't do the test herself. She had a lab technician run a test on a beauty filler. She named Darius's company and started claiming they were involved in human experiments and practically accused them of being responsible for the assassination attempt on Alison Harwood a few days ago."

Alix was stunned and fell back into his seat. Eleanor shook her head in disbelief.

"Your silence speaks volumes, Alix. This is serious, very serious."

"And did the test prove anything along the lines of what she was suggesting?"

"No. The test revealed it was a beauty filler, containing whatever you would typically find in one. I'm sorry; it's not a subject I know much about."

"Seb, I feel completely bamboozled."

"You and me both."

"Can I see this broadcast?"

"Yes, it's all over social media. She's taken it down from her account, but it was too late; it had already gone viral."

Alix raised his arms in disbelief, looking to his wife for any inspiration. "So, let me get this right: a serving MP from our own party has publicly humiliated a company and accused it of wrongdoing without providing any evidence. Is that correct?"

"Well, yes, that's the crux of it."

"Seb, sorry, you're on speaker; I'm looking at Eleanor to see what she thinks."

"I'm shocked, Seb," Eleanor said. "I've never heard anything quite so career-destroying. It's like throwing yourself on a sword. What do you think, Seb?"

"I think you're right, Eleanor. Look, Alix, you're going to face some serious questions. Lord Gatesouth has already been putting pressure on me about this. What she has done raises significant concerns about government officials making such accusations while in office. I just watched a news segment discussing the role of a member of parliament; the fallout is immense. She has gone too far and exceeded her duties. Each year, the number of MPs who have had the whip withdrawn grows. We are losing control of our members, Alix. The opposition is going to have a field day with this."

Alix rubbed his eyes. Just a few minutes earlier, he had been irritated about the questions he would face this coming Wednesday. Now, everything had changed dramatically. "Are we going to release a statement?"

"Not that I've heard of, but we'll need to address this soon. Her position is now untenable as far as I'm concerned."

"You have a meeting with her tomorrow morning, don't you?"

"Yes. If she shows up, to be honest, it was just going to be a severe reprimand for her conduct. However, what she has done today changes everything. I believe there are grounds to remove the whip from her due to misconduct in public office. She should be expelled from the party."

Alix nodded at his wife. "Yes, it does. Yes, it does."

"Look, bear with Seb; I need to think this over."

"Of course, Prime Minister. But please get back to me. We'll need to handle this carefully. At the moment, she is national news, and within the hour, she'll be worldwide news."

"Yep. Yes, she will be. Look, Seb, I'll call you back."

"Okay, I'll speak with you in a bit."

Alix pressed his phone to end the call and leaned back in his chair.

"What are you going to do? I've never heard of anything like this before."

Alix nodded, rubbing his chin in thought. A small smile broke across his face as he waved his index finger. "You know what, my love? This may actually work to our advantage."

++++

David placed the backpack on the rear seat and closed the door. "I'd be lying to myself if I thought you would still be here." He took the seat next to Ryan in the car and shut the door. "Are you okay?"

"Define 'okay'," Ryan replied.

"Well, you're still alive."

Ryan looked into David's eyes. Behind the fake glasses, David's expression revealed nothing.

"The MP and the other two are also still alive. It could have been worse. You did well, as far as I can tell."

Ryan shrugged. "I have no idea what happened back there, but I want to get away from here. I'm guessing you'd like me to start the car?"

David nodded. "We're not going to fly back magically, are we? Do you remember the way?"

"Not especially."

"I had the phones charging in the room. I'll pull up the sat nav and direct you. Remember, drive just over the speed limit, but no more. Don't drive under it, and avoid the bus lanes. Your part in this is almost done."

"Can I speak with my wife?" Ryan asked as he started the car.

David anticipated that Ryan would ask this question; it was reasonable. "Yes, we'll call her as soon as we're on the road," he replied. He needed to speak with Rubin to let him know they were on their way back. If he were honest, he was also eager to hear about the status of Ryan's family.

"Okay, go straight out of here and turn right," David instructed. He glanced at Ryan, who looked seriously ill. David knew he needed to keep him calm during the drive back. He pulled down the visor and checked his reflection in the mirror to make sure that the cap over his ill-fitting wig covered as much of his face as possible. "Once we're clear of this area, we'll call your wife, okay?"

Ryan nodded. "So, what happens next?"

"What do you think is going to happen?" David replied. "We'll continue straight for about a mile, then make our way back to your house. I need to speak with Alpha 2, contact my client, and then we'll be on our way. You and your family can return to your life in suburbia."

Ryan nodded again, but doubt lingered in his expression. "And what about her?"

David shook his head. "Who?"

"The MP?"

"What do you care?"

"Because I have no idea what just happened! You handed me an envelope with instructions printed on the front, telling me to open it only after the test was complete. The results inside were completely different from what I saw in my lab. That's what I'm talking about! And she, the MP, didn't believe a word of it!"

"No, she didn't, but it's done now."

"I have no idea what I'm involved in!"

"You are not involved in anything!" David spat. "You have no involvement here, understand?"

Ryan nodded repeatedly.

"Straight ahead at the roundabout and continue until you see signs for the M25 motorway. Listen to me and make sure you understand this: you are not involved in anything, and you know nothing, okay?"

"Okay, okay! I understand, but the MP looked distraught. There are going to be repercussions from this, whatever it was."

"And as I said, what do you care? She was just a mark."

"A mark?"

"Yeah, a mark, a target, a subject, whatever."

"Because she's a person, a living person just like us. Where's your humility, man?" Ryan slammed his hand on the steering wheel in frustration.

David quickly pointed at Ryan. "You need to stay calm. Focus on the task at hand, and right now, that's keeping us alive on this road." He could see that Ryan was at his breaking point and might lose it at any moment. He reached into his pocket and took out Ryan's phone. "Look, I'll call Andrea. Will that give you some peace of mind?"

Ryan nodded and took a deep breath.

"Alpha 2 has her phone. Just focus on later; this is nearly over." David entered Ryan's code into the phone. "I'm guessing she's in your recent call list?"

Ryan shot a glance at David.

"What? Oh…" David smirked and held up the phone. "I'm guessing 'Fluffy Bunny' is who we're looking for?"

Ryan bowed his head in embarrassment. "Don't you have names for any of your relationships?"

David's expressionless eyes met Ryan's bloodshot ones.

"No. I don't suppose you do. Is it against your code or something?"

"Never you mind," David replied, calling 'Fluffy Bunny'. "What does she call you?"

Ryan almost smiled for the first time all day. "Now, never you mind! And piss off while you're at it."

David grinned and put the phone on speaker, placing it close to Ryan's chin. "Be careful what you say."

Ryan nodded as the call connected after just a couple of rings. "Darling, are you okay?" he asked.

"Yes, yes, we're fine," Andrea quickly replied.

"Where are the kids?"

"They're upstairs playing. I saw the broadcast. Are you on your way back?"

Ryan glanced at David, who nodded in agreement. "Yes, we're heading back now."

"Are you coming straight here?"

"Yes, I think so," Ryan replied, seeking further confirmation. He received it. "Yes, straight back. It should take about an hour at most if the roads are clear."

David pulled the phone away and switched off the speaker. "Andrea, put Alpha 2 on."

Noticing that Ryan's hands were shaking, David pointed ahead. "Keep your attention on the road."

Out of the corner of his eye, Ryan watched David nod as he spoke with Rubin.

"Yeah, maybe around forty minutes to an hour," he said. "What's the sit rep?" He nodded again. "Yes, I know. I'll mention that in a moment. Okay, see you soon."

David hung up and placed the phone in his pocket. "Are you confident you know the way once we get onto the M25?"

Ryan nodded. "Yes, I think so."

"Good. Listen, Alpha 2 raised an important point. At the end of the broadcast, just before it was terminated, the MP said something like, 'Have they got to you?'".

"Yeah, so?" Ryan replied.

"I need you to think about this; it's important. Do you know if any of your staff, neighbours, family, or anyone else has an interest in politics?"

"Eh? What difference does that make?"

"It makes a significant difference. I'm trying to find out if anyone you know may have watched the broadcast or is currently watching it on social media. This is crucial, Ryan; think."

"Um, well, not that I can recall. We don't discuss things like that at work."

"It's essential. If someone believes you are in distress, the police may conduct a welfare check to ensure your safety. Alpha 2 is taking a risk by remaining in your house."

Ryan's eyes widened in shock as he turned his head.

"Don't look at me; keep your eyes on the road. The truth is, it's unlikely anyone will think that. However, you looked highly distressed during the broadcast."

"Did I? I did ask not to be filmed too much."

"Well, they ignored you, from what Alpha 2 just told me. You need to understand what I'm saying. It's more likely they will make a phone call rather than send a unit to your house. If the police call your wife, Alpha 2 will guide her. If they contact you, please stay calm. So, are we cool?"

Ryan nodded; he hadn't considered the possibility of the police contacting him.

"Just stay calm, drive safely, and avoid erratic behaviour. Do you understand?"

Ryan nodded, his knuckles turning white from gripping the steering wheel so tightly. After about ten more minutes of driving, they should reach the M25 motorway, and from there, he would head home.

++++

Ben Tasker couldn't believe what he had just seen. In his living room, he sat on the couch with his wife, and his phone buzzed with activity.

"What do you think we should do?" she asked.

Ben rose to his feet, his eyes fixed on the TV screen. They were so engrossed in the news that he didn't even look at her. With his phone in his left hand, he placed his hands on his hips and shook his head. "I don't know, my love. I've never seen anything like this before."

"But this is all intertwined with everything we're caught up in. Do you think we're safe here?"

"Erm, I…" Ben's phone began to ring; it was senior producer Brian Clement.

"Hi, Brian. Yes, I've seen it, and I noticed that Alison's name was used." Ben turned to look at his wife and nodded. "Yes, we should still run it. Use Alison's stock image. We need to show unbiased reporting. This story has taken a different direction. No, I don't know anything about it," he lied. "Just carry on as best as we can and ensure that full sensitivity is shown when mentioning Alison's name. Check what the press agencies are saying and piece together the information. Parliament is going to be chaotic this week. We'll need to extend our political pieces; there will be legal ramifications from this." He paused to listen to Brian. "Yes, I agree. Please keep me posted. Speak to you later."

"So, has Brian or anyone else heard anything?"

Ben put his phone down. "No, my love. Everyone is as in the dark as we are."

"But she stated what you know live on air! You weren't named, but how many people are aware of what you may know, and by default, what I know?"

"I understand!"

"Are they going to target us next?"

Ben held up his hands. "I don't know, my love. I really don't."

"Well, that's not good enough! We need to know what's going on."

Ben nodded. "I know, and I agree. I suspect we will find out soon enough."

Chapter Twenty-Eight

The constant barrage of abuse on her social media channels was overwhelming, and the aggressive tone of the message Helen received from the Chief Whip was the final straw. She switched off her phone; he had made it clear that she must attend their meeting in the morning, or words to that effect. Scratching her head and closing her eyes in frustration, she knew her career in politics was over; there was no coming back from this, especially with lawyers likely to get involved.

Sitting in the back of a black cab, she felt relieved that the driver didn't recognise her. With her phone turned off, she could use this moment of peace to think. How had Knightark Pharmaceutical managed to do this? What had gone so wrong? Something had changed with Ryan; he seemed scared, or perhaps someone had frightened him. She couldn't prove it, but all the signs pointed in that direction. Had he been pressured? He had previously mentioned that he had a family, and his daughter had broken her leg. She never asked about her well-being, and Ryan had never brought it up again. In any event, were they in danger? She wasn't sure, but what could they do? Did Knightark Pharmaceutical send someone to threaten him or someone close to him? It seemed like the realm of lunacy. Such things didn't happen here, not in this country. Yet, his sudden change in behaviour was suspicious; his actions spoke volumes. Helen's mind raced as she struggled to determine her next move. Should she call the police to check on him or his family? But then what? What if nothing had happened? She knew she would be in even more trouble than she already was if that information became public. She would be labelled a conspiracy theorist, a label already appearing on social media. Memes circulated depicting her in superhero costumes and as a Sherlock Holmes-type character, complete with a pipe, suggesting she was on the brink of solving a great mystery.

The black cab pulled over. "Here we are," the driver announced.

She paid him and grabbed her bags. Given recent events, staying at the other hotel was no longer an option. If people connected the dots and recognised the room from which she had broadcast, journalists would swarm the place in no time. That scenario could lead hotel management to ask her to vacate the property. In London hotels, where many indiscretions occurred, no one wanted a press crew camped outside their doors.

Standing outside her new hotel, she was only about a mile away from the previous one. She needed to remain in the area and faced the decision of whether to attend her meeting with the Chief Whip the following day, as expulsion from the party seemed inevitable. She trudged up the steps and pushed her way through the revolving doors. This hotel was cheaper than the last one, and there were no overzealous door people to assist her with her bags. The reception desk was directly in front of her, but the only attendant was already serving two other guests. Grateful to be free of her bags, she dropped them in the corner of the lounge to her right. Her eyes were immediately drawn to the television; the volume was muted, but there she was on the news channel, centre screen. The image appeared to be a still from her broadcast. Along the ticker tape at the bottom of the screen were the words "breaking news," followed closely by her name, with the strapline "MP accuses pharmaceutical company in bizarre lab experiment."

She swallowed with fear and, noticing that the reception area was now clear, quickly made her way over to the counter.

"Good afternoon. How may I assist you?"

"Just checking in. I'm only booked for one night."

"Let me see. What is your name, please?"

"Um, Lord. Helen Lord."

The receptionist immediately glanced at the TV screen and then back at Helen. Helen offered a brief smile. The receptionist remained professional, saying nothing as she processed the check-in. However, Helen suspected that the receptionist had been watching the news between guests, and she had been recognised before she'd even seen her room. All Helen could hope for was that the receptionist wouldn't alert journalists about their latest newsworthy guest.

++++

"Okay, drive slowly along your road. When you reach your house, back into the driveway."

Ryan nodded. "Why do you want me to slow down?"

David glanced at every parked car they passed. "Because I want to see if any police are nearby."

Ryan looked panicked. "You said a welfare check would be unlikely."

"I know, but it's always good to be prepared." David texted Rubin to let him know they were arriving.

"And you are going to let us go, right?"

"Yes! Now stop panicking. I need to concentrate. We are approaching your driveway, so slow down more." David scanned the road ahead. "Actually, go past your driveway to the end of the road. I want to check the parked cars further ahead."

Ryan saw David pull back his jacket, revealing the firearm. Inside, Ryan was praying there wouldn't be any police and further complications; he was trusting that David would keep his word and that this was all coming to an end.

"Okay. It looks clear. Turn the car around, come back, and then reverse into your driveway, backing right up to the garage."

Ryan followed the instructions, nervously glancing at David, who was scrutinising every car and house they passed. As Ryan reversed up the driveway, he noticed in the rearview mirror that the front door had been opened.

"Okay. Turn off the engine and hand me the keys. We'll leave your gear in here for now," David said.

Ryan's hands shook as he passed the keys after switching off the engine.

"Alright. Remember to stay calm. Now, out you get."

Ryan walked quickly to the front door while David retrieved his backpack and locked the car.

"Daddy!" Annabelle called from the top of the stairs. "I saw you on television!" The young girl beamed with pride, giggling as David stepped into the house. "You still look silly," she teased.

David caught a glimpse of himself in the mirror by the front door. After closing the door, he dropped his backpack and removed his cap, glasses and ill-fitting wig.

"We're playing with my dollhouse. Would you like to play Alpha 1?" Annabelle asked.

David smiled awkwardly and shook his head as he pulled the fake moustache off. He felt a sense of relief knowing the children were okay; leaving them with Rubin had troubled him. There was no telling what Rubin was fully capable of.

When Ryan saw Andrea, he rushed into the front room and embraced her tightly.

Rubin approached David and nodded. "Do you think you were followed?"

David shook his head. "No, it seems clear."

"That broadcast, whatever that was, is everywhere. It's on all the news channels, even young Annabelle just saw it and recognised her dad. We need to get out of here, and fast," Rubin said.

David gestured towards the back garden. "Let's talk out there." The back door was already open.

"Andrea, is Sophie upstairs?" David asked.

Andrea nodded, still locked in an embrace with her husband.

"Good. Keep the girls upstairs. We'll be watching you from the garden."

"Are you going to leave us alone now?"

"Andrea, that's what we are going to determine. Both of you sit tight and don't try to run."

"I believe you have something of mine," Rubin said as they stepped into the garden.

David nodded and handed Rubin's firearm back to him, along with the silencer and spare clips.

"Can you give me back mine?"

Rubin took David's Glock from his belt and handed it to him, along with his car keys and Andrea's phone. "So, I saw the broadcast. How did things go behind the scenes?"

David shrugged. "It looked fine, as far as I could tell. I'll need to contact the client now for further instructions."

"Well, whatever they are, I'll be leaving after this," Rubin replied.

"I know. You've made your feelings clear about that."

"Are you okay? You look like something is bothering you."

David looked Rubin directly in the eyes. "I'm fine, just thinking about a few things."

"Such as?"

"It doesn't matter. We need to clean up. Is the shower area clean? Are the piss bottles and bags still at the end of the garden?"

Rubin nodded.

"We mustn't forget them, along with the towels. I was also in the car for the journey without wearing gloves, so I need to see to that before we head out."

"So, how do you want to handle this?" Rubin asked.

"What do you mean? We're done here."

Rubin laughed and turned around. The couple was sitting on the couch, facing away from them. "We are far from done, and you know it. We need to cover our tracks well, no exceptions. Your car needs to go. I'll be out of the country as soon as I can launder the money. I've cleaned the stair rails, bleached the mugs and sinks, and done everything I can to ensure no fingerprints are left behind."

David nodded, fully understanding what Rubin meant. There was no way the family could be allowed to live. Their faces had been seen, and he suspected Darius would tell him that the family knew too much. "I'll call the client now. We divide the money afterwards."

Rubin nodded and turned back to keep an eye on Andrea and Ryan.

David took his phone from his pocket and stepped a short distance away from Rubin. He dreaded making this call, and the sound of the two girls laughing as they played upstairs didn't help. Lacking a clear understanding of the bigger picture and the situation he and Rubin were involved in, he was unsure how Darius would react to what they had done, mainly if the makeshift lab test produced the results he hoped for. However, the call was answered almost immediately.

"David, I expected to hear from you."

David could tell the phone was on speaker.

"The senior partners and I are delighted."

"That's good to hear, sir. I trust everything was satisfactory?"

"More than satisfactory. The MP took the bait and has made an international embarrassment of herself." Laughter echoed in the background. "I'd say that was a job well done. Please commend your colleague as well."

"Yes, sir, I'll do that," David replied, taking a deep breath and glancing around to ensure Rubin couldn't hear him. "We are almost finished here now. What would you like us to do next?"

There was a pause on the line.

"Sir?"

"I'm surprised you're asking. It's not for me to state the obvious over the phone. You need to complete the task."

"Complete the task, sir?"

"Of course. We can't have anyone else involved."

"But, sir, I can ensure they understand the situation and see the way of things. There are two young girls here…"

"An unfortunate set of circumstances, but your loyalty is to me and this company; everything else is secondary and expendable. Do you understand what I'm saying?" Darius was immediately concerned by the long silence. "David?"

"Yes, sir, I'm here."

"I trust you understand my point. After all, this is your colleague's speciality, isn't it?"

David could hear a couple of snorts in the background as Darius continued.

"Let me make this clear, David. You received a delivery from us, correct?"

David nodded and glanced at Rubin. "Yes, we did."

"And how did you find the contents of that delivery? I trust it was satisfactory..." There was a long pause. "David, there is one and a half million euros in that bag; that amount of cash is not easy to come by these days. I'm sure you'll agree that's far more than your standard rate. The money is for completion; you must have known that when it arrived."

David sighed. "Yes, sir."

"Good! Then complete the task and make merry. I presume the phone line you are using will be deactivated soon?"

"Yes, it will be."

"Good. Please ensure you clean up, leaving no trace behind. We are trusting you!"

"Yes, we'll take care of that."

"Excellent! Outstanding work, David. I will arrange an alternative way for us to communicate in the future, and I will be in touch. I'll contact you via the usual channels when I'm ready. I trust you are satisfied with us as your employer?"

David could sense the grin on Darius's face; he was clearly showing off to whoever else was listening to the call. "Yes, I'm very satisfied."

"Excellent. Then do what needs to be done, and we'll speak again in the future."

The call ended, and David returned the phone to his pocket, closing his eyes.

"So?"

Rubin had noticed him putting the phone away. David turned around and nodded as Rubin removed the handgun from his belt and the silencer from his pocket.

++++

For the past hour, Dr John Farmer had been glued to the news channel. He had received several frantic texts from other junior board members, as their company's name was prominently featured in the news and across all major social media platforms. Sensing the growing panic, he received a group message from Darius. Darius informed them that the company's lawyers would be taking action tomorrow morning and requested that no comments be made to any media, stating that the lawyers would handle all communications. Darius planned to publicly destroy the member of parliament, intending to humiliate her even more than she had already done to herself. He pointed out that there was no evidence to support her claims and assured everyone that business would proceed as usual. Financial markets would be closely monitored, and stock control would track any downturns in business activity. If there was an impact, this would be taken into account in the damages claim against the MP. John suspected that Darius's message had not alleviated the other directors' concerns. They were aware of his plans from the board meeting and recognised that the MP had touched upon something significant, but she had approached it in the wrong way. Now, no one would believe her, and anyone else contemplating making accusations in the future would face similar consequences. Darius would relish the "trial" of Helen Lord, MP, and if he had his way, her downfall would continue to be publicly broadcast.

John reflected on the previous evening when he had a drink with Helen Lord. It was surprising that she attended their event, especially considering what she had planned to do to them today. The lab technician, whoever he was, might also face scrutiny regarding his credibility. John had watched some reruns of the broadcast; the man conducting the test appeared ill at ease and nervous. It seemed he didn't want to be there, which was unusual in itself. Those involved in the news debate questioned who had funded the test: was it the MP or the political party, the same party currently in power? This was a scandal that wouldn't be resolved anytime soon, and somehow, the company of which he was a board member found itself at the centre of it all. If his father were still alive, he wouldn't have supported the new direction that John suspected Darius wanted to take the company. As a medical doctor, John wanted nothing to do with anything illegal. Darius's insatiable appetite for greed and results meant that an addictive beauty filler would only be the beginning, assuming their share price improved. As time passed and profits dwindled, John and the junior board members lost control over the company. If the MP was right, they were shareholders in an enterprise that could potentially put lives at risk.

Suddenly, Lisa's name flashed on his phone screen. None of the other board members had called him, so she must be in a state of panic to warrant a call. He decided to answer.

"John, can you talk?"

It was an unusual opening question, and Lisa sounded nervous. "Yes, I'm at home. Why do you ask?"

"I'm guessing you've seen the news and read the messages?"

"I have the news on screen now. I'm monitoring everything."

"Look, I need to see you."

"Sure, we can catch up during the week. I'm assuming Darius will call a board meeting in…"

"No! Right now. I need to see you immediately!" she pleaded.

"What are you talking about? What's so urgent? Is this related to the news?"

"In a way, but I'm not discussing it over the phone."

John rubbed his head, feeling frustrated. "What's going on? You sound really anxious."

"I'm more than just anxious. I've done something, and…"

"What have you done?"

"I've told you, I can't explain it over the phone. Can you come to my house? We need to talk urgently."

"Bloody hell, Lisa. I'm trying to enjoy my relaxing Sunday, well, I would be, if our name wasn't being blasted all over the news, and I don't even know where you live."

"I'll text you my address. Please come immediately; I can't stress how serious this is."

John had no idea what she was talking about. "Why? Am I in trouble?"

"No, but I think I might be."

John let out a heavy sigh.

"Please, John. This is about to get out of control."

He waved his arms in frustration. "Okay, okay. I'll come to see you. Send me your address, and I'll let you know when I'm on my way."

"Thank you. I really appreciate it. To be honest, I'm not sure what to do."

++++

David quickly put his phone into his pocket, his face a picture of shock. "Wait! What are you doing?"

Rubin, fitting the silencer onto his Smith & Wesson, looked up and paused. "What do you mean?" he shrugged.

"Put the gun away, for God's sake, man! What are you doing?"

"You nodded. This moment had to come eventually. And don't use the Lord's name in vain..."

"No!" David interrupted. "I nodded to confirm that we've reached the end of the task. The client doesn't want them hurt."

"What?" Rubin stepped into David's personal space. "That's a joke, right?"

"No. The client stated they've served their purpose and done what we asked. It's the end of the operation."

"You've got to be shitting me. That's a massive security risk. There's no way I'm letting that happen."

"And I'll remind you, this is my operation, and you are working for me. I'm telling you what the client's orders are."

"Let me tell you something about your so-called client. I'm not an idiot; I can see what's going on here. You switched a vial, and Knightark Pharmaceutical was named in the broadcast. Is that your client? Furthermore, the assassination attempt in London was mentioned as well..."

David looked away, a resigned expression on his face.

"Oh no. You've got to be kidding. That was you!" Rubin practically spat, laughing.

David shrugged. "So?"

"So? You made a complete bollocks of that, from what I've read. Your so-called target is still alive."

David stepped closer to Rubin, their noses nearly touching. "And she shouldn't be. She must have remotely unlocked the car from a distance."

Still holding his weapon, Rubin shook his head, his laughter hollow. "What an absolute mess this is! This is what you've dragged me into! If it had been me, I would have taken out half the bloody block."

"And that's where you and I differ. A target is a target, but I don't believe in getting innocent people hurt."

Rubin's laughter dismissed every word David uttered. "A hired gun with a conscience? That's an absolute joke. This is amateur hour, and I want no part of it. Leaving those people in that room alive shows your lack of judgment."

"We are not killing children!"

Rubin shook his head and sighed. "Okay, they're young. They'll probably forget, so let's take care of the adults then."

"No! Seriously, what's wrong with you?"

"What's wrong with me? What's wrong with you? You've been irritable ever since you came back from London. Think carefully, Alpha bloody 1. They've seen our faces. What are you going to do? Have a harsh conversation with them? Use big boy words and get them to promise not to tell anyone? Because that scenario always works out well!"

"Stop patronising me. That's exactly what I'm going to do. I'll scare them within an inch of their lives, and they will see reason."

Rubin put his hands on his hips and began pacing the garden. Behind him, David noticed the couple in the front room watching them. "Rubin, come here."

"What?"

"Put the gun away, collect the piss bottles, shit bags and bath towels," David's tone shifted to one of authority, growing tired of Rubin's mockery. "I didn't check my car when I returned from London, and I need to make sure it's okay. I'll talk to them while you do a check, and then you can load the car. Once you're done, drive it back here, and I'll meet you with the money."

Rubin shook his head as he put the silencer in his pocket and tucked the gun away in his jacket. He continued to shake his head as he pointed at David. "I'm not happy about this. You are being reckless with our safety. Have you considered the charges we could face if we get caught? Your botched fireworks display in London would come to light as well, leading to an attempted murder charge against you! Authorities must already suspect that someone from our background is responsible for something like that. Seriously, you're attracting attention to all of us. You are being dangerous and careless. This is not how I do things."

David placed a hand on Rubin's shoulder. "You have to trust me. The client is happy, and that's our only concern. I understand that you don't like the situation, but it is what it is. Once we've cleaned up and left the area, I'll drive you wherever you want to go. I'll arrange for my car to be crushed as soon as possible, and we need to keep our contact to a minimum, which means separating the SIM cards from our phones."

"There's no reason for us to communicate any further; my work here is done, and I want no further part of this. I only have one phone with me, and I have calls to make before I return to Nepal."

David stepped back and glared at Rubin. "Oh yes, Nepal, the place where you live a quiet life in worship."

"Are you patronising me? Seriously, what's on your mind? Do you have something to say?"

David shook his head as Rubin confronted him. "Come on, David, tell me what's bothering you, what's going on in that dangerous brain of yours?"

"I have nothing further to say, other than let's finish this up as the operation is over. Will you proceed with the plan I've outlined?"

Rubin stared into David's eyes; they didn't waver. Knowing he hadn't been paid yet, Rubin took a couple of steps back and threw his hands in the air. "You're the boss, and I'm just following orders." He pointed at David. "But I'll tell you this: I respect you because of your background, but I don't like what you're doing. You're being emotional and careless. If I get arrested for anything related to this, there will be no place you can hide. I will find you, no matter where you are!"

David nodded. "I would expect nothing less. Let's gather our things, and I'll go remind the two in the front room of the facts of life."

++++

John unlocked his phone as he started the car. Lisa had texted him her address, and while he entered it into his satnav, he noticed that the drive to her home would take 1.5 hours. Although he didn't know much about his fellow board member, he recognised her as confident, strong, and resolute in her views during meetings. This was the first time he had heard her express any nerves; she didn't seem like someone who would easily overreact. The broadcast by the MP, which named their company and referred to the assassination attempt on the woman from Channel 8, would instil fear in anyone. While he and the other board members needed to handle the situation, all the staff, distributors, manufacturers, and others involved would likely be on edge; effective management was crucial at this time. At that moment, he wasn't sure what role he and the other board members would play in this crisis. The MP had certainly crossed a line with her accusations, particularly concerning the allegation of illegal cosmetic drug manufacturing. He texted Lisa to let her know he was on his way. Whatever was causing her to panic, he was confident they would get to the bottom of it.

++++

Andrea held Ryan's hand tightly as Rubin walked into the front room from the garden. He scowled at them as he passed by and headed into the kitchen. They exchanged worried glances, feeling the unsettling anger emanating from him. David entered the room and took a seat opposite the anxious couple, while Rubin disappeared back into the garden, carrying a couple of empty carrier bags.

David took a deep breath, withdrew his firearm, and placed it on the seat beside him. Ryan's anxiety was palpable; he began to shake with fear. "We did as you asked. You said you were a man of your word!" he exclaimed.

David held a finger to his lips, signalling for them to be quiet.

Rubin re-entered the front room, carrying two heavy-looking carrier bags. "I'll put these in the back of the car," he said, "and I'll grab the towels on the way out; they are already by the front door."

David nodded and held up the car key as Rubin placed the bags down and snatched it from him. Immediately, Andrea coughed and grasped her nose; the smell coming from the carrier bags was overpowering. The three of them sat in silence as Rubin stuffed the wig, glasses, and the moustache into his backpack. "Is this everything? Is there anything else?" he asked.

David shook his head.

Rubin slung the backpack over his shoulder and picked up the carrier bags of excrement. He stepped into the centre of the room and glared at the terrified couple. "My colleague is going to have a little chat with you. Make sure you understand what he says, or I'll be back for all of you."

Andrea gripped Ryan's thigh as Rubin went to the front windows, put the bags down and pulled the net curtain to the side. "It's clear outside. I'll see you in the car, and don't forget the plastic sheet you are sitting on," he said to David before retrieving the bags and leaving the room. The remaining three heard the front door close. David glanced to his right and briefly caught sight of Rubin's outline through the net curtains as he made his way down the driveway.

"He looks angry," Andrea said.

"He is. He's angry with me, and I'm going to explain why." David spoke calmly, maintaining a composed demeanour. "I'll be brief, as I don't have much time. Alpha 2 is upset because he feels you cannot be trusted; therefore, he wants to kill you to protect our identities, which includes your children. I said no."

Ryan immediately flinched and pulled Andrea closer to him.

"Ryan, stay calm. Remember what we discussed," David said, resting his hands on his thighs. "Both of you need to understand that we, as professionals, take our work very seriously. It's crucial that you recognise this, as your future depends on it. Think carefully about this. You won't find people like us online, nor is there a website where you can email to request our services. Protecting ourselves and our clients' interests is paramount, as our clients are extremely important and have significant resources at their disposal. Trust in the private sector is everything; if that trust is broken, someone else will take our place. My client has just instructed me to execute all of you, including Annabelle and Sophie. I lied to Alpha 2 and told him the opposite, that our client said you should live. Alpha 2 is angry because allowing you to live poses a significant security risk for both of us."

Ryan and Andrea exchanged worried glances, but neither of them could find the words to speak.

David continued, "Given the nature of the MP's broadcast and your appearance in it, Ryan, you have now become a person of interest. You need to be prepared for the questions that will come your way. It's also crucial that you remain much calmer than you have been over the past few days. I understand this hasn't been easy for you."

"You can say that again!" Ryan retorted.

"Ryan, be quiet! This is important, and you need to pay attention. Both of you, listen to me very carefully: you need to disappear, and you must do it today."

"What? What do you mean?"

"What I mean, Ryan, is that my client believes you are all dead, and I need it to look that way. However, the reality is that if this were true, and if you don't show up for work tomorrow, this place would soon be crawling with police. Imagine this: you were seen on the broadcast, and then suddenly, your family is found dead. We could make it appear as though it was a suicide, as if you, Ryan, or you, Andrea, were responsible. However, I believe this is not in my client's best interest. A family murdered by their father after appearing on a live feed, for me, raises too many questions that could lead back to us. Therefore, my decision is pragmatic, not emotional, for the sake of everyone involved. My client thinks you are dead, and for now, that is precisely how you need to appear. Ryan, you will be contacted by journalists and others seeking information about your involvement in the makeshift lab test you conducted. As I understand it, you and the MP are prominently featured in the news. You will not be taking any calls, as I will be keeping your phone. In the morning, use Andrea's phone to contact your office and inform your staff that you are taking an unplanned holiday, but do not disclose your destination. Just go. Do not take any photographs or post happy family pictures on social media. All of you need to stay under the radar until this situation calms down. If my client discovers that you are still alive, I will have to address that situation if it arises. Do you both understand the risk I'm taking?

"Um, well. Yes, but where do we go? I'm not..."

"Andrea, that's enough! You stay in the UK and use cash wherever you go."

"Money doesn't grow on trees, you know. What..."

"Andrea, listen!" David picked up his firearm. "All I need to do is place a cushion over the end of this weapon, and it will all be over for you. Do you understand? This is not a negotiation. If I don't believe you right this very second, I'll be calling Alpha 2 back. Trust me, you don't want that; he is not as pragmatic as I am." David leaned back in the seat and placed the gun by his side, his fingers lightly stroking the firearm. "I'm guessing you know that we are former soldiers, right?"

"Um... yes, that had occurred to us," Ryan replied.

"Good. It doesn't matter what regiment we're from, but what do soldiers have?"

The nervous couple exchanged uncertain glances, unsure of how to respond.

"Numbers. We have numbers. You may not like what we've done to you, but I've decided to let you live. You will go and enjoy your lives. Do something good, achieve things, and earn what has been given to you. Do you understand?"

"Yes," they both replied.

"But make no mistake. If you go to the police or let even the slightest thing slip to anyone, there will be severe consequences. As soon as I step out of this door, I will share your names, along with those of your children, with my colleagues. I will also provide your home address and all other information I have about you. There will be no snitching, no running, and no witness protection program. Alpha 2 lives in another country, and his job is to hunt down people like you who have been given a chance and failed. There is nowhere you can hide; we will always find you, and you will never know when or where it will happen. If you fail us, your children will be executed right in front of you, before the blade is turned upon both of you. This is your only chance. Never betray us, or everything and everyone you care about will be taken away, one by one, piece by piece. Do you understand everything I've said?" David picked up the firearm as the couple nodded their heads, tears welling in Andrea's eyes.

"Good. Never forget this day. Do what you are told, and we will never have to meet again. Understand?"

Ryan's quiet response of "yes" was little more than a whisper.

"I have a bag upstairs that I need, and then I'll be leaving," David said. He stood up, tucked the firearm into his trouser belt, removed the plastic sheet he'd been sitting on and headed upstairs to Annabelle's bedroom.

"Hello, Alpha 1," Annabelle greeted him as he entered the room. "Where has your funny, fancy dress gone? I liked you like that; you're funny."

David gave Annabelle a brief smile, folded up the plastic sheet and bent down to retrieve his bag from under the bed.

"Are you going now?" Annabelle asked while her younger sister played alongside her with their dollhouse.

"Yes, I need to be on my way," David replied.

"Will we see you again?"

David paused momentarily. "I hope not." Hearing a car outside, he made his way downstairs, entered the front room, and peered through the net curtain. Rubin was reversing up the driveway.

"Alright, listen to me, both of you," David said firmly as he put on his cap. "Annabelle talks a lot. Make sure she forgets about us, or I'll be back. Do you understand?" He received two nods in response. "Andrea, please see me to the door and bring a cleaning spray and a cloth."

Rubin parked directly behind Ryan's car, leaving the engine running. He was furious with David; his recent decision-making had been unprofessional, and his attitude had seemed off since returning from London. As he glanced over his shoulder, Rubin noticed the front door open as David stepped outside with Andrea. Andrea held a cloth and a spray bottle, following David's instructions to spray and wipe down the passenger door handle. Rubin observed as David handed Andrea Ryan's car keys. He watched over her as she cleaned both the passenger side of Ryan's car and the keys, removing any prints. David returned Andrea's phone, and they had a brief verbal exchange that made Rubin feel uneasy. He pressed against his jacket to ensure his firearm was easily accessible.

With the money bag in hand, David started walking toward the car just as the front door closed behind him. Rubin kept one hand near his firearm; something didn't feel right. There was no good reason for David to be talking to Andrea as much as he had been. He'd better have made things clear; they needed to leave quickly.

As David got into the car, he tossed the plastic sheet and money bag onto the back seat. Rubin immediately locked eyes with him.

"What did you say to her?"

David frowned. "When?"

"Just now, as she was cleaning your prints off Ryan's car. What did you say to her?"

"Nothing of note. I was making sure they understood the facts of life."

"You should have done that inside the house. You'd better be right about this, brother. This is a risk we don't need to take."

"Trust me. They'll be fine."

Rubin put the car into gear and took hold of the steering wheel. "Where to?"

David glanced back at the house, hoping he wouldn't have to return. "Anywhere but here."

Without hesitation, Rubin pressed the accelerator.

As Andrea watched their captors leave through the window, she sprinted up the stairs and rushed into Annabelle's room, falling to her knees. She wrapped her arms around Sophie and broke down in tears.

"Mummy, what's the matter?" Annabelle asked, embracing her mother. Ryan burst into the room, and amidst the flood of tears, they all hugged tightly.

"Here, take Sophie," Andrea said, passing their daughter to Ryan. She then shuffled on her knees towards Annabelle's bed.

"What are you doing?" Ryan asked.

"Something he said to me just before he left," Andrea replied, gasping as she pulled multiple bundles of euros from under the bed. "Oh my God!"

Ryan set Sophie down and stared in shock at the money strewn across the bedroom floor. "What did he say to you?" he asked.

"Something about paying for our silence and helping us disappear," Andrea said, shaking her head. "There must be a couple of hundred thousand euros here!"

Chapter Twenty-Nine

The satnav's calculations were reasonably accurate. It had taken John nearly an hour and a half to reach Lisa's address in Surrey, located on the southwestern side of London. As he approached the security barrier of the gated estate, he slowed; it was evident that anyone living here had to be wealthy.

A uniformed security officer walked up to John's car and signalled for him to stop. Cameras were mounted on the security hut next to the barrier, and the guard was also equipped with a body camera.

"Good afternoon, sir. How may I help you?" he asked while holding his phone.

"Good afternoon. I'm here to see Lisa Wellings; I believe she lives on Chatsworth Rise in this estate."

The security guard nodded and began to scroll through his phone. "May I have your name, please?"

"Dr John Farmer," he replied.

"Do you have any identification?"

John smiled, "Really?"

"Yes, sir," the guard insisted.

John raised his eyebrows, finding it somewhat inconvenient to reach someone's house. One might think the residents had something to hide or were afraid of something. He unclipped his seatbelt and took his wallet from his jacket. "I've got a bank card. Will that work?"

"It will for today, sir, but if you plan to return, a photographic ID would be better, like a passport or a driving license," the guard replied. He took John's card, studied it for a moment, and then handed it back to him. "Your car's license plate has been recorded, which will make your departure easier."

John smiled and put his bank card back in his wallet.

"Go through the barrier; it's the first turning on the right."

"Okay, thank you," John said, feeling bemused by the strict measures in place to enter the upscale housing estate as he re-clipped his seatbelt.

The security guard nodded to his colleague in the hut, and the barrier was raised. "Have a nice day, sir."

"Thank you," John replied. With his company's name all over the news and no idea why he was here, he realised a pleasant day would have to wait for another time.

As he drove under the barrier, it lowered immediately behind him, granting him a clear view of the properties within the gated community. The estate was filled with numerous relatively new constructions. While the buildings were impressive in size, they lacked the character he would have preferred. Nevertheless, it resembled a showcase for millionaires. John smiled to himself at the thought of the phrase "keeping up with the Joneses." Every lawn was immaculate, and each driveway displayed an extravagant collection of vehicles. Lisa's Maserati would have been one of the more affordable luxury vehicles among those he was currently witnessing. He smiled to himself, imagining the local committees gossiping if someone's hedge became unruly.

He turned onto Chatsworth Rise and shook his head. This way of living wasn't for him; it felt like a gaudy display of wealth tucked inside a security bubble. Lisa's house was at number eight, and he recognised her car as he pulled up outside. The security guards must have informed her of his arrival, as her security gates opened immediately for him. He drove through and parked behind her car. She was already waiting for him at the front door, and even from a distance, John could sense her nerves as he stepped out of the car.

"Thank you so much for coming," she called from the front door.

John nodded as he approached her, pressing the lock button on his car remote.

"Don't worry about that too much; it's reasonably safe around here," she reassured him.

"I guess living behind security gates helps with that."

Lisa smiled, "Yeah, you've got me there. Come on in," she said, leading him through to the spacious kitchen. John noticed an open gin bottle on the counter and a few empty tonic cans next to the sink.

"Are you here by yourself?" he asked.

"Yes, my wife is at the gym."

"I didn't know you were married."

"Why should I have mentioned it?"

John grinned. "No, it's just that I don't know much about you."

"And I don't know much about you, either. I keep my private life private. Care for a drink?"

"Sure, but I'm driving," he said.

"You can stay here if you want. There's plenty of room."

John didn't doubt that; Lisa's house was huge. He nodded and walked over to the folding doors at the back of the kitchen. "Lovely garden," he remarked.

"Thank you. Would you like a gin and tonic?"

"Yes, thank you. Maybe you can tell me why I'm here. You sounded nervous on the phone."

Lisa took a couple of cans of tonic from the fridge. "We'll get to that. And yes, you're right; I'm very nervous."

A news channel played in the background, and the MP was still dominating the headlines on television. "I'm guessing this is what it's about," John said, pointing at the screen.

Lisa pressed the mute button on the remote. "Yes, in a way. It's all connected."

"Couldn't we have discussed this over the phone to save me the trip?"

Lisa placed her hands on the kitchen table and took a deep breath. "No, definitely not. Look, I know this may sound like a strange question, but are you recording this conversation?"

"What!" John laughed. "Why would I do that?" He nodded as Lisa handed him a glass, which he took a sip from; she had poured him a generous measure.

"It's just that you're the only person I can talk to about this. I haven't even mentioned it to Becky."

John's puzzled expression indicated he didn't know who she was referring to.

"My wife. I don't even know if I can tell her."

"And why would that be?"

Lisa lowered her glass. "I've done something, and I had no idea what it would lead to… but…"

"And what is it? Go on, what have you done?" John pressed.

"I'm telling you because I believe you share my values. I can't be involved in this."

"Involved in what, Lisa? You're not making any sense."

"What do you mean, what? What Darius and the senior board have been scheming. What do you think I'm talking about?"

Lisa's sudden outburst immediately concerned John. She was agitated, twiddling her hair and struggling to maintain eye contact.

"Look, John. You're a doctor. You can't condone what they are planning to do. It's ethically wrong on all levels."

"I agree, but we haven't been given all the details. I suspect only the four senior board members know the full extent of it. I intend to find out more before making any further decisions about this so-called *'ultimate filler,'*" John said sarcastically, attempting to mock Darius. He took a sip of his gin and tonic and placed a hand in his pocket as he continued, "I must concede that cosmetic surgery is still in its early stages. We don't know what the long-term effects might be, if any. This is potentially a dangerous business from a health standpoint, and I'm well aware of that."

"Yes, possibly, but hopefully, with time, there will be innovations. I'm all for that. I have no objections to people wanting to improve themselves."

"Sorry to correct you, Lisa, but from a doctor's perspective, they are not necessarily improving themselves; they are changing the way they look, or trying to recapture lost youth."

"Yes, okay. You know what I mean, and many would disagree

with you, by the way. But I don't want to be associated with this and what Darius alluded to. Addictive surgery? Come on, what's your take on it?"

John lowered his glass. "I agree with you, I do, but it's complicated. This is my father's legacy. He brought me into the company, and I was only promoted to the board after he passed away."

"Were you aware of the new 'science' they've been developing?"

"No! Of course not."

"Then you are trusted as little as I am." Lisa swallowed the contents of her glass. "I'm thinking of resigning from the board."

"Oh, wait a second. We're all over the news. Stepping down now could be…"

"Dangerous? You must have heard what that MP said; she practically linked us to an assassination attempt!"

John raised his hands in a calming gesture. "I know, I know. I've been thinking about my shares as well."

"And what would you do with them, sell them? That would make you as bad as the rest of them, knowing the epidemic they're trying to create if my worst fears are true."

"It's just that my father had a good relationship with Darius. Although he was much younger than my father, they had an understanding; it was Ronald he was especially close with."

"And if he were alive, would your father have supported this?"

John sighed and set his glass aside. "You still haven't said why I'm here."

"No, I know," Lisa said as she poured herself another measure of gin, adding very little tonic. "Okay, okay," she held up her hands. "Look, on this estate, we have a guy who keeps an eye on things for everyone. He's ex-police and not quite as law-abiding since he retired, but he's the go-to guy if there are break-ins or if people are having extramarital affairs, you know. A lot of that goes on around here; too much money leads to boredom. Anyway, he does a bit of private detective work, and I kind of met with him."

John shrugged. "Kind of? You either did or you didn't."

Lisa ran her fingers through her hair. "Well, you know, last night at Parliament…"

"Yes, what about it?"

"Well, I… I just wanted to find out what was going on. I had already made up my mind to step away from the company. Our senior board, along with those politicians, are up to something. I know it, and you know it. So I thought I'd do a little snooping."

John frowned and tried to make eye contact with Lisa. "What have you done?"

"Well, you know those picture frames I gave to Hawthorne and Gatesouth?"

John laughed as he picked up his glass. "Yeah, those monstrosities," he said, taking a sip of his gin. "What about them?"

"Well, they weren't just picture frames."

"What do you mean?"

"They had pinhole cameras hidden in them; the ex-police guy made them for me."

John's expression shifted to horror as he set his glass down. "You what?"

"Yep. That's what I did. I was just curious, you see. I never could have anticipated what would happen."

"You put hidden cameras in the Houses of Parliament!"

"To be honest, I thought they would just throw them away. They did, but... well... I think you should see. Follow me into the front room."

++++

Seeing a layby up ahead, David nudged Rubin. "Pull in there; I'll take over driving."

They were on a narrow lane with little traffic, over twenty miles away from the Dobey household, and barely a word had been exchanged between them.

Once Rubin pulled over, they switched seats, and David resumed driving. "Where do you want me to drop you off?"

"Back where we first met, by the lake, is fine. I'll make my way from there."

"Alright, that's not far from here."

Rubin noticed the stern look on David's face and sensed the tension during the drive. "What's bothering you? You seem arsey."

"I'm fine."

"If you say so. But I'm telling you, I'm not happy. We should have cleaned up back there, and you know it."

"I told you, it was the client's decision. I wasn't going to overrule them."

"They'll talk once the dust settles and normality returns, and then the cleanup becomes harder. I trust that you've ensured they understand."

David chose to ignore Rubin's comments; he wanted to avoid that conversation again. "How long are you going to be in the country?" he asked.

"A couple of days at most. I need to get to my unit, drop off my gear, sort out the money, and arrange my travel. I don't plan on being back here for a while."

"Well, the money you've earned should be appreciated by your temple and your God-fearing friends."

Rubin grunted under his breath. "And where are you headed?" he asked.

"I'm going fishing. I want to spend a couple of days in peace."

Rubin laughed out loud, shaking his head. "What a waste of time. You go fishing to catch a fish, then release it? You don't even eat it. What's the point? You might as well take up golf, another pointless pursuit for the mindless."

"You have your beliefs, and I have mine. We all handle things differently in this line of work. It's important to take a step back and reflect; it always helps you improve."

"I understand where you're coming from, but honestly, your time could be spent more productively."

"Oh, like you! Worshipping a god to cleanse yourself of your past."

"Seriously, what's gotten into you? What's with all the jabs?"

"I told you, I'm fine. Just reach into the bag in the back and split the money. There's a lot more there than I expected."

"That suits me just fine. I'll need this in case that family back there decides to talk."

David closed his eyes, knowing he'd had enough of Rubin and would be glad to be rid of him. He wouldn't be at the top of the list if he needed assistance in the future.

"When are you ditching this car?" Rubin asked.

"I'm going to contact the breakers later. The car will be crushed, along with Ryan's phone, the piss bottles, and everything else that needs to go."

"Do you trust the breakers?"

David nodded. "I've used them before."

"And what about your little jaunt into London a few days ago with your fubar explosive device? How can you be sure you're clear of that?"

David sighed and glared at Rubin. "I've been doing this job for a long time. It was planned, recce'd, and measures were taken. I don't need to explain them to you, as it doesn't concern you."

Rubin nodded, "If you say so, but it's all connected. If the police get onto you, that could lead back to me."

"I'll never talk. You know that."

"Let's hope so." Rubin leaned over to the back seat and dragged the money bag toward him.

"We're not far away. Can you put your cut in your backpack?"

Rubin grinned. "You weren't joking; there's a lot here. Yes, I'll make space in my pack."

"There's enough there to build a new temple. Nepal, right?"

Rubin immediately stopped counting the bundles. "Why would you ask that? You know it is."

He could sense that David was still brooding over something.

David nodded, "If you say so."

Whatever was on David's mind, his remarks were frequent and

irritating. Rubin chose not to press the issue any further and continued counting the money.

++++

"Please take a seat while I turn on the TV," Lisa said.

John settled onto the plush white leather settee as Lisa picked up the remote and switched on the television. "I had one pinhole camera set into each picture frame, both equipped with picture and audio recording. I paid the ex-copper to keep the picture frames, knowing I'd never get them back. He then matched them to an app on my phone…"

John rolled his eyes. "That's why you kept checking your phone last night."

"Yes, I was just checking to see if they were working. This morning, I downloaded the video file onto the TV. One of the picture frames was tossed into the bin in Lord Gatesouth's office. Although the camera in the bin was still operational, it only recorded the inside view, and the sounds it captured were barely audible. The other picture frame Gatesouth dropped on his desk, which meant it only showed the ceiling, but the audio picked up everything clearly. From what I can tell, Gatesouth was at his desk for a while, working on his computer. You can't see him on screen because of the awkward camera angle, but after some time, he gets up just as someone enters the room. That's when things start to get interesting. You'll need to see it for yourself."

Lisa selected the file on the television and sped it up. "As you can see," she pointed at the screen, "the ceiling looks typical for the Lords. You see a shadow pass by; that's Gatesouth heading to the door. The voices are initially muffled; he offers his guest a drink, and that's where it really picks up…"

> *"Well, do come in, old boy. Care for a brandy?"*
> *"Thank you. A large one is needed."*

An arm passed in front of the camera lens as a drink was handed to the guest.

"Rare for you to be down here, you sure you're not lost!" Lord Gatesouth laughed.

"Owen, I have a favour to ask. You have a very close relationship with Sebastian."

"The Chief Whip? I suppose I've never really thought about it."

"But he admires you,"

A snort of laughter escaped from the Peer. "What do you need me to do, Alix?"

"Wait, who's talking to Gatesouth?" John asked. "Is that who I think it is?"

Lisa nodded and took a seat. "Yes, it's the Prime Minister."

"Blimey!"

"I need her gone."

"Who? Alix, what's troubling you?"

"Helen Lord, I need her gone."

Owen Gatesouth laughed. "She's a pain in your side; I know that much. But why?"

"It's complicated."

"Politics always is, old boy. Try me."

"I want her out of the party. I need you to speak to Seb and set him straight."

"Alix, you're the leader of the bloody party. If you told him, he'd listen to you!"

"I can't risk it. If it ever got out that I was pressuring to have the whip withdrawn from one of our own party members, it would cause significant damage."

"Surely, you can trust Seb. You appointed him, after all."

"These walls have too many ears, Owen. Please, do this for me."

There was a brief pause. Owen let out a deep breath. "Okay, I'll call him tomorrow. However, I must tell you, Alix, it won't be as easy as that. I'm not aware that she's done anything serious enough to have the whip removed, she's just a pain in your ass, and that's all."

"That may be true, but he has a meeting with her on Monday morning, and he needs to take action and push her. Her behaviour draws too much attention and upsets people who are beneficial to us."

"Oh… so it's like that."

"Yes, it's exactly like that."

Lord Gatesouth laughed. "What do they have on you? There's always something in this place."

"I don't want to talk about it."

"We've known each other for years, Alix. What could it possibly be?"

Alix sighed. "No one knows this, not even my wife."

"Okay. I understand. What you share with me will remain confidential."

"It has to, I'm serious, I'm not pissing about!" There was a brief pause before Alix continued. "There was an incident while I was in college, a serious one that involved me. At a young age, my political ambitions were already known, at least in some circles. The incident was significant, people were hurt, and it has scarred me ever since."

"Okay, this is news to me, Alix, but many things happen in college. Boys will be boys, and all that. Besides, it would have shown up on your record in your early days in the party. You couldn't have gotten as far as you have if there were a serious issue."

"Well, that's the problem, and why this is tricky. I was assisted. It was covered up."

"Christ, Alix,"

The camera shook as a glass slammed down onto the desk.

"You know, I was joking when I said, 'What have they got on you?'" There was a long pause. "Honestly, this bloody place… if it's not rent boys, it's payoffs; if it's not cash for questions, it's people trying to buy their way in here, and if it's none of those, we are

sending millions abroad to some bloody pisspot place that no one cares about!"

"As I said, I've told you this in confidence, Owen."

"And it will stay that way! But it sounds like it's being used against you, which means you've got a problem for life. I don't want to know any more about it."

A ping echoed in the background, like an email being received. "What is it now?"

Lord Gatesouth's face appeared on the screen; he looked like he was reading from a computer.

"It's nothing," he grumbled, immediately glancing down. "And as for this piece of crap..."

There was a close-up of a hand moving swiftly, followed by a crash, then the camera and audio cut out.

"And that's when I think the picture frame was thrown in the bin, along with the other one."

John had already set his glass down, and he now had his head in his hands. "Holy shit, Lisa, what the hell have you done?"

"Like I said, I didn't mean it!"

"Didn't mean it? This could potentially incriminate the Prime Minister!"

Lisa waved her hands in the air, stood up, and went to the kitchen to refill her glass. "Do you want another one?"

John's head was still in his hands. "I have no idea."

Lisa quickly returned to the room with a full glass. "I know. That's what I thought when I saw it."

"Do you understand what would happen to you if this became known? You'd have the security services all over you!"

"Well, yes, I figured that out. That's why I didn't want to discuss it over the phone."

"Blimey. You're right to be nervous. This is incredibly incendiary. If this were to get out, the Prime Minister would have nowhere to turn. This could collapse the entire government, a sitting Prime

Minister admitting to being involved in a cover-up." John paused to gather his thoughts. "But a cover-up of what, exactly?"

"I have no idea, and that's why I called you. I have no one else to talk to about this."

"Jesus, Lisa. I don't think you should be discussing this with anyone."

"You can't ignore what you just saw."

"Yes, I can!"

"Gatesouth, who is on our payroll, can be seen on camera. Did you notice that neither our company nor Darius was mentioned at all?"

"So?"

"Well, I'm considering what to do with it."

John stood up. "You mean whether you should do anything with it? This puts you in danger!"

"Listen to me, John. I'm being honest about my decision to resign. What would happen if this were leaked? For many, I've done a public service by exposing this."

"If it leaks, they will know you planted those cameras. It won't take long for Gatesouth to figure it out. He'll remember throwing that picture away."

"Maybe. Maybe not. Look at how much he was drinking last night."

"In any case, I'm not sure this proves anything. You don't see Alix Gregory on screen. He'll claim it's a fake. We don't know what this cover-up is."

"No, you're right; we don't have that information. But Darius does. Don't fool yourself, John. Darius is the person Alix was referring to. Don't you remember? They attended the same college. This recording was made last night, and the Prime Minister even attended our little shindig, and at the weekend, no less. I'm convinced that Darius either invited him or instructed him to be there."

"I don't know, Lisa; this feels a bit far-fetched."

"I don't believe it's a coincidence. Darius has deep connections within the government. He's about to distribute what we suspect is a highly illegal drug, and he's manipulating politicians to take care of his problems. When you think about it, it's perfect. This is why he feels so untouchable and displays such arrogance. If you get in his way, he knows how to handle it. This is Darius in full effect, and he has the bloody Prime Minister of all people cleaning up for him. Just look at what we've seen. That MP we spoke to last night, what's her name again?... Oh, yes, Helen Lord. The footage clearly shows they want to push her out. And why? Because she's a vocal campaigner against what we do, and all of this happened right before she went out on a limb online earlier today."

John grabbed his glass and began pacing back and forth.

"John, listen to me, this is really important. Think about what has happened to the two people who have been the most outspoken against the cosmetic trade. One of them, as we've just witnessed, is being pushed out, and after today's broadcast, she definitely will be. The other nearly died just a few days ago."

John finished his drink, nearly coughing from swallowing it too quickly. "We are not involved in this! We did not know of any of it!"

"But that's not true, is it? The MP mentioned the lab in Brazil, and we know that it was established a couple of years ago."

"Oh, come on! We had no idea what they were doing there."

"I know that, but who will believe us in the court of public opinion?"

John sighed and set his glass down. He glanced at Lisa before starting to pace the room again.

"You see what I mean? We could be implicated in all of this," Lisa added. "I think this needs to be leaked to protect us."

"You think bringing down a Prime Minister and potentially causing a governmental collapse will protect us?"

Lisa pointed at the television screen. "Imagine the consequences if anyone found out we had seen this."

Her nerves were evident as John watched gin spill over the sides of Lisa's glass. "Look! I need time to think about this. We mustn't make snap judgments…"

"How much time do you think we have? We're all over the news, John; it's only a matter of time before journalists and others start trying to contact us. Our names and faces are prominently featured on the company website. I didn't sign up for this, and neither did you! This company is playing dangerous games that are steeped in corruption."

Lisa stopped speaking when she heard her phone sound in the kitchen. "And here it starts!" She paused at the lounge door just as John's phone buzzed in his pocket.

John read the message aloud: "It's a group text from Darius. In light of recent developments, blah, blah, he's essentially advising us not to worry, not to post anything online, and not to speak to any media outlets. Our lawyers are apparently going to start working first thing in the morning to put a stop to Helen Lord, the soon-to-be former MP. The company will release a press statement in the morning. Business as usual."

Lisa nodded. "See what I mean? He's got it all figured out. I need another drink."

Chapter Thirty

Perched on the edge of the hotel bed, Helen had not taken her eyes off the news channel for the last couple of hours. It was still too early in the evening for the channel to show early-release copies of the following day's newspaper headlines. However, judging by the uproar she was currently witnessing, it was likely that she would be featured prominently in the national news, her image splashed across the headlines. Armchair critics were voicing their opinions, and the host was reading their messages. Surprisingly, a few supportive comments had come through, though they were few and far between. She still had Alison's USB drive, containing all the 'evidence,' but she suspected that no one would take it seriously anymore. Was the situation a matter for the police to handle? Possibly, but her actions earlier in the day could prejudice any investigation. There was also the issue of the whistleblower and his disappearance. He had claimed to work in the lab, a fact that could be verified if he was telling the truth, but with his disappearance, she doubted it would even be looked into now.

She turned off the television and buried her head in her hands. Aside from the noise of the busy street outside, this felt like the only moment of peace she would have for some time. Whether she liked it or not, she would have to face the Chief Whip tomorrow. She knew she had to attend; otherwise, her absence would be seen as contemptible, potentially leading to her being ousted from her position. Deep down, she recognised that her actions would probably result in expulsion from the party, and the Prime Minister, along with a few others, would likely be pleased to see her go. A larger question loomed: would she face a parliamentary ban? Her actions could easily be interpreted as bringing the House into disrepute. Whatever was about to happen was now out of her hands. The question for her was whether to act first: change her political party allegiance and "cross the floor," stand as an independent MP, or resign. Changing parties went against her principles and political beliefs. Furthermore, there was no guarantee that any other party would accept her membership at this moment. More importantly, the trial by media and the reaction from her constituents would likely force a by-election, meaning she would have to campaign again. That would be an inevitable disaster, especially considering the comments she had just heard. She could only imagine what her Wikipedia page was saying right now, probably being updated by the minute.

Her thoughts were interrupted by the ringing of the phone in the room. Her mobile had been switched off for some time, and the flashing button on the hotel phone indicated a call from reception. Helen let out a deep sigh; this couldn't be good. Feeling compelled to answer, she picked up the receiver.

"Yes?"

"Helen, good evening. It's John Clifford from the London Definitive. I wondered if you would be interested in an interview."

Helen immediately hung up the phone and went over to the window. Below her, journalists were gathering. The receptionist must have informed the press that she was staying there.

✣✣✣✣

"Would you like another one?" Lisa asked, holding up the nearly empty bottle of gin. "I have another one in the cupboard."

John shook his head. "No, I need to drive back soon."

"I mentioned you could stay. You're welcome to use one of the spare rooms. Becky won't mind," Lisa said, glancing at the clock on the wall. "In fact, she'll probably be back shortly."

"No, thank you. I'll head back," John replied.

"It's up to you, but I'll need to discuss this with her anyway."

"Do you think that's necessary?"

Lisa nodded. "Yes, I believe it is. I'll need her perspective; this could put both of us in the literal firing line."

John looked slightly taken aback. "Well, only if it gets out!"

"Come on, John, it has to come out. We can't keep this to ourselves!" Lisa set the bottle aside and placed her hands on her hips.

"Lisa, you only got that footage by pure chance. You need to be careful and think about your safety. You're not an investigative journalist. What do you plan to do with it? Please don't make the same mistake that the MP did by broadcasting it worldwide for everyone to see."

Lisa laughed, "You know, I just realised something. I guess that means I've now got the Prime Minister by the balls. I wonder what he would do for me?" She smiled as she grabbed the bottle and poured the remaining gin into her glass.

"Seriously, don't even joke about that. I wouldn't want to mess with those people. You'll have spooks everywhere before you know it. They could plant something illegal on your computer and then come in and seize everything. I'm telling you, they have the means to make things happen that never really did."

"Well, they don't have what I have," Lisa replied.

"And that's exactly what worries me about you."

"And you, now that you've seen it," she added.

John sighed, "Oh yeah, thanks for that, by the way. Look, before I head back, what are you planning to do?"

"I've decided to speak to Becky about it. I think I need to. After that, I'm not sure yet."

"I'm not sure if that bottle was full when you started today, but you've had the better part of a bottle of gin. Please do not make any rash decisions or talk to anyone else until you have a clear head. It's easy to feel brave right now, but you might regret it later."

Lisa nodded, "I know. I'm not an idiot."

"I didn't say that. It's just that your nerves seem to have calmed since I've been here, or maybe it's the gin. But please, don't do anything this evening. Our name is all over the news, and this will only add fuel to the fire. If I were you, I'd wait to see what the fallout is from all of this. As it stands, things might settle down in a day or so. If you release that recording, it will drag on for weeks. You need to think about that. You asked me to come over, and this is the advice I'm giving you."

Lisa nodded. "You aren't going to tell anyone about this, are you? I'm trusting you."

"Pah!" John shook his head. "Now I know you're drunk! I'm not sure I want any part of this."

"You've been a board member longer than I have, and your father was a member before you."

"My father was involved with this company long before its focus changed to cosmetic products supporting non-essential surgeries. If he were alive, he'd be furious about the current state of things and the company name being dragged through the mud. In some ways, I'm relieved he's not here to see this."

"Okay," Lisa nodded. "I promise I won't do anything this evening, and as I said, I need to run this by Becky first anyway."

"Alright, I'd be interested to hear what she has to say. Hopefully, she'll talk some sense into you."

Lisa smiled and finished her drink.

"I'd better get going. We'll talk in the morning, yes?"

"Yeah, we can do that. I have no doubt we'll hear from Darius first thing."

John nodded. "I'm certain of it. Just imagine his reaction if he finds out about this!"

++++

MONDAY MORNING

While it wasn't technically a press pack, a considerable number of journalists and photographers were eagerly waiting outside Helen's hotel. They anticipated that she would eventually have to leave, and any photos they captured could be syndicated globally. For the photographers, this could lead to a significant payday. On any other day, Helen would have walked to Westminster, as it was only a short distance away. However, knowing that she would be bombarded with a slew of questions, she decided to call for a taxi. With her phone in hand, she awaited the text message confirmation that the cab had arrived. Standing behind the curtains, she kept a close watch outside. Once the cab pulled up, she planned to make a quick exit. Avoiding the cameras would be impossible. She had thought about slipping out through the rear doors, but that would require careful planning. Since the receptionist or another staff member had likely disclosed her location, exiting from the back would only attract more negative attention if the press were tipped off again. Trying to evade the cameras and then getting caught would only escalate the story. Additionally, she was still wearing the same clothing from the broadcast, which was sure to attract unwanted attention and comments. An hour earlier, she had taken the risky step of turning on her phone, only to regret it quickly. A flood of abusive messages had come in, just as she had expected, some from members of her party and others from journalists seeking a comment. What she really wanted to know was whether the Chief Whip had postponed their meeting, but he hadn't. Joanne, her assistant, had texted to check on her well-being, as her phone had also been ringing constantly. Helen had become the current hot topic, and everyone wanted a piece of her.

A text message from the cab company appeared on the screen. Spotting a black cab pulling up outside, Helen quickly grabbed her bags and hurried out of her hotel room. She chose not to wait for the elevator and instead took the fire exit stairwell, rushing down three flights of stairs. When she reached the door leading to the reception area, she peered through the glass and saw that they were waiting for her. She hoped her near-sprint would catch them off guard. Taking a deep breath, knowing that the next few minutes would likely be all over the news, she pushed against the door, practically threw her hotel key card at the reception desk, and bolted for the main entrance.

"Helen! Helen!" shouted voices from all directions.

Spotting another taxi approaching, she prayed she would get into the right one; getting into the wrong cab would be highly embarrassing and could fuel the headlines about to be written about her. As she dashed toward the cab, shouts erupted around her, and photographers with multiple flashguns illuminated her face. With no door staff to assist her, she had to push past a few of the photographers.

"Helen! Is your position untenable?"

"Are you going to resign, Helen?"

"Accusing a company of criminal activity, what do you have to say, Helen?"

A couple of cameras were thrust into her face, one flash dazzling her eyes. "Please let me pass; I'll issue a statement later," Helen said, but her words did little to deter the eager paparazzi.

"Come on, Helen, can we have an interview?"

She reached the taxi, and the driver's window was already open. "Is this a taxi for Helen?" she urged.

The driver looked perplexed. "Yes, it is."

"Thank God!" she exclaimed as she pulled open the door, threw her bags onto the seat, and quickly slammed the door shut. "Parliament, please, if you would drive quickly." Helen continued to look ahead, trying to maintain a resolute expression as the cameras recorded her. She let out a massive sigh of relief as the taxi finally pulled away. Once they were a considerable distance from the commotion, she turned around to see if she was being followed. They didn't seem to be, and she slumped into the seat, taking some deep breaths.

"So, who are you then?" the driver asked.

Helen looked at him, "What do you mean?"

"I mean, who are you? All the press back there, are you an actor or a criminal or something?"

Helen glanced out of the back window once more; it seemed they were clear of anyone following them.

"So?" he prompted.

"Um, no. I'm a politician."

"Ah, so I was right; you're all bloody criminals!" he joked.

Helen locked eyes with him in the rear-view mirror, but his joke fell flat. He looked away, a bit embarrassed.

"I'm an MP, which is why we're going to the palace. Look, I know it's a hassle, but can you drive me inside? I don't want to loiter at the front gates; I know the taxi will need to be scanned underneath as we go in."

"The meter is running, so no, I don't mind. You want to be dropped off outside Westminster Hall?"

"Yes, please. That would be perfect."

"I was only joking before. When you mentioned Parliament, I figured you might be an MP, but I don't recall seeing that amount of press reporters before, which is why I asked if you were an actor or something. You're famous!" He laughed.

"Not by design." She glanced back as they drove around Parliament Square. Police officers were stationed outside the entrance gates, and the sight of a few photographers made her heart sink. She pulled her identification from her bag. "Hey, there are cameras outside. I know it's tricky, but if you can get us in as soon as possible, please."

"That will depend on the police. Do you have your ID ready?"

"I do." At least the driver understood the protocol; he had probably dropped off MPs many times before. Helen knew, as all politicians did, that many press members, especially photographers, tended to work together. Those waiting outside would already know she was arriving in a black cab. Sure enough, as the taxi pulled in, three photographers surrounded the vehicle. Two of them shouted, trying to elicit a reaction from her. A police officer pushed one photographer aside as Helen held her ID up at the window. The officer recognised her, and the gates were opened, and he waved them through. It could have been worse.

"I mean no offence, but I don't recognise you," the taxi driver said as they approached vehicle control.

"It happens," Helen replied. Just twenty-four hours ago, most people didn't know who she was; only those who followed politics or were involved in her campaign did.

"So, why is there so much interest in you? If you don't mind me asking," the cab driver inquired.

"Oh, I don't know. I might have accused a pharmaceutical company of being drug peddlers," she said casually.

As they came to a stop at vehicle control, the cab driver turned around, his eyes wide in disbelief. "You did bloody what?"

One of the security officers at the search control gave her a slight smile as he walked around to her side of the taxi with a search mirror. Helen couldn't tell if his smile was patronising or not, but she knew she wouldn't be seeing too many of those today.

++++

Helen had walked the length of Westminster Hall almost every day since being elected as the member of parliament for Shrewsbury in Shropshire. Today, however, the sheer size of the hall felt overwhelming. Everywhere she turned, she sensed the weight of scrutiny; every whispered comment seemed directed at her. Though she wanted to head straight to her office, the thought of navigating the bustling hub of Portcullis House filled her with dread. At this early hour, the floor would be teeming with people working on the estate. Still, she felt a strong urge to get her meeting with the Chief Whip over with. After passing through Central Lobby, she made her way towards the library. Sebastian's office was just a short distance away. As she walked past a sign for the Prime Minister's office, she couldn't shake the feeling that he might be questioned later that day about her actions. Whether it was paranoia or reality, the tension in the air felt palpable as she arrived at Sebastian's door. Adjusting her bags on her shoulder, Helen took a deep breath and confidently knocked three times.

"Come in."

As much as she dreaded this moment, part of her was relieved that he was already inside. Helen pushed the door open. Sebastian was seated behind his desk, accompanied by two individuals, likely his research assistants, whom she didn't recognise.

"Ah, Helen. You're early. We weren't sure you were even going to show up."

"I thought I'd arrive early to give the firing squad plenty of time."

Sebastian smiled and nodded at the two others in the room. "That will be all. Thank you." Once they left, he picked up his phone and noticed a new message had arrived. He read the text from Lord Gatesouth before placing the phone back on the table. "Take a seat, Helen."

She set her bags next to the chair in front of his desk and sat down.

"That was quite something yesterday. It's all anyone is talking about; in fact, world affairs seem to have been temporarily forgotten, such is your impact. I don't think I've ever seen anything like it."

Helen sat up straight in her chair, unsure of how to respond.

"So, I'm a little confused, actually, we all are," Sebastian said, waving his finger. "Are you a member of parliament or a private detective?"

Helen took a deep breath. "That's not funny, Seb, and you know it."

"You'll address me by my full name in my office! You've been causing too many problems and bringing disrepute to this place. In that regard, I must ask you this question: Are you recording this conversation?"

Helen shook her head.

"No? I'm going to ask you again. Just in case you are: Are you recording this conversation?"

"No, I'm not. Are you?" Helen responded.

"No, I'm not. I don't think anyone wants to remember this conversation for posterity," he replied, tapping his fingers on the arms of his chair. "As I said, this is quite something. Making false accusations against a party donor, no less. How's that for gratitude? This campaign of yours needs to stop. Let me get this straight: the 'death of beauty' I…"

"I never called it that, and neither did Alison. You know, Alison, who was nearly killed last week!"

Sebastian paused, his tone becoming more sombre. "Of course. I keep up with the news, just like everyone else who knows you are sitting in my office this morning."

Helen swallowed, sensing the underlying threats.

"It simply won't do. This is a terrible situation, and you've dragged this house into it. The oldest parliament in the world should be a place where people can trust and have confidence that their leaders are acting in their best interests. Your ongoing campaign is tarnishing this institution! Your job is to look after your constituents. It's astonishing, you've become worldwide news as a backbench MP! What would you do if you were in my position?"

Helen shook her head. "Um, well... I'd start by getting my facts straight. The Althing in Iceland is the world's oldest continuously operating parliament. But I could be wrong about that, too."

"Jesus," Sebastian said, shaking his head in disgust as he tapped his fingers on the desk. "That was a rhetorical question, and I don't need to hear another word from you. No one needs to hear from you any longer. You've said enough. You know the lawyers for Knightark Pharmaceutical will come after you with everything they've got, and my job is to ensure this does not affect the party or the government. For that reason, you are now a rogue, an outcast, and you are alone. You are finished. Do you understand me?"

"In my defence, Sebastian, there…"

"I couldn't give one shit about your defence. You're done. I'm removing the whip from you, and you are expelled from the party with immediate effect. Furthermore, I will recommend that you be expelled from Parliament. I'm sure many others will support that! Your actions have consequences, and you will not drag us into your little games. How dare you accuse a company, any company, of what you did without a shred of evidence? You are an embarrassment to the political establishment."

Helen bowed her head.

"I could say that you should do the decent thing and resign, but I'm not going to give you that chance. The best option for you is to run for a by-election, but let's be honest, the fair residents of Shrewsbury are appalled, or so I've heard. You have no support. It's going to become very lonely in your world, Helen Lord." He paused, continuing to tap his fingers on the desk. "A statement will be released to the press and party officials within the hour. However, you are not banned from the parliamentary estate, yet. But if I were you, I'd disappear. I understand the press is eager to have a little chat with you, and I wouldn't recommend that. You have enough problems heading your way as it is. Do you understand me?"

Helen nodded.

"Good. Now get out of my office!"

Helen stood up, gathered her belongings, and quickly made her way to the door. Sebastian's actions were hardly surprising, but as she stepped into the corridor, he was right about one thing: she needed to get out of there.

✢✢✢✢

Sitting in his garden with a mug of coffee in hand, David felt well rested after a peaceful night. The last few days with the Dobey family and Rubin had been exhausting. For the past hour, he had been searching online to see if any news outlets had reported anything about Ryan and Andrea. While there was extensive coverage regarding the lab technician and his involvement in the botched test with the MP, no significant information was reported about them. David made a point of checking their social media accounts. Previously, their profiles were public, but their settings have now been changed to private. He found some confidence in this; it seemed like a positive sign they might be heeding his instructions. Only time would tell, and if they made a mistake, it wouldn't just be the police on his trail but also his client, Darius. Despite his garden's overgrown state, he planned to spend a couple of days fishing, believing it would give him the time he desperately needed to think. Rubin occupied his mind; he didn't doubt for a second that Rubin would have executed the family. However, doing so would have created an entirely different set of complications, and complications like that were not easy to manage. There was still work to be done, and while he would later prepare his fishing tackle and bait, finding new transportation took priority. He needed to get to the car breakers.

David took a sip of his coffee. Everything he planned and every action he took worked in phases. His phone was about a mile from his home, switched off, with the SIM card removed and hidden. He would first need to check the area before retrieving the phone, just in case it had been tracked at any point. Darius had said he would arrange for a new phone, as he often did, with a new, unregistered line. He intended to use it until his next assignment was complete, regardless of where it might take him or what it might involve. The online portal he and others from his regiment used was a private-sector facilitation hub. There was no need to venture into the dark web; communications were kept simple, with nothing ever disclosed. It served merely as a resource centre for arranging meetings. All you needed was a secure VPN router. If anyone were to look for him, they'd find him in Mongolia or elsewhere, not at his disused farm in rural Kent. David finished his coffee and walked into the kitchen. On the kitchen table lay the money bag. Rubin had taken his share, which was a substantial amount for the work they had done. However, David was concerned about Rubin's true motivations; he didn't believe for a moment he was funding a temple in Nepal. Along with the money he had already given to Rubin, he now had around three-quarters of a million euros. The money David left for the Dobey's came from his share, and he regarded it as an investment, protection for everyone involved. Fortunately, his contact at the car breakers accepted euros.

As for his firearm, even though it hadn't been used, he didn't want to take any chances and planned to dispose of it later in the usual manner. Once all the phases were complete, he planned to take a couple of days for himself by a peaceful lake.

++++

Despite her earlier reservations, Helen assessed her situation and decided to go upstairs to her office in Portcullis House. Although she had been banned from the political party, as the Chief Whip informed her, she had not yet been barred from Parliament. As uncomfortable as it felt, going into hiding served little purpose and would only exacerbate her problems and speculation.

"Hi, Helen," Joanne said, turning around as Helen entered the office. Her loyal assistant looked shocked. "To be honest, I wasn't expecting to see you."

Helen dropped her bags and slumped into the chair opposite Joanne. "To be honest, I wasn't expecting to be here. Where's Tobias?"

"Oh, he called. He doesn't want to come in. He feels that being associated with a discredited politician wouldn't benefit his resume." Joanne wore an awkward expression.

Helen laughed and kicked off her shoes. "Not to worry. He wasn't that impressive anyway."

"Helen, I'm concerned as well."

"Go on," Helen prompted.

Joanne took a deep breath. "It's almost difficult to put into words."

"Please try. We've known each other for a couple of years now. You've always been loyal, and I have been to you, so please say what's on your mind."

"Well, okay. There has been an email circulated by communications stating that you've been expelled from the party."

Helen ran a hand through her hair. "Well, they didn't waste any time."

"I'm almost compelled to ask if it's true, but I'm guessing it is."

"Yes, it is."

"God, Helen, what are you going to do?"

"Honestly, I'm not sure yet."

"The phones just won't stop ringing. A journalist with a press pass knocked at the office door this morning. You're the lead story everywhere. I assume you've seen the newspapers today?"

"I haven't, to be honest. I didn't want to check."

Joanne nodded. "I see. How was it downstairs?"

Helen shook her head. "Awful. When I came up the escalator from the old part of the palace, there were sneers, laughter, everything, you name it. Everyone stopped as I walked across the main floor to reach the elevator. It felt like a thousand eyes were on me. I feel sick."

"And I feel that way for you, and if I'm honest, for myself too," Joanne replied.

"Please don't worry; nothing is going to happen to you. I'm not quite sure yet whether I'll run as an independent candidate; it's too early to tell. But in any case, if I do lose my seat, I'll write to the party members and recommend you. You'll keep your job here at the palace. What's the feedback from the constituency?"

Joanne tried her best to smile. "Trust me, you don't want to know. You may need to keep your head down for a bit. But on the positive side, everyone has now heard of Shrewsbury; you've put it on the map."

Helen laughed. "I appreciate your attempt at humour, but Shrewsbury was the birthplace of Darwin. I think it was already on the map."

Joanne smiled. "Would you like a coffee?"

Helen shook her head. "I've been in these clothes for a couple of days. I need to clean up and change. Can you keep an eye on things for me? I'm not available for interviews, no matter who they are."

"Sure. Do you have any idea what you're going to do next?"

"No. However, I have the facts, and they cannot be ignored."

Joanne immediately looked away. Her loyal assistant now doubted her. Helen took a deep breath, realising she was utterly alone.

++++

Lisa's name lit up on John's phone. After the footage she had shown him the previous day, he had been expecting her call.

"Hi, John. Can you talk?" she asked.

"Yes, I'm at home. What's happening? What are you planning?"

"I've made a decision. I discussed it with Becky last night, and she agrees with me. But first, have you told anyone about what you've seen?"

"That's a joke, right? You must be kidding. If anyone knew what you did, your house would be crawling with the law right now."

"And that's why I'm calling. Do you have much planned for today?"

"Not particularly. I had some consultancy work scheduled, but with everything that's happened, especially your escapades, I cancelled it for today. It probably won't surprise you to hear that I didn't get much sleep last night."

"Mmm, I, on the other hand, crashed out. Must have been the gin. Look, I need to ask you a favour..."

"I'm not sure I want to get involved in your favours."

"Look, I know you're apprehensive, but I've made up my mind. I'm going to resign from the board. I want no part of what is happening, and Becky agrees with me."

"Have you told Becky everything? Has she seen the footage?"

"Yes, that was all we talked about last night."

"Well, okay. I respect your decision, but resigning now isn't going to look good for you."

"I'm not concerned about appearances. I'll say it was due to all the negative press. But, John, listen, this needs to stop. Darius and his cronies can't be allowed to succeed with their plans."

"So, what do you intend to do?"

"Well, this is where I need your help. Have you seen the news, specifically the breaking news?"

"I've had the TV on, yes. Why?"

"The MP, Helen Lord, has been expelled from her party because of the broadcast she made yesterday."

"Of course she has. That was inevitable."

"And that's why I'm thinking of her."

"Thinking of her for what reason?"

"Giving her the footage."

John buried his face in his hands, stunned. "Now I've heard it all!"

"She's perfect; she has nothing to lose. Let her run with it. It keeps her and the story alive. They mustn't be allowed to get away with this!" Lisa paused, waiting for a response. "John?"

"Yes, Lisa. I'm here."

"Look, you are not implicated in any way. The company, Darius, or any of the board members aren't mentioned. This is a cover-up right at the heart of the government. We can't let this go… John?"

"Stop! Please, stop. I'm trying to think about what you're saying."

"Well, you can't honestly say you want to be involved in this. Aren't you planning to resign as well?"

"I haven't made any decisions yet. Remember, this is my father's legacy. I intended to wait and see how things unfold before making a decision, not prematurely or under pressure from you."

"Okay, I hear you."

"Besides, it seems like your mind is already made up, so why are you even telling me this?"

"Because, like you, I'm monitoring the situation closely. You've probably seen the joint messages that Darius is sending us. He's currently focused on legal matters. This will catch him off guard."

"But as you pointed out, he isn't directly named."

"That's true, but he has used his influence to buy his way into the government. This could put a stop to his plans and take him down a peg. Even if this new so-called filler is ready for distribution, it might still hinder him. We need to do the right thing!"

"We?"

Standing in the car park outside her office, Lisa glanced around. "Yes, we. About that favour, I wanted to ask you, now is the right time, and I mean right now, before this product goes into circulation. For all we know, it might already be in the country."

"And?"

"Look, I'm stuck at work; there's no way I can get away. I have the footage on a drive, and I don't want to risk emailing it to her. Could you collect it from me?"

"Lisa, I don't want to be in possession of that."

"It would only be temporary. I'm going to call the MP, and I was wondering if you could drop it off for her?"

John burst into laughter.

"Please, John. You're the only one I can trust. I can't get away from here!"

"You do realise that if this is broadcast, Lord Gatesouth will be seen in the footage?"

"Yes, well, he's a money-grabbing creep anyway. So what?"

"So! When he sees it, there's a good chance he'll figure out the footage came from that picture frame you gave him."

"He binned it. The cleaners would have emptied the bins by now, so he won't be able to prove anything. It's Monday; that incident happened on Saturday night."

"I'm well aware of that. But you don't work at the palace, and the bins may not have been emptied yet."

"And so what? What's he going to do, send people after me? We need men like him out of that place anyway. This could lead to major reform. How could you disagree with reforming the entire system?"

"I'm not disagreeing. I'm just saying they might figure out that you did it, and that could lead to serious consequences for you."

"Arrogant, self-serving, entitled men aren't going to bully me. It's bad enough being the only woman on the board as it is. This is no longer a man's world, and with what I have in my pocket, we can bring about change. All I'm asking is for you to pass this to her. No one will ever know. Once it's done and whatever the MP decides to do with it, I'll resign."

"Christ, Lisa. I don't know."

"You must agree that it has to be done now. There may not be another opportunity, and we can't let that filler make its way onto the streets, do you hear me?" Lisa could hear a large sigh. "Well?"

"Look, I don't know. I need to think about it. If Darius, or anyone else, ever found out that I had given it to her, I shudder to think of what might happen."

"Trust me, it won't come to that. Just meet her in a safe place, somewhere away from cameras or prying eyes. It'll only take a few minutes."

"Then there's the small matter of getting into London, which you seem to be forgetting."

"Will you? Please."

"Look, I don't know. I need to think about it first. You should call her and see what she has to say. Then we can go from there."

Lisa breathed a sigh of relief. "Thank you, John. I'll do that now. I'll be in touch."

As Lisa's number disappeared from his phone screen, he sat in silence. She was right; what she had could bring about change. Whatever he decided, no one could ever find out that he had been involved with it.

Chapter Thirty-One

"Office of Helen Lord MP"

"Good afternoon. Is Helen there, please?"

"I'm sorry, but Helen isn't taking calls at the moment."

"Could I ask who I'm speaking with?"

"My name is Joanne, and I'm her research assistant. May I ask who I'm speaking to?"

"This is Lisa Wellings. I met Helen on Saturday evening at a reception in the House of Lords. Is it possible to speak with her? I noticed you didn't answer my question about whether she's there."

"As I mentioned, Miss Wellings…"

"It's actually Mrs Wellings."

"I apologise, Mrs Wellings, but she's not taking calls at the moment. It's quite impossible."

"Well, given the news, that's hardly surprising. However, she will want to speak with me. Please let her know it's Lisa from Knightark Pharmaceutical; I'm on the board. I trust you've heard of us?"

Joanne briefly pulled the phone away from her ear in surprise. "Yes, I've heard of you."

"I think everyone has, especially right now. The reason for my call is that I support her. I assure you, I'm not calling to reprimand her or anything like that. I have information that will be helpful to her. Could you tell her that, please?"

Joanne paused before responding, "Mrs Wellings, could you please hold?"

"Of course."

Joanne put the call on hold, rose from her seat, and knocked on Helen's door. Since their earlier conversation, Helen hadn't left her office.

"Yes, come in," Helen called out.

Joanne opened the door. "Helen, you have a phone call, and it might be one you want to take."

"I'd be surprised. Who is it?" Helen asked.

"She claims to be Lisa Wellings, a board member from Knightark Pharmaceutical."

Helen sat back in her seat, a deep frown crossing her forehead. "Are you sure? It could be a journalist pretending to be her."

"She mentioned that she met you on Saturday night, downstairs in the Lords."

Helen nodded. "I recall meeting someone who said she was on the board. A lot has happened since then. What does she want?"

"I don't know. She claims to support you and mentioned that she has information that could help you; those were almost her exact words."

"I doubt that. It's probably a trick. Have you been monitoring my emails? I've already heard from their lawyers."

"Yes, I've seen that. I didn't want to bring it up with everything else going on. Do you want me to tell her you're busy, or should I take a message?"

Helen swallowed and chewed on her lower lip. "No. Put her through. Let's hear what she has to say for herself."

"Okay, if you're sure."

"Yes, please connect her. Would you mind closing the door?"

Joanne nodded, closed the door, and took the call off hold. "Mrs Wellings, Miss Lord is now on the line. I'm just going to put you through."

"Good, thank you." Lisa took a deep breath; she had no idea how this call would unfold.

"Lisa, this is Helen."

"Helen, hi. Thank you for taking my call…"

"I'm somewhat surprised to hear from you," Helen quickly interrupted.

"To be honest, I'm surprised to be making this call," Lisa replied.

"So, apparently, you have some information?"

"Yes, I do. This is a bit unusual, and I won't be able to discuss it in any detail over the phone, but I have some footage that you may find useful."

"Footage? What footage?"

"From Saturday night. It's a covert recording, and I won't say more about it at this stage."

"Lisa, you're speaking in riddles. I'm still not sure why you are calling." She could hear Lisa take a breath; she sounded frustrated.

"Helen, because this could lead to significant changes, very serious changes! I'll arrange for it to be delivered to you. What you choose to do with it is up to you."

"But…"

"Understand this, Helen, and it's essential: you never got this from me. The same applies to my colleague who will be delivering it to you. You need to keep us out of this. You're in enough trouble as it is. This may very well, how shall I put it, revive your career."

"Well, Lisa, I'm intrigued, but can't you just email it to me?"

"Definitely not. This must be delivered by hand, with no exceptions. So, what do you say?"

Helen paused, "How do I know this isn't a trap? I've already heard from your lawyers. Are you trying to entrap me?"

"No! You have to believe me. We are on your side. What's happening needs to stop. Now, I'm not sure if this call is being recorded, but I've said enough. I'll need your mobile number to pass to my colleague. He will call you so you can arrange a meeting place."

"Look! I can't prove it, but I suspect my friend Alison got on the wrong side of you, and look what happened to her."

"I don't know anything about that, I assure you. Just make sure to meet in a public place, one that doesn't have cameras watching."

Helen scratched her head. "That might be a bit difficult in this current climate, cameras are everywhere."

"Well, that's how it is. I have a pen ready; can I have your phone number?"

"Just give me a moment." Helen needed to think. She had publicly named their company during the broadcast in an attempt to shame them, only to end up shaming herself in the process. She wasn't comfortable with the situation; it felt entirely unexpected. Moreover, she wasn't sure if she was genuinely speaking with Lisa.

"Helen, are you there?"

"Look, okay, I'll take a chance. Here's my number..."

++++

"John, great news! Helen has agreed to the meeting."

John could hear the excitement in Lisa's voice. "Well, good for you, but I didn't!"

"Look, I know, I know, but she's given me her mobile number. She doesn't know your name, I promise. I only mentioned that you're a colleague. It's just a drop-off."

"She'll recognise me from Saturday night. I was right next to you, remember?"

"I know, but even if she does remember you, the understanding is that she must never divulge our names to anyone. Besides, I was the one who obtained the footage, not you; you didn't even know about it. I simply can't get away from work, or I'd do it myself. John, we need to act quickly. We can't just sit on this."

"You mean you can't sit on it, Lisa. I'm very uncomfortable about this, no matter what you say, whether I'm just the delivery boy or not. I don't think Darius and the board will see it that way."

"Okay, I hear you. Look, what if I assured you and gave you my word that if this were to come out, I would take full responsibility, including the drop-off? I refuse to live in fear of these suited bullies; there's no way they'll ever find out what happened."

"And I'm just supposed to trust your word? We don't know each other well enough for that."

"Listen, I earned my position on that board through hard work. Many people trust my word, and I wouldn't be where I am today without it."

"Even if I agreed to this, I'm not going anywhere near Westminster. There are cameras and security everywhere. Why can't she come to your workplace or meet around the corner from you?"

"For the exact same reason. There are cameras everywhere in this area."

"I don't know..."

A slight smile appeared on Lisa's face; John was starting to come around. "I understand, and that's why I suggested a neutral location. Don't forget, she's very nervous right now, not just because of her actions, but also because of what happened to her friend. We still don't know who was behind that."

John paused for a moment. "Does she know what's on the footage?"

"No, I wouldn't tell her. I just mentioned that it was something significant."

John sighed. "It's definitely significant."

"So, what do you think?"

"Fine. Send me her number; you owe me one."

++++

"Hello, Ronald. I trust you are well. You must be tired?"

"You could say that, Darius. Yesterday was a long day, all things considered."

Darius could hear the exhaustion in Ronald's voice and turned up the volume on his phone. "I'm sorry you had to go to the secure facility as well. I had the other senior board members with me; there's much to do, but we are on schedule."

"That's good to hear. Is it still just the two of us who know the address of the secure holding?"

"Yes, and I want to keep it that way, at least for now. I didn't hear back from you. I trust everything was satisfactory?"

"Completely. The unit is fine, and the shipment is secured and safely in cold storage."

"Excellent. How many made it through?"

"The special projects team sifted through every box. I must say, even with their keen and trained eyes, it took a few hours."

"I can imagine. Any suspicions?"

"No, I explained the product's value, and it was simply a packaging error that required the individual boxes to be separated. It was quite tedious, but we only encountered a few minor breakages. Overall, we did well, and the stock count is as you hoped it would be."

"Around nine thousand vials?"

Ronald laughed, "If you say so; I wasn't going to hand-count them."

Darius grinned, "That's good, my friend. Very good."

"So, when are you planning the rollout? I've seen what's happening in the news; there's a lot of fallout. Darius, I need to be honest with you: having our name used in the public eye like this concerns me. I can only imagine how it's affecting our staff and distributors."

"Don't worry, my friend. I've got it under control. I spoke with Human Resources earlier, and this is just a temporary slip-up that's being managed. Everything has gone according to plan, and the troublemaker has lost her credibility. I also learned that she has been expelled from her political party due to her actions. We won't be hearing from her again."

"Okay, we trust you, Darius, if you're sure."

"I trust all of you as well. I plan to let this situation die down a bit, and then we will move on to the next phase and distribution. Nothing can stop us now."

++++

John had been in possession of Lisa's USB for about fifteen minutes. Aware of the significance of what he was carrying, he felt the weight of every moment and looked forward to being free of it. A couple of hours had passed since Lisa's initial call. After agreeing to deliver the USB to the MP, he drove into central London and met Lisa outside her office in Clerkenwell, located in the southwestern district of Islington. Although she was incredibly grateful, John clarified that he would not be doing any more favours for her in the future. With this in mind, he changed her initial plan. Although Lisa had provided him with the MP's phone number, he hadn't called her, ensuring that only Lisa would communicate with the MP. He wanted to keep his number out of her call logs. Lisa contacted the MP and informed her that the USB would be delivered later. She also promised to call back when they were nearby. At John's request, Lisa also chose the meeting location.

After receiving another call from Lisa, Helen was heading to the Farringdon area of London in a black cab. Lisa had instructed her to bring a laptop and mentioned that the meeting place was located on a road called Bowling Green Lane. There was a pub on the left-hand side, and the USB drive would be handed to her outside the pub. During the cab ride, Helen frequently glanced over her shoulder and kept an eye on the traffic around her. Lisa's instructions were vague and cryptic, which made Helen feel quite anxious. Her phone, now switched on, was inundated with calls and messages; the volume was relentless, and even the driver had commented on the noise. If he recognised her, he kept it to himself, and she was relieved about that. She silenced her phone but kept the screen on, torn between two choices: should she ask the driver to wait and take her back to Westminster, or should she pay him and let him go? Though she felt alone and uncertain about what she was stepping into, having the driver with her could provide some reassurance and a sense of security. On the other hand, if he did recognise her, he could take a photo of her and whoever she was meeting and sell it to the media, something she had read about happening before. However, she had promised to attend the meeting alone; clearly, whoever the courier was did not want to be seen by anyone else. Helen was placing significant trust in Lisa, someone she barely knew.

"Just pulling into Bowling Green Lane," the taxi driver said. "Where would you like to be dropped off?"

Sure enough, there was a pub up ahead on the left. A well-dressed man, probably in his early forties, was standing outside. Helen recognised him but couldn't quite place his name. "Could you drop me just outside that pub, please?" she asked.

The taxi driver pulled over. As Helen saw the man up close, she remembered where she had seen him. He had been at the Lord's reception a couple of nights ago, standing next to Lisa. Though she couldn't recall his name, she felt she had to take a leap of faith and let the taxi driver leave.

"Here's fine. Thank you," Helen said. She paid the driver, collected her bag, and stepped out onto the road. The man was looking her up and down, but didn't say anything or approach her until the taxi had pulled away.

"I know you, don't I?"

"We've met briefly," he replied.

"I'm sorry, but I don't remember your name."

The man responded with a forced smile. "Are you recording our conversation?"

"No, why would I do that?" Helen replied.

"The reason will become clear when you see what's on this," he said, holding up a USB drive. "Be exceptionally careful with it. Please ensure that I, or anyone else, is not mentioned. It came into your possession, and that is all. It was sent to you in the mail. Do you understand?"

Helen swallowed and nodded. "What's on it? Have you seen it?"

"What I've seen is irrelevant. You need to understand the conditions before I hand this over to you."

"Yes, I promise."

The man lightly tossed the USB drive to her, and she barely caught it with her trembling hand.

"You have a lot of enemies at the moment, Helen. Once that's out, you'll have enemies in very high places."

Helen swallowed in fear as the man turned and walked away.

++++

The man who had handed over the USB device walked down the narrow side street next to the pub. Helen still couldn't recall his name, but his face was familiar. She recognised him from their brief meeting on Saturday evening and her research on Knightark Pharmaceutical. She was convinced she had seen his image among the board members on their website. He may have even mentioned it that night. So much had happened since then that her memory was clouded. As he reached his car, he glanced back at her before getting into a black Jaguar and slowly driving away in the opposite direction. Once he disappeared, Helen propped herself against the side wall of the pub, her shaking hands adjusting the laptop bag on her shoulder. She had no idea what she had gotten into; the intrigue web was expanding by the minute. Putting a hand to her chest, she took a deep breath. Having never been in this area before, Helen took a moment to study her surroundings. Bowling Green Lane was a busy road lined with offices and workplaces, with cars constantly passing by. Leaning against the pub wall and with her picture all over the news, she needed to regain her composure. With the USB drive in hand, she needed to find a place to review its contents immediately. There were no benches or seating areas outside the pub, and since it was late afternoon, the café across the road was reasonably busy, making it an unsuitable option as well. After taking a few steps away from the wall, she peered through the pub's windows. Only a few people were inside; it had already been a trying day, and a glass of wine wouldn't hurt. She pushed through the doors and went straight to the bar. Three suited men were standing further down, and an older man read a newspaper at the far end of the bar, his dog asleep on the floor next to him.

"May I help you?" asked the young lady behind the bar as she approached her directly.

"Yes, thank you. I'd like a glass of wine, please."

"Would you like white, red, or rosé?"

"White, please."

"And would you like a small, medium, or a large glass?"

"A large, please."

Lisa recognised the cheap, branded bottle from which the lady poured. The wine was likely to be terrible, but it would suffice for now. Helen glanced to the left side of the bar, and her pulse quickened instantly. "Oh, excuse me. Would you mind changing the TV channel? I don't think anyone is watching it."

The lady nodded and handed Helen the remote control without looking at the screen. Helen immediately pressed the button to switch to the next channel, letting out a sigh of relief when sports appeared on screen; her face had just been on the previous news channel. A glass was placed in front of her.

"That will be thirteen pounds fifty, please."

Helen accepted the extortionate London prices with a nod.

"Oh, you like American football, do you?" the lady asked.

Helen rummaged through her purse for cash. "Sorry, what did you say?"

"On the TV. American football. What's your favourite team?"

"Oh, um, the blue one. Do you accept cash?"

The lady looked a bit confused as she took the twenty-pound note and went to the till. "Here is your change," she said, returning to Helen.

Helen noticed the barmaid's frown as she received her change. "Thank you," she said. Quickly snatching her glass from the bar, Helen walked over to a seat by one of the windows. After taking a large gulp of wine and grimacing at the taste, she placed the USB drive on the table and took her laptop out of her bag. Opening the computer, she inserted the USB into one of the side ports and waited. The wine tasted somewhat better on her second mouthful. "Come on, come on," she muttered as a file appeared on her screen. It was a video file. Looking around the bar, unsure of what she was about to watch, Helen rummaged through her bag for her earbuds. After finding them and connecting them to her laptop, she picked up her wine glass and took a deep breath as the video began to play.

The video was filmed from an unusual angle, aimed at the ceiling. The ceiling design looked familiar; perhaps it was one of the offices in the House of Lords. The quality of the recording indicated it had been obtained surreptitiously and was clearly covert. For some time, nothing of interest happened, and then the scene changed. Muffled sounds, possibly drinks being poured, followed by a voice that she recognised. Fascinated, Helen shook her head and took another sip of wine. As the conversation became clearer, her hands began to shake. "It can't be," she whispered, covering her mouth in shock. Helen gasped when Lord Gatesouth's face appeared on the screen. "Holy fuck!" She yelled at the top of her voice, and she immediately looked around. The men at the bar turned to stare at her, the woman behind the bar frowned with concern, and the dog at the far end of the room awoke. Its owner picked up his newspaper, flipped it over to check the front page, and then glanced directly at her. Flushing with embarrassment, Helen awkwardly smiled, removed her earbuds, and slumped into the chair. Her hands shook uncontrollably, and her right leg bounced under the table. This was unprecedented. She stared at the still image of Lord Gatesouth on the screen, tears welling in her eyes as she realised the power she now held in front of her. This was serious leverage. If she had seen this footage twenty-four hours earlier, things might have turned out differently, but that moment had passed. She had been kicked out of the party, and there was no changing that.

By the time Helen finished her wine, she had watched the footage three more times. Now, she knew exactly what to do. It was time to reset the balance, and she knew just the person who could help her with that: Mr Ben Tasker, the Chief Operations Officer of Channel 8 Television.

++++

BOARD ROOM, CHANNEL 8 TELEVISION

"Can you run me through the schedule again?" Ben asked.

Sharron Broadhurst, the senior broadcaster and news anchor, picked up her notes. "Ben, we've already covered this."

"I know, but where do we stand with the Lord story?"

Senior Producer Brian Clement responded, "Ben, the segment is ready. The researchers and co-producers have done their best. Helen's phone is either switched off or ringing endlessly. A couple of us have spoken to Joanne, her senior researcher, but she won't engage in any conversation. The MP has gone off the radar."

"Well, that's hardly surprising given the circumstances. However, since I spent time with her recently, I thought she would have spoken to us," Ben replied.

"The whip's been removed from her, Ben. Her story will be old news tomorrow."

"Okay. Sharron, please make sure to add that we tried to contact Helen Lord for a response, but our requests were ignored."

"Will do. With pleasure," she said.

"In the piece, can we also provide an update on Alison's condition? We are hoping to get words from her soon, as she's apparently in recovery. I'm going to visit her in the hospital after this meeting. And can we also..." Ben paused and broke into a fake laugh. "Well, speak of the bloody devil."

Brian noticed Ben looking at his phone. "What is it?"

"Would you believe it? The soon-to-be former MP is calling."

"You're kidding! Keep her talking, put her on speaker, and I'll get a camera in here," Sharron said quickly as she left the room.

Ben answered the call and set the phone on speaker in the centre of the table. "Helen! It's so good to hear from you. I'd say you've put the town of Shrewsbury on the map!"

"What? Oh, yes, by the way, Shrewsbury was the birthplace of Charles..." There was a brief pause. "Never mind. Can you talk?"

"For you, Helen, absolutely," Ben replied.

Helen could detect the sarcasm in his voice. "Good. Now, take the phone off speaker and move to a quiet place."

Ben looked around the room. Brian shrugged, and Jennie Upland, their head of social value, gestured to encourage him to listen to what Helen had to say. Ben nodded, picked up the phone, and held it to his ear. "The call is off speaker now, Helen. What is it?"

"Go to another room and make sure you're alone."

"Jesus, is that really necessary?"

"And don't try to record this call," she added.

Ben turned around and rolled his eyes at his fellow board members. "Okay, I'm going to my office." As he left the room, he noticed Brian shaking his head. "You're a bit paranoid, aren't you, Helen?"

"So would you be if you knew what I know."

Ben rolled his eyes again and entered his office. "Alright, I can talk now. What's on your mind?"

"Can you get me on the seven o'clock news?"

Ben couldn't help but look surprised. They had been trying to contact her all day. "Helen, we have a full broadcast planned. We were just discussing the segments; all the pieces to camera have been filmed and edited."

"Yes or no, can you get me on?" Helen insisted.

"We've been trying to reach you all day. Why would..."

"I have an exclusive. A world exclusive, and I'm offering it to you," she interrupted.

"And why would you do that?"

"For Alison."

Ben nearly choked with laughter. "Forgive me for not believing you are sincere, Helen. But what possible exclusive could you offer? I'm sorry to say that interviewing you, even after the stunt you pulled, doesn't qualify as a world exclusive, a national exclusive. Yes, I'll concede that..."

"Listen, I'm coming to you first..."

"Yes, I suspected that's why you used the word 'exclusive.'"

"Will you stop patronising me? Now listen, I'm trying to address something important. Our friend was seriously hurt, and you lost millions on that ill-fated Beauty Beach program. Do you want to get your channel back in the game? Yes or no?"

Ben paused for a moment; she had captured his interest. "Where are you, Helen?"

"I'm outside a pub, just a couple of miles outside of central."

Ben smiled. She may have been drinking. This could be television gold. "Okay, so what do you have? If it's interesting, we might be able to fit you into the broadcast."

Helen laughed. "You really don't understand, do you? This isn't about fitting me in; it's the whole bloody program."

"Helen, it's a live one-hour broadcast! There are other world events to cover besides just you. So what do you have? I'll be leaving soon, so please talk me through it."

"No. I'll show you. What if I told you I have footage of the Prime Minister involved in a cover-up?"

Ben nearly rolled his eyes, but his journalistic instincts were curious. "Okay, you have my attention. Can you email it to me?"

"Absolutely not. It's not safe. I'll bring it to you, and you will watch it on my laptop, not anyone else's, understand? Those are my terms: take it or leave it."

Ben had to admit that the maverick MP sounded sincere, and if she was telling the truth, it could lead to a major story. "Wait, did you say there's footage? Was it filmed without people's consent?"

"Yes, to be blunt. It's a covert recording."

"Did you do the recording?"

"No, someone else did."

"Will you tell me who that was?"

"Never. I will not reveal my source. As a journalist, you must respect that."

"I do, but it's not that simple. Is the footage verified? What's its provenance? Filming without consent, regardless of the circumstances, is a precarious area that could lead to lawsuits if the footage is published. I would need to run it by legal; that could take time."

"You don't have time. Trust me, it's indisputable. Once you see it, you'll want to take the chance and run with it."

"Helen, we can't air this live until I've had a chance to review it, along with a few others."

"I understand. That's why I'm willing to come and show it to you so you can make an informed decision."

"Alright. But what are you looking for in exchange for this exclusive?"

Helen looked slightly surprised by his question. "What do you mean? Money?"

"Yes, that's exactly what I mean. And I have to say, I think you might be on the verge of unemployment, which is why I want to know your motivation."

"You say that, but this footage will change everything. So, do you want to take a chance, Mr Tasker?"

Ben nodded; of course, he did. "Okay. Do you need me to send a car to pick you up?"

Chapter Thirty-Two

After postponing his visit to see Alison in the hospital, Ben waited by the front desk, having been informed that Helen's arrival was imminent. After her call, he sat down with the producers and the production team for their news program. He had been as honest with them as possible; apparently, the MP had some "evidence" regarding the Prime Minister's involvement in wrongdoing. Following Helen's political downfall the previous day, which was a consequence of her actions, it was an understatement to say that everyone was sceptical. Jennie, their head of social value, expressed her concerns about broadcasting a film obtained surreptitiously, and her opinion was supported by some team members. They had all been in the industry for a long time, and given their loss in the legal case concerning The Beauty Beach, they decided to proceed with caution, if at all. If the MP wished to appear on live television and make a fool of herself, that was her choice, and it would certainly boost the ratings. In the highly competitive world of news broadcasting, another channel held a significant lead in viewing figures and had been winning nearly all the journalistic awards for news coverage. If Helen has what she claims to have, it could potentially boost their advertising revenue and viewer numbers.

Ben quickly approached the front doors as the channel's pool car arrived outside. He checked his watch; they were going live at seven, and time was running out.

When Helen stepped out of the car, she sensed his urgency. She walked briskly and shook Ben's hand. "Okay, where should I go?" she asked.

"First, let's head up to my office so you can show me what you have," he replied.

As they approached the elevators, Helen noticed several people staring at her, and Ben saw it too. "It seems you're quite famous," he said with a slight smile.

"Not for the right reasons," Helen muttered as they entered the lift.

Ben pressed the button for his office floor, and the doors closed. "Your broadcast yesterday was bound to attract attention, regardless of the outcome. By the way, have you spoken to the guy who was your lab assistant, the one who appeared on the broadcast?"

"No, I tried calling him earlier. His phone is off, and his office said he's taken some time away. They didn't know when he would be back."

"Fair enough," Ben said as the lift door opened and he pointed the way. "Would you like a drink?"

"No, let's just get this over with."

Ben led Helen into his office. "Please close the door behind you if that would make you more comfortable." It clearly did, as he noticed Helen quickly shut the door.

"Right. A USB drive came into my possession…"

"How?"

"That doesn't matter right now. Please don't interrupt; we're short on time. A USB drive came into my possession." Helen opened her laptop and handed it to him. "I've downloaded the contents onto my desktop. Do you see the video file icon?"

"Yes," Ben replied as he put the laptop on his desk.

"Open it and press play. The volume is already turned up to full."

As the video started to play, Ben asked, "Who's this?"

"It will all become clear in just a moment. Listen very carefully to the words."

Ben nodded. "Is this filmed in Parliament?"

"The House of Lords."

Although Ben could hear the words clearly, he tilted his head toward the screen. "So, that's Alix Gregory speaking. Who's the other one?"

"Lord Gatesouth."

Ben's eyes widened. "Okay..."

As the conversation continued, Ben looked up in shock. "Did he just say what I think he said?"

Helen nodded and began to pace the room anxiously.

"Holy shit, Helen. This is huge! But it's just voices; you can't see anyone. Oh wait... Oh my God. That's Gatesouth on screen!"

The video finished.

Ben took a seat, his face clearly reflecting his shock. "I have to listen to that again." He replayed the recording. "Do you mind if I take this to production and run it through some filters? We need to see if we can make the sound even clearer."

"No. Now that you can see the value of it, you can do as you wish, as long as you give me what I want in return."

Ben paused the video and leaned back in his chair. "And what is that?"

"I want you to broadcast the footage you just saw in its entirety. After that, I will be interviewed live. Then post the recording online immediately across all your social media platforms, websites, and other relevant channels. You should send it to every outlet and agency. If you want to brand the footage with your logo as an exclusive, I have no objections. However, you are responsible for distributing it. In about an hour or so, it will start spreading on its own, as everyone will want to share and watch it. You understand the implications of that recording, don't you?

Ben nodded. "Potentially, this could spell the end for our Prime Minister. He's definitely going to have some questions to answer. What do you think he has done?"

"That's for you to investigate. Your journalists should be able to dig into this; it will keep you all busy for a while. He won't be able to hide from it. He'll likely claim it's fake or that it's AI-generated or something similar."

"Certainly, if Gatesouth's face weren't on the screen, it would complicate matters. But he's clearly identifiable." Ben leaned back further in his chair and clasped his hands behind his head as he considered his options. "Look, if we give you the interview, you need to acknowledge that the footage is yours. Honestly, it's probably a weak legal stance from our perspective since we are the broadcasters. However, if the footage turns out to be fake, you must take full responsibility. After all, you brought it to us."

"I'm fine with that, and trust me, it's not fake."

"You say that, but you're not explaining how you obtained this or who provided it."

"I'm not."

"But Sharron, our news anchor, will ask you that question on air. You know how tough she is."

"That's okay. I'm prepared for that."

Ben rubbed his chin and glanced at his watch. "We've only got a few minutes if we're going to include this."

Helen noticed that Ben was deep in thought. "What's the matter? What is it?"

"I'm just considering the legalities, Helen. Is there a potential breach of human rights here? There's no entrapment, and I'm sure of that; there's no sub judice since there's no legal case."

"You can sort out the human rights issues and everything else later. Besides, who's going to pursue you? The two parties involved will know this is a true and honest recording. What you just saw on the screen actually happened."

"And when did this take place? There's no time code or date stamp."

"Saturday night."

"And how do you know that?"

"I saw them both at a Knightark Pharmaceutical social event on Saturday night."

Ben laughed, "The same company you claimed was involved in human testing."

"The very same."

"Okay. Here's what we're going to do. Do you have the USB drive with you?"

Helen tapped her jacket pocket. "Yes."

Ben closed the laptop and handed it to Helen. "Then follow me."

++++

Ben rushed off to speak with the production team, leaving Helen in the green room. She anxiously checked her watch as each minute passed; time was against them. Her hands shook as she held a cup of water. If they were going to broadcast and follow her instructions, she needed to be prepared for the interview. Any display of nerves, such as shaky hands, would be perceived as a weakness and could undermine her credibility. Her critics, both online and in the press, would seize any opportunity to capitalise on that. According to Ben, the biggest challenge they faced was legal. With so little time left, he would likely have to decide on his own. As she sat in silence, she knew that phone calls were being made, but how could they possibly pass up this opportunity? They had to proceed with the broadcast; it had to go on. Sharron Broadhurst was known for being a tough interviewer, especially with politicians, and she often interrupted responses mid-sentence. Given the disastrous lab test from the day before, which millions had already seen, Helen knew Sharron would not make it easy for her. She would take full advantage of the situation to press Helen for answers.

A young woman entered the room and introduced herself as a runner for the channel. She informed Helen that it was time for her to follow her into the studio.

"So, does this mean they are going to broadcast?" Helen asked.

"Yes, I think so. Production had a quick meeting, but I wasn't a part of it. I heard from someone else about what you brought in; it sounds incredible. Please wait over there, behind the cameras. Ben will join you shortly."

As Helen took a deep breath, she noticed that several members of the production crew were staring at her. This was a tremendous opportunity that had unexpectedly come her way. To her left, Sharron appeared with notes in hand. She might need to refer to them, as the autocue may not be ready in time due to last-minute changes before the broadcast. Spotting Helen, Sharron quickly approached her with a smile.

"Hello, Helen!" she said warmly.

Helen didn't trust her for a second.

"It's been a while since I've interviewed you. We've been trying to reach you all day," Sharron continued.

"I've been a little busy with one thing or another," Helen replied.

Sharron maintained her smile. "That doesn't surprise me. What you did yesterday was quite bold, and what I just saw upstairs is truly remarkable. I'm looking forward to speaking with you about it." Sharron walked off and placed her papers on the news desk, then walked to the side of the room to change her jacket and shoes.

"Helen!" Ben called as he approached her. "Here's the situation: we're working hard to clean up the audio in the recording, but we need to be cautious not to alter it in any way. With your permission, we would like to add our logo to the corner of the footage. Overall, I wouldn't consider it broadcast quality, but it will have to suffice."

"And what about the interview?" Helen asked.

"Yes. Sharron will introduce the program at the beginning of the broadcast. She will then inform the audience that we have an exclusive story. The footage will be shown first, and afterwards, she will come to you for an interview. To be straightforward, you were already part of our initial broadcast this evening, given yesterday's events and your expulsion from the political party today. Some segments from the original broadcast will be kept. Do you have any issues with that?"

Helen shook her head. "I pretty much expected it. What has happened has happened. Now we need to focus on what we can do together for the future, and tonight is all about that. The campaign Alison fought for will not be forgotten. Everything is connected."

"But you can't prove that. As far as I know, no one can."

"We'll see."

"Well, okay, but go steady. Sharron might have to cut you off if you start making unsubstantiated claims without evidence. I will be communicating with her through her earpiece throughout the broadcast. I'm taking over this segment because I need to take responsibility for it. After we finish, the program will return to the other planned news features. However, can you stay a little longer? There will be questions afterwards, and we might set up a web chat with you. Depending on the feedback, we may feature the recording again at the end of the broadcast."

Helen nodded and glanced at her watch. "We don't have much time, but yes, I can stay for a bit."

"Okay, great. We need to get you mic'd up." He called someone over and instructed them to connect the remote microphone to Helen. "Helen, I need to go upstairs. I'm taking a major risk putting this on. Have a good interview."

Helen took a deep breath as a member of the production team approached with a microphone.

"Hi, Helen. We need to attach this to you; it should go here. Please clip this around the back. Let me know when you're comfortable, and we'll do a mic test."

Helen followed the instructions, spoke into the small microphone and glanced over at Sharron, who was reading her notes.

"We are about to go live, so please take a seat next to Sharron. A chair has already been prepared for you."

Sharron nodded at Helen as she settled into her seat. A glass of water was placed in front of her.

"Here you go; we're about to go live," said the crew member.

"Okay, everyone!" a producer yelled from behind the cameras. He silently counted down for Sharron before pointing at her.

Helen watched a screen to the side as a picture segment played over the news programme's generic broadcast music, featuring a short clip from the recording.

Sharron looked up from her notes and addressed the camera. "Scandal at the heart of the government as a secret recording surfaces, featuring the Prime Minister and Lord Gatesouth. We will speak with Helen Lord, MP, the disgraced Member of Parliament who has exclusively brought this recording to Channel 8 News. What's next for the Prime Minister? Also coming up..."

Helen swallowed as the other news items were read aloud, quickly reaching for her glass of water. She was taken aback that the word "allegedly" was not used; instead, the Prime Minister was named directly. Her hands trembled as she hastily set the glass down, then hid her hands beneath the desk to keep them out of view. The opening music faded away.

"Good evening. Tonight, in a world exclusive, we report that the Prime Minister is now at the centre of controversy following the emergence of a secret recording. In this recording, he demands the removal of a member of parliament from the government and discusses involvement in a cover-up related to harm done to individuals. In a moment, we will speak with Helen Lord, the MP who was targeted by the Prime Minister's demand. Yesterday, she conducted a broadcast in which she claimed, without evidence, that a pharmaceutical company was involved in human experiments and addictive cosmetic surgery. Helen Lord has since had the party whip removed and has been expelled from the party. Before we speak with her, we will show the complete unedited film."

++++

PRIME MINISTER'S RESIDENCE, 10 DOWNING STREET, LONDON

Alix took a sip from his glass of rum and laughed. "Larry, how did you get in here again? I bet you've seen some sights in this place over the years. Come on, come and say hi. Darling! The cat has gotten into my room again!" Alix shouted as he heard footsteps approaching his door quickly. Eleanor burst into the room.

"Darling, has Larry been fed?"

Eleanor quickly grabbed the remote control for the television.

"What? What is it?"

"That bloody MP again!"

"Which one?"

"Helen Lord!"

The television was switched on, and Eleanor went straight to Channel 8 news.

"What about her? I took care of her earlier," Alix said.

"I don't think you did!" Eleanor snapped, her hands shaking. Alix noticed the worry etched on her face. "I was in the kitchen with the news on in the background when the presenter mentioned you and a covert recording. She said it was an exclusive and hinted at a cover-up." Eleanor turned up the volume as Alix stood up to face the television.

They both began watching the short, low-quality recording.

"That's the Lord's, isn't it?" Eleanor asked.

Alix nodded, his expression filled with worry as the footage continued to play. Eleanor covered her mouth with her hands and let out a scream of shock, looking directly at Alix.

His face was horrified. "What the hell have you done?" she yelled as the glass slipped from Alix's hands and shattered on the floor. Alix held his head in his hands, the colour draining from his face. "Oh my God!" was all he could say as Larry tore out of the room.

++++

As the recording concluded, Sharron turned her attention to the camera lens. "The footage you just watched was provided to us by the Member of Parliament involved in a major controversy. This footage will raise additional questions about MPs and their connections to business and outside interests. However, before we delve into that, the exclusive footage we received includes what we believe to be the spoken words of Alix Gregory, the Prime Minister. The individual you saw on screen was Lord Owen Gatesouth. Now, let's turn our attention to Helen Lord, the now-disgraced Member of Parliament who, just yesterday, took it upon herself to conduct a live laboratory test on YouTube. Helen, how did you obtain this footage? Were you responsible for it?"

"No. Good evening. It was delivered to me."

Sharron shrugged. "Delivered how?"

"It appeared in my mailbox."

"Email or traditional post?"

"It came through the post, at work, at Westminster."

"And how was the footage, which we now have in our possession, sent to you?"

"In an unmarked envelope on a USB drive," she lied.

"An unmarked envelope was dropped in your parliamentary post box. That suggests it was left by someone working at Westminster."

"That's your interpretation, Sharron. I'm not aware of that at this time."

"And when did this footage become available to you?"

"Today."

"And when was it filmed?"

"Saturday evening, in the office of Lord Gatesouth."

"Who filmed it?"

"I do not know, as I say, it was sent to me."

"How can you be sure this footage is authentic? Could it be fake?"

Helen shook her head. "Definitely not. The comments the Prime Minister makes are specific, and you can clearly see Lord Gatesouth's face. It is now up to them to deny it."

"In the footage, the Prime Minister names you and calls for your removal from the party, something that happened earlier today. Are you attempting to damage the Prime Minister out of a personal vendetta?"

"No, not at all. I was not aware of the footage's existence until today."

"But you didn't place the hidden camera?"

"No, I don't have access to that office."

"Maybe a friend or a staff member arranged this?"

"Look, Sharron, I can see where you're trying to take this, but I assure you that I did not know of it."

"Your credibility is questionable after the stunt you pulled yesterday when you accused a pharmaceutical company of serious malpractice. Many would argue that your claims were outrageous and unscientific. We won't name the company, as you provided no evidence to support your allegations. Your broadcast has made international headlines. Is this really what's happening here? Is this all about you?"

"No, far from it. This is about Alison Harwood, a friend of mine who was the victim of a violent attack last week in our nation's capital. I believe that trained professionals carried out the attack under the orders of others because Alison knew what I know."

"And what is that?"

"Because we have corruption at the heart of the government. Those in power are being bribed. I was shown evidence indicating that some cosmetic surgeries contain addictive properties. Most individuals who undergo cosmetic surgery have little idea of what is being placed inside their bodies."

"We checked earlier, and the police have not provided any further updates regarding last week's explosion in London, where your friend was seriously injured. I understand that Alison's condition has improved, and she is now speaking with the police. The man who assisted you in your so-called lab test is called Ryan Dobey..."

"Please address him by his title: Dr Ryan Dobey."

Sharron raised a conciliatory hand and nodded. "Dr Ryan Dobey. We have been trying to contact him, but have been unsuccessful so far. We have spoken to the camera team that filmed you, and they have decided not to provide any further comments. You're all alone in this, aren't you?"

Helen shook her head with a somewhat incredulous smile on her face. "I think you are missing the point of what you have just broadcast. This vindicates me. It shows that my questions and efforts to uncover the truth have exposed people for who they really are."

Sharron lightly tapped her earpiece. "Maybe the Prime Minister wanted you removed because of what you have done?"

"This was filmed the night before the lab test, so it has no bearing on the matter. Until this very moment, the Prime Minister wouldn't have known about the existence of this recording."

"This still feels like it's about you."

"No, you're missing the point." Helen turned to the camera. "I know you are watching, Prime Minister. What do you have to hide? What has been covered up? I am aware that the researchers for this programme are already investigating you. In the next hour, investigative journalists from across the country will scrutinise your actions. What have you done, and who knows about it? Who has driven you to the edge of corruption? What are you trying to conceal, and whom are you trying to protect, Prime Minister?"

The camera shifted away from Helen's face as Sharron received instructions in her earpiece. "We'll return after a commercial break."

++++

Eleanor snatched a chair and placed it in front of Alix's desk. She sat opposite him, desperate for answers. "What the hell have you done?"

Alix had his head in his hands. "Oh my God, oh my God, how did this happen? What am I going to do?"

"Do? Do! You're finished. There's no escaping this. We've spent years working towards this, and I've supported you every step of the way. You fucking idiot!"

Alix remained still, not responding.

Eleanor took a deep breath. "I have no idea what you're talking about in that footage. Who has something on you?"

"Darling, please. I don't want to talk about it; I need to think."

"You have to talk! You either fight this or you'll be forced to stand down."

Alix slumped in his seat, his face pale and his body trembling. "Do you think I can claim it's fake?"

"I don't know, Alix. I really don't. I can hear it's you. That conversation took place, didn't it?"

Alix nodded. "Can't we still say it's fake, like some AI-generated thing or something?"

"Owen was clearly in the picture. Channel 8 must have thought the footage was authentic, or they wouldn't have aired it; now they have a world exclusive. And who announces it, of all people? That bitch Sharron Broadhurst, she's had it in for you from day one!" Eleanor slammed her hand against Alix's desk in frustration. "The story this evening was supposed to be about Helen Lord, and now she's completely flipped it. God, you're such a..." Eleanor threw her hands in the air in exasperation. "What is it? What do they have on you?"

"I don't want to tell you, okay? It's better if you don't know. If I tell you, it'll be harder for you to maintain any form of deniability."

"Alright. Let me rephrase that. Who has something on you?"

Alix took a deep breath and looked up at the ceiling. "Darius."

"Darius! Darius Neath? That insufferable, verminous man. I always suspected he was too close to you. I wouldn't trust that smug idiot as far as I could throw him." Eleanor's eyes widened as she sighed in resignation. "Oh no, that's why he's always around; that's why his company has financially supported you all this time. He needed you to repay the favour, whatever that might be, so that he could have people in the heart of government, including you!"

Alix gritted his teeth and closed his eyes. "He wouldn't have done this."

"Of course he didn't. He has you right where he wants you. Clearly, Gatesouth didn't do it either, since he's implicated just as much as you."

"Hardly. But that video was filmed in his office. I should call him."

"Do you think that's wise? Your calls will be logged. It could look like a panicked reaction."

"Journalists aren't monitoring my calls. They're more cautious now after the phone hacking scandal."

"All the same, Alix, listen to me. If this all comes out, are you going to name Darius?"

Alix opened his eyes, filled with worry. "I can't."

"Why not? Why shouldn't he take the fall as well?"

"Because I need him to keep quiet! We'll respond by saying it was a private conversation, that nothing significant was said, and we'll keep the focus on my comments about trying to get Helen Lord removed."

Eleanor turned around, hearing movement and phones ringing outside the room. "Alix, you were heard pressuring Owen to remove her. Seb was mentioned too."

Alix picked up his phone from the desk, which had been set to silent. He saw two missed calls from Sebastian, along with several others. "Darling, could you check the windows? How does it look out there?"

Eleanor got up and cautiously looked outside. A photograph of her, looking concerned from a window at Downing Street, would be newsworthy and marketable. She turned back to Alix, "It's not good. They're starting to gather outside, and cameras are being set up."

Alix nodded. "I'm going to call Owen. The video was filmed in his office. No matter what happens, I need to find out who is responsible for this!"

++++

Darius turned down the volume on the television and began stroking his chin. This was not part of the plan. How could Owen and Alix have been so reckless? He closed his eyes to collect his thoughts, reflecting on what he had just seen. Thankfully, neither his name nor his company's name had been mentioned, which could have made things much worse. Nonetheless, this was an unwelcome disruption to their plans. His phone vibrated on the desk. A glance at the screen revealed that William was calling; he must have seen the news as well. William was the calmest and most level-headed of the three senior board members. Alone at home, Darius answered the call and switched his phone to speaker mode to speak with the senior American board member.

"I take it you've seen it?" Darius asked, hearing noise in the background.

"You could say that! I'm at the hotel bar, and it's playing on the screen. I asked them to turn up the volume, and now it's all anyone can talk about. How does this affect our plans?"

"I hope it won't have any impact. We weren't mentioned, and he won't say anything if he knows what's good for him."

"If you say so. It's highly annoying, though. He's useful."

"Mmm, I suspect he's not anymore. It's regrettable considering our investments in him."

"Do you think there's any way he can manoeuvre? Can he steer his way out of this?"

"No, it's as clear as it can be, given what we know. The only way he could change the course of this situation is to shift the focus onto us. It wouldn't make sense for him to do that; I suspect Alix will still be removed from office. He'll receive a good pension, and we'll take care of him for keeping his mouth shut."

"That sounds expensive, especially if there's no value to us. What if there's an outcry for an investigation? I heard a cover-up was mentioned."

Darius nodded thoughtfully. "You know, my friend, they might push for that. However, there needs to be some evidence of criminal wrongdoing, and that will be impossible to establish. Even if Alix were to confess, it happened so long ago that uncovering anything would be difficult. I took appropriate steps at the time. The best thing for him to do is step down and disappear from public service. In time, it will all blow over; these things always do."

"As you Brits say, it seems like a bloody shame."

Darius laughed. "We do have a different vocabulary, but I'll find a way to use him at a later stage. He'll do as he's told, but never mind. Politicians come and go; sometimes you back the wrong horse."

"And what about the other one?"

"Owen? I think he's also on a sticky wicket, but not as much as Alix."

"The footage looks like it was filmed in Owen's office."

"Definitely. I was gathering my thoughts when you called. I need to set things in motion, and my very next call will be to Owen. But let me tell you this, my friend: whoever is responsible for this will pay a very heavy price."

✢✢✢✢

"So, what's the wager for tomorrow?" Lord Owen Gatesouth asked his house guest.

"I don't know, you old bugger. You always stiff me," Lord Charles Hawthorne replied with a snort.

Owen laughed and noticed his phone ringing. "Oh God, what is it now? It's bloody Alix calling."

"Get rid of him," Charles said. "You've done what he asked of you."

"My intervention was unnecessary, as it turned out. That Helen Lord character made a complete fool of herself; her downfall was her own doing."

"Are you going to answer?"

"He'll only pester me if I don't," Owen sighed as he answered the call. "Yes, Alix?"

"We've been fucked!"

Owen quickly pulled the phone away from his ear in shock. "Don't you use that language with me! Don't forget who you're speaking to. I don't care if you're the bloody Prime Minister!"

Charles hadn't heard what Alix had said to Owen, but he was surprised by Owen's reaction.

"Owen, something serious has happened. Have you seen the news?"

"No, why? I'm with Charles. We have a golf day tomorrow, don't you remember? I invited you..."

"Trust me, you won't be going to golf. You and I are all over the news!"

"Why, old boy? I haven't publicly involved myself with you for ages."

"This wasn't public; it was private! Our conversation in your office on Saturday night was filmed."

"What? That's impossible! I would never allow something like that in my office."

"It's all over the news. Owen, you have to believe me."

"I've already told you, Alix, there are no cameras in my office. I don't believe in such things. It's bad enough that the public sees as much as they do in that building. Hold on. Charles, the remote is over there. Can you turn on the TV and find a news channel? Apparently, Alix is in a spot of bother."

Charles rolled his eyes and turned on the television.

"You misheard me, Owen. We are in much more than just a spot of bother!"

"Okay, calm down, old boy, you're practically spitting your words. Can you turn that up, Charly?"

Owen froze as he watched the headline revolving at the bottom of the screen.

Charles turned around in surprise. "Owen, your name is on the screen. It says that secret footage was filmed in your office. What's going on?"

Owen walked toward the television, his mouth falling open in disbelief. "Alix, are you still there?"

"Yes, and I'm telling you, our conversation was recorded!"

"Hold on." Owen's expression was one of worry as he saw a still image of his face on screen. "Oh no," he whispered as Charles turned to him, alarm evident on his face. "Owen, what is the meaning of this?"

The phone slipped from Lord Owen Gatesouth's hand as he raised his hands to his face and swallowed. "Charles, I've been fucked!"

Chapter Thirty-Three

Charles took a seat, watching as his fellow Lord paced back and forth in the living room. "Owen, what are you going to do?" he asked.

"I don't bloody know! How the hell did a camera end up in my office? This is a major security breach, and I'll have someone's head for this!" Owen exclaimed, kicking a chair across the room in frustration.

Charles shook his head. "I'm trying to gather my thoughts. This is truly shocking, but from my perspective, Alix is the one in trouble. He's the one who asked you to speak with Sebastian, right?"

"But I'm still implicated!" Owen flailed his arms in anger. "You can clearly hear Alix mentioning a cover-up, and I didn't report it; I just went along with it, dismissing it as an everyday event."

"But there's nothing for you to report," Charles replied. "Just say he has a drinking problem and that he makes ridiculous statements sometimes."

Owen paused and waved a finger. "That's not a bad idea."

"It's about self-preservation from now on. You need to distance yourself from Alix to protect your reputation. This happens often in that place. Think about everyone who's come and gone; we are survivors. You didn't bully the Chief Whip; you simply asked him to review Helen Lord's position, didn't you?"

Owen finally stopped pacing and nodded. "I did communicate it via messages, though." He quickly picked up his phone from the floor. The Prime Minister's call had long since disconnected, and the screen had a small crack from the fall, but it was still functioning.

"What did you say?"

"I'm just scrolling through messages. Hang on, Charly. Oh, wait. I called him yesterday, but I messaged him this morning. My message said, 'Remember our conversation from yesterday.'" Owen let out a massive sigh of relief.

"Okay, quick damage control. That doesn't mean anything. Your call won't have been recorded, so there's no evidence."

Owen nodded. "But I didn't tell anyone what Alix said about there being a cover-up."

"Like I said, you could claim he has a drinking problem, so you didn't take his comments seriously. Running the country is a stressful endeavour; look at the number of politicians we know who end up buried in a bottle. I think this will all blow over for you."

"Easy for you to say. It won't blow over for Alix, though, will it?"

"Certainly not. Questions will be asked about you, and you need to distance yourself from him."

Owen's phone rang as he glanced at Charles. "Darius is calling."

"He's a good man to know in a crisis. I'd take the call if I were you."

Owen nodded. "Okay." He put the phone to his ear. "Hello, Darius... yes, I can talk. I'm at home here with Charles; no one else is around... Alright, I will do that. He wants me to put the call on speaker," Owen said to Charles.

"Can you hear me, Darius? You're on speaker; Charles is listening."

"Yes, I can hear you clearly," Darius replied. "This is a most unpleasant situation, gentlemen. I'm most displeased about what I've seen in the news."

"Well, so am I, old boy. My bloody name is all over the headlines," Owen responded.

"I'll choose my words carefully over the phone, but in the news footage, Alix was filmed saying something about a cover-up. Do you know anything about that, Owen?"

Owen glanced at Charles and swallowed. "No. You can hear me say I don't want to know anything more about it. Charles and I were just discussing it, and I need to keep my distance from Alix."

"Alix's career in politics is over! But that's not my main concern.

I'm interested in how a recording took place within your private office. That interests me a great deal."

"I have no idea, Darius. Could a journalist have gained access in some way? Many reporters have press passes for the palace, though I'm not sure why I would be of interest to warrant such effort."

"Alright, let's talk this through. If you turn to Channel 8 right now, they mentioned they were about to rerun the footage; they are currently interviewing an opposition MP via a web link."

"Charles, could you please select Channel 8?"

As the picture appeared on the screen, Owen tutted in annoyance. "That bugger always shows up when there's political capital to be gained," he said, pointing irritably at the television. He was not on speaking terms with the MP featured on screen.

Charles snorted in agreement with Owen's comment.

"Alright, here we go," Darius said.

Glued to the television, Charles and Owen remained silent as the footage replayed.

"Pause the live TV if you need to. Observe every tiny detail you can see on screen," Darius added.

Charles nodded, holding the remote in anticipation.

"Okay, look, you're now on screen," Darius said. "It seems like you picked up the camera from your desk."

"Can you pause it?" Owen asked Charles as they both examined the low-quality image of Owen displayed on the screen.

"What did you pick up?" Charles inquired.

"I have no idea. I was checking emails, and to be honest, I'd had a few drinks."

"Think hard, Owen," Darius demanded.

"Why would there be a camera on my desk? I never would have allowed it."

Darius rolled his eyes. "It may have been hidden inside something. It looks like you picked something up and then discarded it, possibly into a bin or something."

Owen scratched his head, looking uncertain. "I… I'm not…" He suddenly paused, glancing at Charles with surprise. "What happened to your picture?"

Charles frowned, clearly confused. "What do you mean, what picture?"

"The picture we were both given…" Owen started to say.

Darius interrupted, "What pictures are you talking about?"

"That dreadful picture of the palace," Owen said to Charles.

"Oh, that dreadful monstrosity. I gave it to you, didn't I?" Charles replied.

Owen looked thoughtful, closing his eyes as he recalled the moment. "Yes, I remember. I threw it in the bin!"

"What pictures are we discussing, gentlemen?" Darius asked again.

"I…I... yes, that's right. I received an email! I leaned over the desk and you heard me say something like, 'and this bloody thing,' before tossing it away. It was the picture frame!"

"My Lords, I'm not fully understanding. Are you saying someone gave you both a picture?"

"Yes, my God, Charles! There must have been hidden cameras inside them!"

Charles nodded vigorously and stood up. "Are they destroyed?"

"I threw them both in the bin, Charles."

"Could they still be there?" Darius asked urgently.

"No, not a chance. The office bins would have been emptied by now. They'll be long gone."

"Okay, Owen. Now I need you to think. Who gave you those picture frames?"

"Well, that's the strangest thing, old boy. You gave them to us."

"What do you mean? I haven't…"

"Not you specifically. One of your board members, the woman. Sorry, I can't remember her name. She's the only woman on your board."

Darius froze in shock. "Are you saying that the same woman gave both of you a picture?"

"Yes, that's exactly what happened. It was early on Saturday evening. I dropped it onto my desk, and not long after that, Alix showed up at my office." Owen paused. There was silence on the other end of the phone. "Darius, are you still there? Charles is nodding along with everything I've said. Are we thinking a board member is behind this?"

Darius had been developing his plans for over two years, taking pride in his ability to consider every possible outcome and swiftly deal with any unexpected obstacles. However, this situation presented a challenge he hadn't anticipated. "My Lords, does the name Lisa Wellings ring a bell for you?" he asked.

"Yes, that's her!" Charles responded eagerly.

"That's right, old boy. She's the one who gave the picture to each of us," Owen added.

Darius closed his eyes for a moment. "Okay, thank you both. I'll take care of this. I'll be in touch." He gently set his phone down on the desk, took a seat, crossed his legs, and swung his left leg back and forth. He knew this matter needed immediate resolution. Owen and Charles could potentially be mistaken, so he needed to seek clarification before taking any further action. For Lisa's sake, he truly hoped she hadn't betrayed him. He decided to call his phone expert from the special projects team to start investigating and see where it would lead.

++++

"And we are off the air. Thank you, Sharron, and well done, everyone. It's amazing how quickly we were able to put that together. How are we looking?" Ben asked one of the production team members.

"Immensely well, frankly. We're going viral; our broadcast is now being rebroadcast worldwide. The viewing stats must be off the scale."

"Incredible!" Ben grinned and clapped his hands together as he looked around the studio. "Where is Helen now?"

"She's in the green room."

"Okay, I'll go and see her. I mentioned a possible live webchat with her, but I've changed my mind. I think we've said enough for now. If all of us could keep an eye on things, please update me on any fallout from this and any official statements from Downing Street. I have a feeling this is going to be a very long night."

Ben started to make his way toward the green room and stopped to shake hands with Sharron as he reached the door. "Well done, that was great."

"I enjoyed that. It's great to have an exclusive again. How are we looking?" Sharron asked.

"Let's just say everyone now knows about it."

Sharron smiled as she walked away.

Ben opened the green room door. "Helen, there you are. How are you feeling?"

Helen was sitting alone, studying her phone. "I think we've created quite a bit of attention."

"You could say that; you did very well," Ben said as he sat beside her. "So, what are your plans now?"

Helen put her phone down. "Honestly, I don't know; I've never been in this position before."

Ben smiled. "I don't think many have."

"I'm still being labelled a maverick online."

"Is that really a bad thing? It shows you have the courage to stand up for your beliefs."

Helen looked Ben in the eyes. "You've changed your tune," she said with a slight smile.

Ben leaned back in his seat, unbuttoned his shirt sleeves, rolled them up, and took a deep breath. He nodded a few times, still smiling. "I've had some time to think things over, Helen. Just yesterday, you were sunk, trapped in a political hole that even the very best could not escape from. But now, I'm not so sure. From a legal perspective, some would argue that I should have had you sign a release agreement and that you should take as much responsibility as possible for that recording. However, we broadcast what you provided us. To be honest, I don't think a signed piece of paper would hold much value for us if everything goes wrong. I've taken a significant risk with you, Helen. If that footage turns out to be fake, we could find ourselves in a lot of trouble."

"I agree. However, I'm sure it's not."

Ben leaned forward in his chair, a smile spreading across his face. "But you didn't tell the whole truth, did you?"

Helen looked at him in shock. "About what?"

"I don't believe that USB drive arrived in your mail. I think it came from somewhere else."

"Are you recording this?"

Ben laughed and shook his head. "No, but I don't blame you for being paranoid after everything you've been through in the last twenty-four hours."

"There's a camera above me," Helen pointed out.

"I know, but it's just a security camera for safety in the green room. I assure you, this is a private conversation. You know, I was planning to see Alison this evening, but it's too late now, and I suspect a few of us will be here for most of the night. I will visit her tomorrow. I'm sure she'll be proud of you; she might even call you now that we've heard she is talking again."

"I could come with you."

"I wouldn't."

Helen was surprised by his response. "Why not?"

"I'm going to give you a little bit of advice based on my journalistic experience. Whether you take it is entirely up to you. Here it is: you need to ride this out."

Helen scoffed. "Sharron gave me a hard time."

"Of course she did; that's her job. She rode you hard, but I've seen her be much tougher. You handled her well, and that's my point. Look at where you were yesterday. You made a complete mess by accusing a company of wrongdoing without any evidence. What you claimed was scandalous, but it was based on hearsay. I know what you and Alison found, but there wasn't enough evidence to justify your actions, and you didn't protect your backside. Despite that, you took the information and ran with it. No one would doubt your intentions, but you crossed the line. You were right to have the whip withdrawn from you. Now you're still in the news, but from a different perspective. The real question is, if you were still a party member, would you have allowed us to broadcast what you received?"

"Um. I'm..."

"It was a rhetorical question. Honestly, the best thing for you right now, if you don't mind me saying, is to go home. Return to your constituency. You won't be welcome in Parliament anyway.

I'm sure what happened tonight will spell the downfall of a Prime Minister. It could also lead to a governmental collapse, and you are right at the centre of it. So, in that regard, just ride it out. Consider crossing the floor to another party or standing as an independent MP if you haven't had enough of politics."

They both laughed.

"But in all seriousness, Helen, no one believed what you said yesterday. People might react differently now; you may be surprised by how they respond to you." Ben rose to his feet. "And of course, if that fails, you could always find a job in the media." He waved his hands in the air. "I can see it now: Helen Lord, political correspondent!"

Helen smiled briefly.

"Your career is far from over; you've only just started, Maverick!" He grinned as he handed her the remote control for the television. "We can only hope the police are successful in their investigation and catch the individuals responsible for the attack on Alison. Considering everything that has happened over the past few days, I do not doubt that those responsible will now go to ground." He paused briefly to gather his thoughts. "Right, I need to get back to it, but feel free to check our competitors' news channels. What I'm saying will all make sense. You know where to find us if you need anything. I trust you can find your way out when you're ready."

As Ben headed toward the door, he added, "Oh, and by the way."

Helen looked up.

"I knew that Shrewsbury was the birthplace of Charles Darwin."

As Ben left the room, Helen decided to sit quietly, letting her thoughts drift rather than turning on the television. Perhaps Ben was right; her career might just be beginning.

✢✢✢✢

The old grandfather clock ticked steadily in Darius's office, the only sound breaking the silence. As he sat at his desk, his mind raced; events had unfolded in ways he hadn't anticipated. Every decision he made now was crucial to keeping their plans on track. The recent attempt on Alison's life had failed, buying him some time but little else. David Needham had assured him that the only evidence from the initial lab test involving Ryan Dobey had been destroyed. Darius had no choice but to trust David's word as he reflected on the events that had transpired. The first lab test had returned a positive result for the heroin derivative, which was fine. Alison and Helen were always going to go public; while David's intervention had ultimately failed, it had at least delayed their plans for the time being. The MP had taken the bait and gone it alone. Just yesterday, she had been labelled a rogue; now, Darius wasn't so sure. People might start paying more attention to her. The covert recording between Alix Gregory and Lord Gatesouth was unfortunate. While he was confident that Alix would never talk, he knew he might have to take the fall for it. If Alix didn't step down, Darius might need to find a way to encourage him to do so. Journalists would now investigate the Prime Minister's background in an effort to decipher his comments on the recording. However, he was confident they would not uncover anything of significance. Nonetheless, he had lost leverage with Alix's probable departure, which was a costly setback. While he still had allies in parliament from the main opposition parties, the modern dynamics of Westminster made business considerably more challenging. Each year, new MPs entered parliament through by-elections triggered whenever a member fell ill, or, more often, fell from grace; this was as inevitable as the rising sun. These new MPs didn't adhere to the traditional ways of the political game, and everything had become more transparent, with every transaction documented and all declarations made public. This was the new way of running parliament, and it was detrimental to business.

Rubbing his eyes and massaging his forehead, he knew he needed to address this new problem immediately. The thought of one of their own betraying him was unexpected, unethical, and deeply frustrating. Lisa Wellings was outspoken and often a thorn in the side of some board members, but not to him. He appreciated her tenacity, as she had rightfully earned her place on the board. He hoped that Owen and Charles had made a mistake, but deep down, he doubted it. The two men from the Lord's enjoyed his financial support, yet they lacked common sense, despite being intelligent. Earlier, he had enlisted the help of his phone expert from the special projects team to monitor the calls made and received by Helen Lord, John Farmer, and Lisa. The overhead costs of the entire operation had skyrocketed, primarily due to expenses from the special projects team and additional costs incurred by David and his colleague. At least David had managed to silence the family involved in the lab test, which was one less concern. Although he didn't pry into David's methods, there had been no media coverage regarding the family, and he had confidence that David had handled the situation professionally.

Now, a new dilemma emerged: with Alix's exposure, would Helen Lord resume her efforts to undermine them? What actions might she take, along with her wound-ridden friend? Nine thousand vials were already in the country, ready for release, to be hidden in plain sight among their standard fillers. What would the member of parliament do? Attempt to buy all the stock? That seemed unlikely, as she might soon be out of a job and could hardly expect financial backing for her unorthodox and maverick pursuits. It would be reckless for her to try. The chances of her coming into contact with one of the new vials were minimal, and they would plan accordingly. The UK would serve as their testing ground, with additional vials added with each batch. Once their fortunes improved, they would shift their focus to the Far East and the lucrative American market as their next targets.

Darius's phone vibrated on the desk. It was Geoff, his phone expert, calling. He picked up the phone, hoping he had gathered some useful information.

"Good to hear from you," Darius said, his voice filled with anticipation.

"That's okay, Darius. I have the information you requested."

"That's good to hear. I'm trying to determine if there's a common link between the phones you've been monitoring."

"Understood. You want to know if they have been in contact?"

"Yes, exactly."

"Well, the short answer is yes. They have been communicating."

Darius's heart sank. "Please, continue," he urged, shaking his head.

"Yesterday, Lisa's phone called John's phone. After that, they met in the Surrey area. I've tied their phones together and confirmed they met at Lisa's home, as her phone is registered to that address. John travelled to meet her, and they were together for a couple of hours."

Darius nodded. "Okay, what happened next?"

"Nothing happened until earlier today when she contacted him again. The data indicates that she then contacted Helen, after which Lisa got in touch with John once more. Additionally, another call was made from Lisa's phone to Helen's. A couple of hours later, I matched the locations of Lisa and John's phones in the Clerkenwell area, suggesting they might have met; this was only a few hours ago. I checked, and Lisa has offices in that area. According to the phone data, John then moved on without her; while I don't have the exact location, it appears he went to the Farringdon area of London."

"Did John have any phone contact with Helen Lord at any point?"

"No, I haven't found any evidence of that. However, I've linked their phones in Farringdon, which suggests he met with her."

Darius closed his eyes, realising everything was coming together quickly. "Was Lisa with them?"

"No, I don't think so. To clarify, her phone was in the Clerkenwell area. That doesn't necessarily mean she wasn't present, but based on the data, her phone was located in Clerkenwell."

"Okay, Geoff. So, if I understand correctly, only John met with Helen?"

"That seems to be the case, according to the data."

Darius couldn't believe what he was hearing. "Right. I need proof of their meeting. I need to confirm whether Lisa was also there. Do you know if there are any CCTV cameras in the area?"

"I honestly don't know," came the reply. "But it shouldn't be difficult to find out. It depends on whether the Metropolitan Police control the cameras in that area. If private security contractors monitor the area, it might be trickier. Obtaining footage from individual sources, such as shop cameras, can be a time-consuming process. Sometimes, those people need a bit of 'encouragement' to release such footage, if you know what I mean."

"Yes, I understand. Just give me a moment, will you?"

"Of course."

Darius pulled the phone away from his ear and rubbed his eyes. He knew this situation needed to be handled quickly, but he wouldn't take any action without solid proof, especially when it involved board members. He lifted the phone again. "Okay, can we find out if there are cameras in the area first? That's the priority. You also need to pinpoint the exact location where they met. Is that possible?"

"How quickly do you need to know, Darius?"

"Now."

There was a hint of a forced laugh. "How did I know you were going to say that? Well, look, if the Met controls the cameras, that shouldn't be a problem, especially since the events occurred today. That's the first thing we need to confirm. If that's the case, we should be able to obtain some footage. If the cameras are controlled by someone else, like a private security company, we'll need to address that once we have more information."

"Understood. So, you're confident that if it's a police camera, you can access it?"

"Of course. But, as you might expect..."

"Go on. How much is it going to cost?"

"I don't know," was the straightforward reply. "I'll need to do some fact-checking first. If there is a police camera, I know a couple of people who can help. It will also depend on when they are on shift. It will have to be paid in cash, and it will be expensive. If I can locate a camera, would you like me to obtain a quote first?"

Darius shook his head. "No. Please proceed, but listen, Geoff. No one else can know about this; leave no traces. This is vitally important. Do you understand?"

"Of course. I'll be in touch, but it may be quite late by the time I get back to you. This isn't just about making a couple of calls, as I'm sure you understand."

"Don't worry. I rarely sleep anyway. My phone is on for you."

"Okay. I'll call you as soon as I have an update. But Darius, there may be nothing there. Although the area is designated as central London, it's not exactly like Oxford Circus. You may need to prepare yourself for disappointment."

"I understand, but please try your hardest. Talk to you later."

"Goodbye, Darius."

As soon as the call ended, Darius fell back into his seat. It was unbelievable. Although he didn't know Lisa very well, John's father had been a senior board member. John had the pedigree; his lineage was tied to the company.

Darius rubbed his eyes in frustration, knowing that he had been betrayed.

++++

Darius's phone rang, and a glance at the clock showed it was 2:16 AM. Having sat at his desk for hours without moving, he felt a wave of relief upon seeing that his phone expert, Geoff, was calling.

"Hi, Geoff. How are we looking?" Darius asked.

"This hasn't been easy, but I believe I have what you need. There are a couple of police-controlled cameras in the area. One of my contacts helped out. They weren't on duty and had to make a special trip to retrieve the footage I've managed to obtain for you. Just to confirm, you have your own secure network, correct?"

"Yes, that's correct."

"I'm going to text you an email address. You'll need to set up an account with it. Once you've done that, I will email the file from my secure network to yours. After you receive it, delete the email address immediately. There won't be any trace back to you. Just to be clear, this is for you, and you alone. Once you've viewed it, delete it, and it will be scrubbed from my end as well. My colleague captured the footage, and I had to collect it from them as they wouldn't risk sending it to me directly."

"I understand," Darius replied.

"My colleague took some risks to obtain this information, and I'm sure you can infer the line of work he's in."

Darius nodded; Geoff had excellent police contacts. "I appreciate your efforts; you've done exceptionally well given the timeframe."

"The footage isn't perfect, but I managed to get a more accurate lock on their phones. It shows a general view of a road called Bowling Green Lane in Farringdon. There's a pub there, and I believe that's where they meet."

"You believe?"

"Yes. I'm unsure about John; I've only seen his picture on your website. However, Helen is definitely in the frame; her face is highly recognisable, especially since she's all over the media at the moment. I'm confident it's her."

"You mentioned they meet outside the pub. Do they go inside?"

"No, they only spend a brief moment together outside."

That should be enough for a handover, Darius thought.

"My colleague managed to zoom in with the camera, but the image isn't crystal clear. Still, it may provide the information you need. Has the email address appeared on your phone?"

"Hold on… Yes." Darius checked the text and pulled his keyboard closer. "Just give me a moment while I set it up."

"Not a problem. I can wait."

"I've never seen an email address like this before."

"No, it's not a standard Gmail or anything similar. Just let me know when you're ready to receive it."

"Alright, I think I'm in."

"Sending now. I'll wait while you verify."

"A file has arrived. Hold on." Darius opened the video file. "You're right; it's not very clear. Can you see John arriving in this?"

"No, it's just a quick grab of footage. At the beginning, he's outside the pub. If you could confirm that it's your subject."

"Just a moment." Darius studied the footage, needing to be sure. It could be John. A black taxi pulled up alongside him. A woman got out, her back toward the camera. She approached the man as the cab drove away, then she turned around. "Yes, that's her, alright."

"What about him? Is that the man you are looking for?"

"Hold on." Darius focused as best as he could. It appeared that the man was holding something up. Whatever it was, it looked small. Then, he threw it toward the member of parliament. It could be a USB drive.

"My colleague was able to zoom in a bit more at this point, but the quality of the picture became less clear."

The camera zoomed in. Darius swallowed and closed his eyes. He was sure it was his fellow board member.

"Is this what you were after, Darius?"

Filled with rage, Darius practically spat his words, "Yes, it is!" In the recording, he saw John walking away, while the MP remained standing outside the pub as the footage ended.

"Darius, I monitored his phone. He left the area and didn't return."

"Do you know if he went to visit Lisa?"

"No. He left London entirely and headed towards Kent. Is this all you need?"

Darius took a deep breath. "Yes, I think this clarifies things. How much do I owe you?"

"I'm not sure. I told my colleague to wait around, just in case you needed something else. Is there anything else?"

"No, you've done an exceptional job, my friend. Can you find out how much I owe you? I'll arrange for a bag drop."

"Of course. Can we do this within the next forty-eight hours, please? I want to keep my colleague happy in case we need his assistance again."

"That won't be a problem. Thank you once again."

"Darius, please remember what I said: delete the footage and the email address."

"I'll take care of that immediately."

"I'll say goodnight then. I'll message you with the exact amount owed as soon as I have it."

"Thank you, Geoff. Goodnight."

Darius closed his eyes and tilted his head toward the ceiling. He began to take deep breaths as the weight of betrayal settled in; it was undeniable. Turning back to the screen, he ignored Geoff's instructions. He deleted the email address but kept the footage, knowing he would need to rewatch it. Sitting in silence, he felt his anger building and slammed his hands on the desk, furious that his plans had been jeopardised. John and Lisa had likely cost Alix Gregory his job, implicated Lord Gatesouth, and supported the disgraced MP. Years of work, research, and money had been invested in this venture to restore the company's profitability, and this was the thanks he received. It would not stand. Betrayal had no place in business. He would reflect on it overnight, but for now, he had to consider that there was more cleaning up to do.

Chapter Thirty-Four

TUESDAY MORNING

KNIGHTARK PHARMACEUTICAL UK HEADQUARTERS, LONDON

"Mr Neith, Mr De La Roche is here to see you."

"Thank you. Send him in." Darius adjusted his suit jacket and moved to the office door to greet his senior board member. "Thank you for coming into the office, William."

William stepped into the office and quickly closed the door behind him. "Your call sounded urgent. I'm only here for a couple more days before I head back to the States."

Darius nodded. "Would you like some tea or anything else?"

William shook his head as he glanced at the television screen. "What's the situation with your Prime Minister?"

"It's too early to tell. For now, he has gone to ground, but he won't be able to hide for much longer. The press smells blood, and he is right in their crosshairs."

"I'm concerned, Darius. I know Ronald is, too. You sail too close to the edge."

"My friend, everything is under control."

"I don't doubt your resourcefulness, but you can be quite cavalier at times."

Darius smiled. "Let's talk. Follow me." He opened the door that led to his private balcony. From the twelfth story, it offered a prime view of the city of London.

William set down his bag and stepped outside.

"I'd prefer to talk out here. As you are aware, I've become

somewhat cautious about what I say in my office these days, particularly regarding a matter I need to bring to your attention. Please close the door behind you."

"That sounds serious. What's going on? Is it something to do with the PM?"

Darius shook his head, glancing across the city. "No, he's contained for now. It's something else. I need to discuss it with you, and then we can decide whether to inform Ronald and Hugh. I'm trusting you with this."

William turned to Darius and leaned on the railing. "So, what is it?"

"As you know, a covert recording was obtained inside Westminster, specifically in Gatesouth's office. I know who placed it there."

William's eyes widened with curiosity. "Who was it?"

"I regret to say, my friend, it was someone close to us. Someone who didn't share our beliefs and didn't understand the bigger picture."

"And?"

"It was Lisa Wellings."

William's mouth dropped open in shock. "You can't be serious; she's one of our own. Why would she do that?"

"Because she's a non-believer."

"Wait a second, Darius. How do you know this? How can you be sure?"

"I spoke with Gatesouth and Hawthorne. They both received picture frames from Lisa at our reception on Saturday evening. Inside each frame was a covert camera; what seemed like a thoughtful gift was actually a trap."

William's laughter sounded far from genuine.

"You're right to be in shock, my friend. So am I."

"But what was she hoping to gain?"

"I'm not entirely sure, but her actions, and those of John Farmer, sadly seem intended to undermine us."

"No. John too? I know you've been keeping an eye on them. Are you certain?"

"It's confirmed. Lisa obtained the footage, informed the MP, and John personally delivered it. I have a CCTV recording on my laptop if you'd like to see it."

William shook his head. "No, that won't be necessary." He began pacing along the balcony. "I just don't understand, Darius. I'm at a loss! Does this mean our plans are on hold? Should we abort?"

Darius nearly burst out laughing. "Absolutely not! Too much has gone into this. We are not bailing out now."

"But two board members have betrayed us. If we don't take action, they will continue to undermine us. This is very serious!" William's voice was filled with anger.

"Yes, it is, my friend. Yes, it is, and that is why you are here. We need to assess our current situation. Alix is out of the picture, but he won't say anything..."

"How can you be so sure?"

"Because he's implicated in a crime. You don't know the details, but trust me; he doesn't want that information to come to light. He has no choice but to stay quiet. Eventually, he will have to fold and step down. When the time is right, we can bring him back to our side. He still has useful connections that we can leverage for our benefit, so it's not a total loss."

William's expression showed disbelief as he put his hands on his hips. "I don't understand how you can remain so calm about this."

Darius raised his hands to help William steady himself and maintain his composure. "First, there's Alison Harwood, our main nemesis. Regardless of what happens next, she will be frightened, wounded, yes, but scared. I suspect she won't be as brazen with her rhetoric moving forward. Secondly, there's the MP. I believe she will still face a parliamentary ban for her actions. Although she released the covert recording, I suspect she will continue to hold a grudge against us. Even if she continues as an independent MP or calls for a by-election and somehow wins, her resources will be minimal, which isn't a concern for us. Let's not forget that she embarrassed herself on an international stage by making unsupported accusations against us.

Our lawyers have already initiated legal action against her and will pursue all of her assets, including her home, savings, and even her pet dog, if she has one. We will break her spirit, and sooner or later, she will give up. The wheels are already in motion in that regard."

"However, even if everything unfolds as you expect, there are still many assumptions being made, and that doesn't address our board issue."

Darius nodded. "No, it doesn't." He turned to face William. "I called our asset earlier, but the call went to his voicemail, which doesn't surprise me. He has been quite busy for the last few days. I'm hoping he'll return my message."

William let out a deep sigh and began scratching his head. "God, I almost forgot about that and the lab guy's family. I haven't seen anything about it on the news." He started pacing the balcony, shaking his head in dismay. He pointed at Darius. "This was supposed to be a single operation, and now we have a body count. Seriously, how much is all this costing us? Covert assets are always expensive."

"It's substantial now, my friend. But we're in too deep. And to clarify, there are no bodies at this point."

"What do you mean, 'at this point'?"

"This is the final cleanup to eliminate any obstacles. I'll explain all of the costs another time. It will require some creative accounting, but I'm on top of it."

"Wait, hang on. You said you called the asset." William looked Darius directly in the eyes. "Oh no, you can't be serious!"

"Is there any other way?"

"You want to eliminate two of our board members? I don't think that will go unnoticed! May I remind you that our name is being widely broadcast on social media and in the press? It was bad enough to authorise a public execution in the first place, and a failed execution at that, since she still lives!"

"It's true, my friend. What happened was unfortunate, but we still have control over the situation. However, we need to silence both of them."

"Darius, listen to me. We have a long history together, built on a foundation of enormous respect and trust. But this, this is crossing a line."

"Hear me out. I'm talking about setting an example. Don't think for a second that I like this any more than you do, but our hands are being forced by their actions and betrayal. Starting with Lisa, she's married, lives in a gated estate, and has offices in London. Any attempt on her life would create a bloody mess and be difficult to cover up. On the other hand, John was the one who delivered the film to the MP. He lives alone and works from home."

"And so?"

"And so, I'm thinking about sending our asset to him."

"Jesus, Darius," William said as he began to pace back and forth again. "This situation is getting worse and worse."

"We have been betrayed by two of our own. They have already gone to great lengths, and it will only escalate from here. We need to address this now."

"And what about Lisa? What do you plan to do with her?"

Darius shrugged. "Nothing."

William crossed his arms and started tapping his left foot. "Nothing, you say?"

"That's right. Nothing at all. I suspect she will resign soon, and when she finds out that John has disappeared, it will likely push her to leave the company."

"So, you intend to make John disappear?"

"Correct. No evidence. Passport gone. He vanishes."

"I don't know, Darius; that sounds a bit flimsy to me."

"What would you rather do: tamper with his car brakes or stage a botched break-in at his home? Both options take time and leave a trail of evidence. This way, there will be nothing. He'll become a modern-day Lord Lucan and simply go off the radar."

The American board member frowned, "Who is Lord Lucan? Is he another one we pay off?"

"What? Never mind. The point is that a complete disappearance is the only solution I see. We need to clean up our house. I'm telling you, Lisa will resign once she realises he's gone. And seriously, what can she do? Run to the police with what evidence?"

William rubbed his head. "I don't know, Darius. This could get messy."

"If handled correctly, it shouldn't. Even if the asset gets caught, he's only ever been paid in cash, and our communications are encrypted. I already have a new phone ready for him. You need to trust me, he's military. Men like him never talk, and we don't use torture in this country to get answers. He'll never break. Do you have a better suggestion?"

William crossed his arms as he leaned against the balcony. "Why am I here? Why are you telling me this?"

"Because you are my right-hand man, and I want this to remain between us. If we are to advance this business, we must be fully aware of all the facts and every aspect involved. If anything were to happen to me, I would like you to take over the management of this company. That's why you're here."

William nodded with a slight smile. "I've never heard you say that before."

"Well, you're hearing it now, my friend. Now, are you with me or not?"

William clenched his jaw as he considered the implications. "No mess?"

"No mess. No trace."

"That seems like a shame. I liked his father."

"So did I, my friend. So did I."

✢✢✢✢

"Good God!" David Needham exclaimed as he sat on the edge of his sofa after switching to a news channel. Covert footage of the Prime Minister mentioning his involvement in a cover-up dominated the broadcast, along with replays of Helen Lord's interview. It was an astonishing situation. After an early night and abstaining from television, this was the first he had heard of it. "Bloody MPs," he muttered. Snippets of the lab test were replayed, and the studio's 'experts' debated the story. Their main discussion revolved around whether Helen Lord's actions were justified or irresponsible. In any case, David thought, it must have been a cunning journalist who planted that covert camera; someone was in for a hefty payday. Lost in contemplation, he sipped his coffee. This was all a bit too close for comfort. How on earth did Helen obtain that footage? He was relieved there was no mention of Ryan and his family. That thought reminded him of his appointment with the car breakers. He finished his coffee, fed the fish in his tank, grabbed his binoculars, and locked the front door of the old farmhouse. It was a short walk to the car. The phone he had been using was hidden nearby and would be disposed of today, along with the vehicle.

After a fifteen-minute walk, David nestled himself into a hedge. Further down the overgrown lane, he spotted his parked car. Carefully concealing himself, he removed the lens caps from his binoculars and scanned the area around the vehicle. He was concerned about the possibility of professional military surveillance, but police surveillance did not worry him as much. In his experience, police typically operated from their vehicles, which made them easy to spot, especially in rural areas like this. Military personnel, on the other hand, were more skilled at working long hours and adapting to various environments. From his observation point, he scanned the surrounding bushes for any signs of activity, such as freshly cut branches in the trees above or anything that appeared out of place. With so much foliage in the lane, it would be difficult to spot any hidden cameras. Satisfied to some extent, David put the binoculars away and leapt over a stile into a farmer's field. As he walked along the hedgerow, he kept an eye on the ground for boot prints and checked the hedgerow for any signs of disturbance. He continued moving forward, passing the car without stopping. After navigating through the farmer's field, he reached the next stile. As he stepped over it and onto the tarmac, he looked up and down the lane. There were no signs of movement, no dog walkers, and everything seemed clear. He decided to take a chance and approached the car. The sooner he could dispose of it, the better. The vehicle was lodged firmly against some bushes, and he felt it prudent to check for anything unusual before pulling out the key from his pocket. Until he revealed the key, he would appear to be a curious passerby, wondering why someone had abandoned a car here. It was a story he had rehearsed countless times before. Seeing nothing suspicious, he felt reassured, unlocked the car, and drove away quickly. As he made his way to retrieve the phone, he remained vigilant for any vehicles following him and scanned the sky for drones. Everything seemed calm; he appeared to be in the clear. The phone was concealed in a plastic bag hidden beneath some rocks halfway down the next lane. In this quiet rural area, not many people passed by. He kept it simple for one night, ensuring the bag remained hidden. As he approached to retrieve the phone, he checked that the area in front, behind, and above him was clear. He quickly pulled over, jumped out of the car, and rummaged through the patch of rocks covered in weeds. He found the phone bag with the SIM card nestled between two discarded bricks off to the side. Rushing as quickly as he could, he jumped into the car and drove away. After travelling a mile, he pulled over. Feeling confident that he wasn't being followed, he inserted the SIM card and turned on the phone. David sat patiently, tapping the steering wheel as he waited to see if he had any missed calls. Only Rubin, another client, and his primary client, Darius, had this number. David rolled his eyes when a message arrived; it was Darius asking him to call. Ensuring no one was around, he called Darius. What Darius wanted was anyone's guess, as he had done enough for him over the last few days. He planned to head out with the fishing rods later, once he had a replacement vehicle. This call about potential additional work was highly irritating.

"David, thank you for returning my call. Can you talk?" Darius asked.

"I can, for now. What's on your mind?"

"I have another job for you, and it's urgent."

++++

The golf day had been cancelled, and Charles Hawthorne had already left Owen Gatesouth's house. With hardly any sleep, Owen felt relieved to see Darius's name appear on his phone. Hopefully, he would have some answers.

"Owen, can you talk?" Darius asked.

"Yes, I can talk to you. I'm inundated with calls and bloody emails; this is a fine mess!"

"Not necessarily for you. I know this is tricky..." Darius began.

"Tricky? I'm all over the bloody news, old boy!"

Darius could hear the frustration in Owen's voice. "I know, but look. This is all going to come down on Alix, not you. You haven't done anything wrong, and what Alix said to you, you didn't take it seriously anyway. That's why you didn't report it. You don't know anything. I'm calling because I'm handling it."

"And how are you doing that? This isn't going away any time soon."

"That part is true. The ball is now in Alix's court, but I can't share too much over the phone. Just know it's being taken care of, but I need you to do something for me."

"That's a bit bold, especially when it was one of your board members who set me up."

"Like I said, it's being handled. You won't hear from her again, I assure you. Has the Prime Minister called you today?" Darius asked.

"No, not yet, but I suspect it's imminent."

"Good. Here's what I need you to do. He will want to know how a camera got into your office, and I need you to say that you don't know."

"What? But I know exactly how it got there!"

"Yes, I understand that you and I know the truth, but no one else does, except for Charles and the person who placed it there. To protect yourself and your reputation, it is essential to distance yourself from Alix. When you take the call, I need you to say that you suspect the camera was placed there by someone working undercover, perhaps a journalist. Do you understand?"

Owen let out a heavy sigh. "And why should I do that?"

"It's quite simple. How much money have I paid you over the years?"

"Darius, don't be like that. We have an arrangement…"

"And I intend to honour our working agreement moving forward. You need to tell the PM what I just told you; doing so will stop the questions and redirect attention elsewhere. This is important: my company has innovations on the horizon, including products that have been in development for a couple of years. We can't let this issue continue; we need to resolve it. If you follow my instructions, it will deflect attention from us and keep everyone in the clear."

"This sounds like self-preservation to me, Darius."

"In part, yes. But this company is about to turn its fortunes around, and I want you to be part of that journey. There will be significant rewards, and I've always taken care of you without asking for much in return."

"I don't know. I can't have my face all over the TV screens!"

"And I will make sure that doesn't happen. So, will you do this? It's a matter of loyalty, Owen. Does your loyalty lie with me or with the Prime Minister?"

"Darius, honestly…"

"Well, what's it going to be? I promise I'll make it worth your while."

"My loyalty lies with you, Darius; you know that. But I don't want to see that woman again. How dare she put that in my office!"

"Her resignation is imminent, I assure you," Darius stated confidently.

"And what if she talks? What if she gets involved with that Helen Lord? Where will we be then?" "I have plans in motion; you know

I can make things happen. Plus, I'm going to double your monthly retainer as a gesture of goodwill for informing the Prime Minister about what I just told you."

There was a brief silence on the other end of the line. "Well, okay," Owen finally grumbled.

"Do you give me your word?" Darius pressed.

"Yes, Darius. I give you my word. I'll inform Alix when he calls. I'm surprised I haven't heard from him already, now that I think about it."

"Excellent. I'll keep you updated on developments, and we'll meet when all of this blows over."

"Let's hope that happens very soon! I really can't bear for this to drag on any longer."

"Goodbye for now, Owen," Darius concluded.

From the balcony, William nodded at Darius. "That sounded like it went better than I expected."

Darius smiled. "He's always been motivated by money, just like many others. He'll do as he's told."

✢✢✢✢

David held the phone in his hands and exhaled deeply as he contemplated his options, including whether he should complete this latest assignment presented by Darius. Although he was well compensated for his work, that money would mean little if everything came crashing down around him. Over the past week, he had taken significant risks, sailed into dangerous waters, and pushed his luck. This new assignment was also highly risky, as it required immediate action. For reasons he didn't fully understand or concern himself with, it seemed that Knightark Pharmaceutical had a problem with a rogue member on its board of directors. This board member now had a price on his head, and David had quoted the required amount. However, this task was not straightforward. A quick kill is generally simple, but Darius also wanted the body disposed of, leaving no trace evidence, so it would have to be a swift in and out. The board member lived in a large property in Kent, and according to Darius, he had some security measures in place, though nothing particularly sophisticated. David noticed a lack of confidence in Darius's words when he made his statement. The individual lived alone and had no immediate family members, which alleviated some concerns. He worked from home as a consultant. David had agreed to take on the work, contingent upon a predicted successful outcome, and he indicated that the task required two people for a quick clean-up. Given the limited timeframe, he had no choice but to contact Rubin, assuming he was still in the country.

The target was Dr John Farmer.

++++

Over the course of the morning, Owen Gatesouth had walked around his garden several times. Throughout his years of public service, he had managed to avoid controversy, in stark contrast to some of his counterparts. Although his image appeared frequently in the media, it was not as prominent as that of Alix or the bloody, troublesome Helen Lord. He hated the attention and felt nauseous. For now, it was out of his control. His fellow peers would judge him, but as a seasoned politician, that concerned him little; he believed he could weather the criticism. What troubled him most was the court of public opinion. The world and the political system were changing; further reform was imminent, and the Lords would undergo transformation.

He glanced at his phone and immediately slowed his pace. Alix was calling. Owen closed his eyes, knowing that this call was inevitable; it was only a matter of time. He would have to lie to the Prime Minister, as his loyalties lay elsewhere. He couldn't jeopardise his relationship with Darius; Darius knew too much and had just offered him a pay incentive. The sooner Owen's name and picture were out of the media, the better. Alix would have to take the fall.

Taking a deep breath, Owen answered, "Hello, Alix."

"I nearly hung up! You took so long to answer!"

"Suffice to say, you're not the only one calling today. What's happening? What's your position?"

"There is no position. I'm being briefed constantly and have advisors everywhere I look. I can't even make a move without it being questioned."

Owen smiled briefly. "I can well imagine, Alix. How can I help, if at all?"

"We are fact-finding, Owen, but we need to understand how that camera ended up in your office. You didn't place it there since you are in the footage. Can you offer any guidance or thoughts on this?"

Owen scoffed. "Of course I didn't bloody put it there! Why would I have a camera in my office?"

"Exactly, but it seems you picked up the camera and then discarded it. It looked as if it had been thrown aside, possibly into a bin. I have people looking into it."

Owen felt his heart rate increase, relieved that this was not a face-to-face meeting. "I don't know, Alix. I've been trying to figure it out myself. The only assumption I can make is that a journalist or someone else must have placed it there."

"But who has access to your office?"

"That's not the issue, old boy. I often leave it unlocked, as do many others in the Lords. We engage in politics differently than you do; I don't leave state secrets sitting on my desk."

"I have the Serjeant at Arms' department investigating it. They're reviewing the camera footage inside the palace. So far, we haven't seen anyone enter your office except for me. You can see how this looks. We are all confused. I must ask you, and please answer honestly: Was that camera yours? Did you leave it on your desk? Was there another purpose for it?"

"What!"

"Please, hear me out, Owen. This is important. You won't be in any trouble, but we need to conduct an investigation. We can't have covert cameras in the palace. I need to know if you did this, even if it was an accident. Please be honest with me."

"I assure you, Alix, that is not the case. Why would I do that?"

"Okay, okay, but you picked it up, whatever it was or whatever it was hidden in. Where did it go?"

"Um, I'm not sure. I might have thrown it in the bin."

"And that's what we suspected, which is why we're now going through all the rubbish collected since the weekend."

Owen froze upon hearing this. "Is it possible that it could still be found?"

"Doubtful, to be honest."

Owen let out a sigh of relief.

"Owen, we've known each other for a long time. Do you have any additional information that could help us with this? That's why I'm contacting you personally. We are friends. Please think carefully, can you remember picking up anything from your desk that you might have thrown away?"

"Prime Minister, since this has been broadcast worldwide and I'm in the footage, I've thought about little else."

"Alright, okay. I'll have to take your word for it."

"My word has always been good, Alix."

"I know. I know."

"What do you think is going to happen?"

"It's too early to tell, but I'm under a lot of pressure; the press and the opposition are calling for my head."

"Do you think you'll give in to them?"

There was a long pause. "It's not looking good. Please help me if you can."

Owen's face was filled with guilt. "But of course I will."

"Thank you. It wouldn't surprise me if you get called by the Serjeant at Arms department or the police."

Owen closed his eyes, filled with worry. "I'll do whatever I can, old boy."

"Right. I must go now; we'll talk soon."

"Thank you, Alix. Good luck with everything."

Alix murmured something as he hung up.

Owen took a deep breath and resumed walking around his garden. If they uncovered the picture frame, they might realise that he just lied, and if that unravelled, it would lead them straight back to Darius.

Chapter Thirty-Five

Thankfully, David's phone still had around seventy percent battery life and plenty of data. He had parked the car a short distance away to take some time to sit, think, and strategise for Darius's latest assignment. Given the extensive news coverage of the Prime Minister and Helen Lord earlier, it was reasonable to assume this new task was somehow connected to those developments. The assassination of a board member was something he could never have anticipated, but it wasn't his place to ask questions. However, if Darius's actions became reckless and he displayed signs of instability, reprisals would be unavoidable and police involvement certain, potentially jeopardising David's safety. As he reviewed Darius's instructions on his phone, the urgency was unmistakable: this needed to be carried out immediately. Planning such actions could take weeks or even months. Mistakes were likely to occur without meticulous preparation; operational phases were essential to ensure his and the client's safety. He entered the board member's home address into Google Maps and reviewed the surrounding roads, including a view of the front of the house. David rubbed his chin and exhaled loudly as the map loaded on the screen. This was going to be a challenging task. Dr John Farmer lived in Bickley, an affluent neighbourhood in Kent. The properties in the area were expansive and indicative of wealth. He resided on a road called Woodlands Rise, a short cul-de-sac with a small turning area at the end. Every property on this road likely costs millions, indicating that most houses are probably continuously occupied in some form. The gardens were well-maintained, either by the owners, who might have a talent for gardening, or by professional gardeners. As David viewed the street, he noticed a mix of high-end luxury cars and several affordable vehicles in excellent condition parked in the driveways. This observation suggested that young drivers likely resided here, possibly having obtained their cars with their parents' financial support. There were only eighteen houses in the cul-de-sac, but he suspected that people frequently came and went. John Farmer's home had a sizeable driveway and a security gate at its entrance. The street view on his phone was clear enough for him to spot a mounted camera next to the security gate. However, there were no cameras at the road entrance, though that may have changed since the mapping application captured the images. The doctor's house was situated halfway down the road, partially overlooked by both sides. The house directly opposite could pose a problem. Darius wanted to leave no trace evidence, making a distant kill impossible. As he examined both the front and back of the house, it became clear that the task would not be straightforward. They would need to drive the car right up to the front door, and the good doctor would have to be placed in the back. David lowered the phone, contemplating the critical phases ahead. He felt relieved that he hadn't disposed of the car yet; he would need to take care of that immediately afterwards, leaving the doctor inside to be crushed with the vehicle. He never risked putting weapons or explosives in the crusher; those would be safely disposed of on the way there. Given the location and the necessity for a quick escape, this assignment required two people to work together. He needed Rubin. Additionally, Rubin's handgun had a silencer, which David didn't currently possess. He also had some unresolved matters to discuss with Rubin. He had little choice; they needed to enter through the front gate. It wasn't ideal, but it was unavoidable. Breaking into the house through the back could leave trace evidence, and a house directly behind the doctor's garden would make undetected access even more challenging. Darius was clear: nothing could be left behind; their target had to disappear entirely. It would have to be a "kill and grab," hoping there was no one else inside the house and that the occupants of the house opposite didn't see anything. The CCTV at the front gate would be the main obstacle. The mapping tool didn't indicate whether the house opposite had cameras further up their driveway. They also needed to locate the doctor's phone and passport. The phone would be relatively easy to find, but the passport was a different issue. That detail was frustrating and could be time consuming. Once the doctor was reported missing, the police and customs officials would scrutinise airports and ports. He half-expected Darius to instruct him later to make sure the passport was used in a manner that would leave a trace of its journey. This would involve departing from a private airstrip and landing at a small, foreign airport where corrupt customs officers could be found. To anyone investigating, it would appear that John Farmer had simply taken a vacation somewhere off the beaten path. He cleared his phone screen and called Rubin, surprised that the phone rang as Rubin was supposed to keep his phone switched off until it was disposed of.

"Hello, brother," Rubin answered. "I didn't expect to hear from you so soon."

"I thought your phone was supposed to be off?"

"It has been at times. I'm still trying to clean my spoils, if you catch my drift."

David understood; Rubin meant he hadn't laundered his money yet. "Yes, I understand. I thought we were meant to be careful."

"What's your phone doing on then?"

"Something came in. Are you available for another job before you head out?"

"That depends on the numbers."

"I'll make it worth your while, similar to before."

Rubin smiled; over the last week, David had paid him very well. He could do a lot with that money, and another similar amount could be put to great use. "Okay, you have my attention," Rubin said, "When is it for?"

"Today."

"Today? That's a bloody fastball. I have other things to take care of," Rubin stated.

"For what I'm offering, you can change things. Just imagine what you could do for your temple," hearing his own words, David shook his head and rolled his eyes.

"Well, when you put it that way… what time and where?" Rubin asked.

"Can you meet me at the lake again, the same one as before?"

"I can get there."

"Where we're going is only a twenty to thirty-minute drive from there. Can you arrive by three p.m.?"

"I can do that."

"Also, bring your work bag, just like you did before. Don't forget to bring all the necessary accessories; they will be essential. We need to maintain silence."

Rubin understood exactly what that meant. It sounded like a hit was being planned, and he would take that any day over the babysitting duties they had to deal with last week. "Yes, I understand. I'll be there at three p.m."

"Good. I'll see you then." David hung up the phone. When Rubin hears the details later, he won't like them. A quick hit with so little planning meant he would have to deal with Rubin's constant critiques about professionalism. But for now, he was committed, and the next step was to figure out how to handle Dr Farmer's CCTV.

++++

David kept a close watch on the roads, glancing overhead occasionally, but he saw no signs of anyone following him. With his phone switched off and the SIM card removed, he was taking a calculated risk, but he needed equipment for Darius's latest task. Time was of the essence; he needed to act quickly, gather what he needed, and get back on the road.

After parking outside his farmhouse, he hurried upstairs to retrieve his firearm and two loaded magazines. Ensuring his home was securely locked, he then headed to the garage. There, he chose a fishing rod designed for long-distance casting. He rigged it with a heavy line, attached a large single hook, lowered the rear seats, and carefully fed the assembled rod into his vehicle through the boot. He loaded a box containing an unopened self-inflatable dinghy for children, a large bag of gravel, some rope, and two breeze blocks into the back of his nondescript family hatchback. As a medium-sized car, it would likely need to be rearranged to accommodate the doctor as well. He could cover the doctor's body with the towels they had taken from Ryan's house. Once the car was loaded, he gathered his green fishing hat, an unbranded fishing jacket, sunglasses, disposable PVA bags, and flesh-coloured disposable gloves. Putting on the gloves, he carefully cleaned his Glock to remove any fingerprints, then placed it in the glove compartment. The drive to the lake would take approximately thirty minutes, followed by an additional twenty to thirty minutes to reach the doctor's house. To avoid running out of fuel while transporting a corpse, he opened the car's fuel cap and quickly added several litres of petrol from his large fuel tank. After securing the garage, he put on his sunglasses and fishing hat before setting off. If all went according to plan, he should arrive at the lake with plenty of time to spare.

++++

Rubin stepped out of the car and paid the driver. "Keep the change," he said as he picked up his bag and slung his backpack over his shoulder. The driver nodded in thanks and drove off. Watching the car disappear from view, Rubin walked beside the trees that lined the large lake. Through the gaps in the foliage, he saw David sitting alone on a bench next to a bend in the lake. Rubin shook his head in dismay when he saw the same car they had been using parked in a nearby lay-by with its windows slightly open. Whatever David had planned needed to be done quickly; using the same vehicle was careless. From behind the trees, Rubin could see they would not be alone. Other anglers were scattered around the lake, clearly in for the long haul, with various green dome-shaped tents set up at different spots.

David sat upright as Rubin walked over and dropped his bag next to him.

"Are you still carrying all the money you earned in that bag?" David asked.

Rubin lowered his backpack and sat beside David on the bench. "I haven't been able to place it yet. Why is your car still here? I thought it was going to be crushed."

"I pushed that back until after we've completed the task," David replied. "I'm surprised you're still carrying all that money with you."

"Why? What kind of idiot would try to rob me?"

David nodded. "Fair point."

"Sloppy work, brother, still moving around in that car. It must have been picked up by ANPR cameras everywhere."

"Possibly. However, the police will only investigate if there's something to investigate. As far as I know, there isn't anything at this time. The family has gone underground; they heeded my advice."

"Still dodgy, if you ask me. So, what needs to be done?"

"We have a target. A doctor needs to be removed without leaving any trace evidence."

"Okay, how much time do we have?"

"Today."

Rubin's eyes widened, and his laughter sounded forced. "You're kidding, right? You've done the recce's and the workups?"

David anticipated Rubin would ask these questions; he would have if the roles were reversed. "It's a quick in-and-out. It's a private home, a large property on a private road. We need to get him into the back of the car, and he'll be disposed of in the crusher along with the vehicle later."

"Why can't you handle this yourself? I appreciate the work, but couldn't you have done it on your own?"

"There's an issue. There's a camera outside the house, positioned next to the security gate. We can only access the place from the front..."

"Why?"

"Because my client wants to leave no signs of foul play, just a quick hit and into the back he goes. There's also a house opposite, so our target's house is overlooked."

"Do they have cameras?"

"I don't know."

"You don't know? Haven't you even checked out the area?"

"No, it's a fastball. I only had time to research online."

"Wow," Rubin shook his head. "So this is completely unplanned, that's what you are saying; it stinks of compromise. Anyone could show up, and if that happens, your car won't be big enough to fit them all. What's happened to you? You're taking way too many risks for this client. It's unprofessional."

"That's the business we're in. Sometimes, you need to act quickly. I trust you brought your silencer, right?"

Rubin nodded.

"And your fake police ID?"

Rubin laughed, knowing what was coming next. "You want me to try to gain entry to his place by speaking on camera?"

"It's the only option I have, given the short timeframe. We can't risk breaking in. There's a large garden at the rear, but it borders someone else's property, and there's no vehicle access."

"What about the camera footage?"

"We can delete it from his phone. My client has a contact who can hack the mainframe. I can arrange for the footage to be deleted remotely and strip it from the servers when we know what type of camera and system it is."

"And I'm supposed to trust that?"

"Do you have any better ideas?"

"Yes. I would have done a recce for a kick-off. This is fubar."

"We can do a quick recce upon arrival. We'll abort if we don't like what we see, and the car will go to the crusher. If it doesn't work, it doesn't work. All I know is that this needs to be done immediately."

"So, if it's a no-go, we can withdraw. That's what you're saying?"

"Yes, that's exactly what I'm saying."

"And what about my payment?"

David sighed internally. With Rubin, it always came down to

money. "You'll still be paid, but it will only be twenty percent if the task isn't carried out."

Rubin turned away to consider David's proposal. Twenty percent for doing nothing sounded like a fair deal. They would probably cancel it anyway. "So, what else is needed?" he asked.

"Needed?" David replied.

"Yes, how is he going to vanish into thin air?"

"We need his phone and passport."

"Oh, here we go... How do we find the passport if he's dead? That could take hours. What if he has a safety deposit box or something?"

"I know, but this is the card we've been dealt."

"Does he have any family? Could anyone else be there? How can you be certain about these things?"

"Because my client knows him very well. He has no children and, to our knowledge, no partner."

"So why does he live in such a big ass house?"

David shrugged. "I guess it's because he can."

"Mmm. I don't know; this feels sketchy."

"Will you come along for the recce and give me your thoughts? Remember, there's twenty percent for just taking a look." David felt confident he was now speaking Rubin's language.

"And you have this money with you?"

"No, it's at my home. We'll go there afterwards," David replied.

"The car needs to be disposed of immediately. You can't take it anywhere near your house."

"I have an arrangement with the owner of the vehicle crushers. Whenever I drop off a car, I always pick up something new. There are no cameras in that area, which is one reason why I prefer to use that breaker's yard. Besides, I'm sure I'm not the only one who uses it for similar arrangements. I always pay cash, no questions asked. So, do you want to come along or not?"

"For twenty percent, I'll take a look. But if it looks like a certain compromise, I'll bail."

David stood up. "That's fair. Let's put your things in the car and head out immediately."

++++

"What's going on here?" Rubin asked, noticing the fishing rod and other accessories as he dropped his bag and rucksack into the back of the car.

"I'll explain on the way," David replied.

Rubin took a seat in the passenger side and immediately opened the window to its fullest extent. "It absolutely bloody stinks in here," he remarked, glancing back at the bags of excrement still in the car. "No wonder you left the windows open," he added. As David started the car, he glanced at Rubin. "We're going fishing afterwards."

"You might be; life is too short for that shit," Rubin scoffed.

The car pulled out of the side lane and entered the main road. "I think you misunderstand. I'll show you how I handle weapon disposal afterwards, before I take the car to the crusher," David explained.

"With a fishing rod?" Rubin scoffed again.

"I never put weapons in the crusher. I don't take that risk."

"Why not? It's not like they're going to discharge or anything!"

"All the same, it's not a chance I'm willing to take."

"Well, alright, fair enough. So, what are the breeze blocks and the dinghy for? At least you still have the plastic sheet from the other place; I'll fold that up tightly and take it in with me."

"Because you're right, I'm going fishing afterwards. I need to rebuild part of the bank I like to fish from, and the dinghy is for when I'm fishing. I like to place my bait under overhanging trees. I push myself out on the dinghy and drop my hook by hand since it's too difficult to cast without getting the line caught in the trees. Some people use a remote-controlled bait boat, but..." David noticed Rubin yawning. "Anyway, there you have it. I'll be putting everything in the new car afterwards."

Rubin pulled down the visor, shook his head, and looked out the window. "Okay, tell me this: what's the point of sitting out for hours, often in the cold, to catch something only to put it back? Where's the sense in that?"

"I told you before, it's my solace, my escape from the real world. Besides, as a man of God, you should understand the desire not to kill something. I don't see why that doesn't apply to you when it comes to people."

"It's different."

"How?"

"Because I use my money to do good."

"Oh, right, for your temple in Nepal."

Rubin immediately looked at David. "Why did you say that in a patronising tone?"

David met Rubin's eyes. "Because I can't see the good you're doing." He turned the car to the right, following the signs for Dartford; Bickley wasn't far from there.

"How can you possibly see? You're not a believer."

"Fishing allows me to think and clear my head; it's also how I keep my conscience clear! How do you justify the work you do?" David snapped. "Does your God forgive you because you give back? That sounds like a bribe to me!"

Rubin could hear the anger in David's voice. "Where is all of this coming from?"

"Because you take the money to Nepal, right? And then what? You give it all to the monks?"

"That's right, and you know it's for Nepal," Rubin replied, his voice rising with anger. "They use it for the temple, and it helps sustain them."

David struggled to keep the car steady, his frustration mounting as he processed Rubin's words. "Seriously, what's gotten into you? My conscience is clear because I give back."

"Yeah, I bet you do," David shot back.

Rubin punched the dashboard in anger. The impact caused the

glove compartment to swing open and reveal David's Glock. "Oh yeah? What do you plan to do with that? This isn't the Wild West out here; there are consequences for shooting someone. We're a long way from the field, my brother!"

David took a deep breath, trying to remain calm. He needed Rubin with him for this final ride. "Close the glovebox, will you?"

Rubin slammed it shut. "So, we're just going to show up at this doctor's house, kill him, and stuff him in here with all your fishing gear? Is that the plan?"

"Yeah, that's pretty much it," David replied.

Rubin's laughter mocked the seriousness of their situation. "Absolute bloody jokes. Have you ever seen that Tom Cruise film where he rides around in a taxi? He gets out and starts shooting up a nightclub, without a disguise, in full public view. Breaks the bad guys' bones, probably shoots a dozen people, and just walks away. Can't remember what the movie was called, but..."

"Collateral..." David interrupted.

"Yeah, Collateral. Anyway, he does all that without any disguise or concern for reprisals. There'd be CCTV everywhere. People don't get away with that shit in the real world, you hear me, David?"

There was a brief moment of silence between them. David took a deep breath as they entered the outskirts of Dartford. "I actually quite like that film."

Rubin turned to look at David. "Yeah, it was pretty good as it happens, but you get my point, right?"

David took a left turn at a roundabout, heading towards Sidcup.

"Did you see him pull off the Mozambique drill on that guy who tried to rob him? Straight off the hip: double tap to the heart, and then one to the head, fraction of a second," Rubin finally managed to smile.

"Yeah, I read he trained with live ammo."

"I've carried a rifle for over twenty years, and I can't perform the Mozambique drill as quickly as that."

David laughed. "How do you know?"

"Because after watching that film, I practised."

David glanced at Rubin with an eyebrow raised, "Are you telling me a bloody actor is better with a handgun than you?"

Rubin looked back at David and laughed. "I didn't say that. I bet you wouldn't fare any better."

"I've never really thought about it; I have better things to do with my time."

Rubin laughed again. "Yeah, like going fishing."

David smiled, relieved that the conversation was back on track. There was no time for a Rubin meltdown. "Right, once we pass through Sidcup, we'll head toward Chislehurst. It's not far from there."

"Fine. Pass me the address; I may as well take a look at it first," Rubin said.

David entered the passcode on his phone and read the address from Darius's message.

"Well, well, well," Rubin said, looking at the street view on his phone. "This is how the other half lives. I don't think even with you paying me in full, I could afford to live here."

"Yep, it's highbrow, alright," David agreed.

"David, seriously, given the value of these properties, I would expect to see cameras everywhere."

"I couldn't see any at the entrance to the road in the pictures you're looking at."

"Mmm, since it's a cul-de-sac, it'll be difficult to do a casual walk-around first. Are you sure this car is going to the crusher immediately, no matter what happens, and that it's on cloned plates?"

"One hundred percent."

"Okay, we'll need to check if you can park at the beginning of the road, as long as it's not too visible, or find a spot on one of the side roads. If I'm satisfied after driving through, I think we'll need to do a traditional door knock."

"So, you're thinking you will use your ID again?"

"It's a Met Police ID, and through the camera, he shouldn't be able to tell that it's fake. Besides, how would a doctor know that a police ID is fake anyway? I assume he's a doctor of medicine, not a forensic scientist or something similar?"

"No, he's in medicine. I checked him online."

"I'll need to come up with an excuse to get him to hand over the passport. If I can pull that off, I'll take him out, call you over the radio, and then you can drive in. I also need to figure out how to open the security gate. If you see anyone pull into that road, message me immediately; we may have to abort."

"What's your story for wanting to speak with him?"

"I'm not sure yet. How long until we get there?"

"About fifteen minutes, give or take," David said, tapping his fingers on the steering wheel as he thought. "I think I have a plan. Yes, this could work. The doctor is associated with Knightark Pharmaceutical; he's a member of their board. If you say you're investigating claims made by the MP about the company, that might be plausible."

Rubin nodded in agreement. "That could work. What was her name again?"

"Helen Lord," David replied. "She's the MP for Shrewsbury in Shropshire. This approach might convince him to let you through the gate."

"If he does that, I'll let you know as soon as I see the gate opening. However, that doesn't solve the camera issue, does it?"

"No, it doesn't. I've been thinking about that. From what I can tell, the camera looks modern. If it were older, I would have brought my old Polaroid camera and placed an image of the outside over the lens once you were inside. My concern is whether there's a control station monitoring it. If it's a network camera that only syncs with his phone, it shouldn't be a problem. Hopefully, our drive around the property will provide some answers. Many large properties like this often advertise the security company they use."

"That will have to do then. When we get close, I'll change my appearance."

"You're not going to wear that long wig, are you?"

Rubin laughed. "No, of course not. I have a shorter one."

"Alright. We should be in his area in about ten minutes."

Chapter Thirty-Six

Dr John Farmer had just finished an uncomfortable and challenging conference call regarding his position on the board of Knightark Pharmaceutical. Except for Darius Neith, the CEO, no other individuals had been mentioned in the press concerning the scandal. News channels were broadcasting the covert footage and Helen Lord's interview while awaiting an official announcement from the Knightark Pharmaceutical board. The company he consulted for was alarmed and sought reassurance about his position, the pharmaceutical company's standing, and whether he could continue to focus on his work. Although he managed to provide his client with some peace of mind, personally, he felt anything but reassured. Lisa's footage had gone global, truly shaking up the political landscape. Thankfully, the MP took responsibility, and there were no disclosures regarding how she obtained the footage. Presumably, the authorities would question her at some point. There were still calls for her to be banned or, at the very least, suspended from the House of Commons. However, from what he observed, the maverick MP seemed to have garnered some support. Nevertheless, he had delivered the footage to the MP; it had been in his possession. Although he was careful not to contact her directly, it worried him. The story was of such significance that, if the pundits and headlines were to be believed, the Prime Minister's resignation was only a matter of time. Here he was, sitting in his kitchen with a coffee in hand, aware that he was part of it all. With so many facets to the story and lawsuits just beginning, this situation and the name of Knightark Pharmaceutical would remain in the public spotlight for some time to come. He had messaged Darius earlier for an update, but had received no response. Darius was likely busy, gritting his teeth over the next phase of legal challenges aimed at crushing the MP. Hearing the doorbell buzz, John felt his nerves jangle; he wasn't expecting anyone. He hoped it wasn't a journalist. If it were, he would send them to Darius. John set his coffee down, walked to the front door, and glanced at the camera. A man stood at the end of the driveway with no car in sight. The man wore glasses, had a short bobbed hairstyle, a moustache, and appeared somewhat scruffy. John hesitated before answering the door, waiting until the doorbell rang again before he decided to respond. He rubbed his eyes, irritated by the persistent visitor. The man didn't seem well-groomed enough to represent a security company; he must be a journalist. Reluctantly, John pressed the intercom button.

"Yes, what is it, please?" he asked.

"Good afternoon," the voice responded. "Is this Dr John Farmer?"

"Who's asking?" John inquired, watching as the man pulled something from his pocket and held it up to the camera, which immediately blurred his face.

"I'm Detective Michael Dashwood from the Metropolitan Police. I wondered if I could have a moment of your time?"

John recoiled from the intercom, his heart racing. Did they know he had passed the video file to the member of parliament? How could they possibly know? He placed a hand against the side of the intercom to steady himself. This didn't seem like a regular police officer; he was likely from a special department of the Metropolitan Police, especially since the Prime Minister was involved. The buzzer sounded again.

"Um, yes. How can I help?" John asked.

"Dr Farmer, I was wondering if you could open the gate. I'd like to have a chat with you."

John closed his eyes, unsure of what to do. "About what?"

"It's regarding Helen Lord, MP."

John bowed his head in disbelief, wondering if he had done something wrong. How could they know about this? If he refused to let the officer in, others might come, likely with a warrant, and he would be the subject of gossip in the area. At least this officer was alone, and since he was a detective, he wasn't in uniform.

"Um, yes, come in," John said, pressing the button to release the gate and quickly putting on his shoes. When the officer stepped onto the driveway, John noticed him using a radio. That didn't bode well, perhaps he wasn't alone after all. John opened the front door, his hands trembling. The last thing he wanted was to be arrested. He had read conspiracy theories about secretive police departments and had dismissed them, but the man approaching him looked intimidating and very capable. It was only when they were up close that John noticed the officer's facial scars.

"Dr Farmer, thank you for welcoming me. May I come in? It's a sensitive matter," the officer said.

"Uh, yes," John replied, flustered. "Of course, I'm in the kitchen." He pressed the intercom button to close the gate. The police officer followed him inside but remained silent. Out of the corner of his eye, John saw the officer looking around the house and at the floor. John turned down the television volume and noticed the officer glancing at the MP's image on the screen.

"So, are you alone, Dr Farmer?" the officer asked.

"I am, yes. But what does this have to do with the MP?" John asked, distracted by the sound of his phone bleeping in the next room. "Bear with me for a moment; I just want to see who that is."

The officer nodded but remained silent as John walked into the front room to retrieve his phone. John read Lisa's message asking if everything was okay. He considered replying that the police were present, but when he turned around, he noticed the officer following him into the room. He decided to respond to her later.

"This is a big house. Do you always live alone?" the officer asked.

John walked past him and returned to the kitchen, and placed the phone on the counter. He couldn't shake the feeling that the officer was observing his every move. "That's a personal question, but yes, I chose to live alone a long time ago."

"That's not what I meant," the officer clarified. "Do you have housekeepers or anyone else in the house? This is a private matter."

John shook his head. "Not today. I have work to do. Could you tell me what this is about? Do I need to call my lawyer?"

A hint of a smile appeared on the officer's face. "No, that won't be necessary. We are talking to individuals who may have had involvement with the member of parliament."

"I don't have any involvement with her."

"But you are associated with Knightark Pharmaceutical, aren't you? I'm led to believe you're a board member."

John swallowed. "Well, yes, I am a junior board member."

The officer nodded. "I see. Can you tell me if your passport is up to date?"

"Passport? That seems like a strange question."

"It's simply a matter of procedure. Due to the accusations made, we are checking that everyone we speak to has a passport. We also want to remind them not to leave the country."

"Leave? Why would I do that?"

"As I mentioned, Dr Farmer, it's just procedure. May I check your passport?"

"Can't you look that up at work?"

The officer smiled slightly. "Of course. However, everything must now be formally requested, which takes time. If you show it to me now, I can avoid that process."

"That still seems a bit unusual to me. Dashwood, didn't you say your name was?"

"I did. If I can check your passport, I'll be on my way. We are just making a social call to those involved with the MP."

"I told you, I have no involvement with her! What is this really about?"

"The allegations of human experiments and so on. I've never encountered something like this in my career."

John swallowed again. The officer had a point; the MP had made those accusations, so it was only logical for them to investigate. "Okay," John said, raising his hands, "so you're not going to take my passport?"

"No, I just wanted to make sure you have a valid one and to advise you not to travel while we conduct our investigation."

"So, I'm not under arrest for anything?"

"Only if you refuse to comply with my request, that would be considered obstruction, Doctor."

John took a deep breath. "This seems strange to me. Surely, I need to be arrested and charged for you to impose passport restrictions." He sighed, "Hang on, it's in the safe."

As the doctor left the room, shaking his head, Rubin pressed the talk button on his radio twice to inform David to stand by. He took out a pair of disposable gloves from his pocket, put them on, then pulled out the large, folded plastic sheet from under his shirt and placed it on the kitchen island. Rubin moved cautiously along the length of the kitchen, stepping carefully on the vinyl floor, and peeked into the next room. The doctor had his back turned as he sifted through papers in his safe. Rubin noticed a substantial stack of money inside the safe but didn't move any closer, not wanting to risk leaving boot prints on the carpeted area outside the kitchen. Quietly, he turned around, returned to the centre of the kitchen, and laid the plastic sheet on the floor on the other side of the kitchen island.

"I've got it," Rubin heard from the other room as he took out his handgun and attached the silencer. He concealed the weapon behind his back just as the doctor re-entered the room.

"Here you are," John said, holding out the passport.

"Thank you, Dr Farmer. Could you please place it on the kitchen island in front of me?"

John smiled slightly as he moved forward. "You know, I think I should call my lawyer because—"

Before he could finish his sentence, Rubin grabbed John by the shoulder with his left arm and pulled him forward just as two distinct popping sounds echoed through the room. John's eyes rolled back as he tried to speak; two bullets had struck him in the chest, causing him to lose his balance and fall against Rubin. Supporting the doctor's body, Rubin quickly dragged him to the other side of the kitchen island. He checked to ensure that neither bullet had exited John's torso before laying him down on the plastic sheet. Although he felt relieved that John's body had absorbed the impact without any exit wounds, Rubin felt a surge of anger as he noticed blood on his jacket from where the doctor had fallen against him. Noticing that John's feet were a similar size to his own, Rubin placed the weapon on the plastic sheet, quickly removed John's shoes, and put them on his own feet.

"Alpha 1 receiving?" he said into his radio.

"Send."

"Proceed, out."

"Received."

Rubin sprinted to the front door, pressed the gate release, and opened the door slightly. He quickly returned to the kitchen and began wrapping the plastic sheet around John's body. He paused for a moment. Despite the blood on his jacket, he was not soaked; it was contained and not dripping. He stood up, double-checked to ensure no blood was falling from him, and then ran into the next room. The temptation of the money in the safe was too strong to resist. Hearing a car pull up outside, he hastily stuffed the money into his pockets and, using his elbow, closed the safe door and elevated the handle to lock it. He gripped the combination dial between his elbows, turned it slightly, and then returned to the kitchen, where he could see David standing at the front door.

"Stop. Don't come in," Rubin said. David hesitated momentarily. "There's carpet everywhere. I've got his shoes on; I'll come to you."

"What's the damage? Any spillage?" David asked.

"No. Two rounds to the chest, neither went through; he went out like a light." Rubin replied, handing over the doctor's phone and passport.

David tucked them into his pocket, opened the car's boot, took out the fishing rod and propped it against the side. "Are you sure you can drag him across this white carpet?"

"Yeah, he's not bleeding much. It's mostly on me from when he fell against me."

"Are you sure there's no spatter?"

"Positive." Rubin made sure the plastic sheet was wrapped entirely around the body before bending down to grab the doctor's legs to begin dragging him.

David noticed Rubin panting as he dragged the lifeless body towards the front door.

"Keep an eye outside. Are we still clear?"

"Yep." Their earlier drive-by of the area showed that the house across the street had no visible cameras, except for a doorbell camera that was positioned out of sight from the doctor's front door. David quickly checked the camera system the doctor had been using. "The camera system is web-based. I notice there's another camera above the door. We can erase the footage."

As Rubin reached the front door, David stretched and grabbed the legs wrapped in plastic. Together, they lifted the doctor's body from the ground and placed the corpse into the boot of the car.

"Don't forget your boots," David reminded him as he put the fishing rod back into the car and covered the doctor's body with the towels. "Make sure to leave footprints from the doctor's shoes and wipe away any that could be yours."

Rubin hurried back to the kitchen while David glanced at the internal security panel. He noticed a key rack next to the door and grabbed the first set, which had five keys attached. David tried each key in the front door lock until he found that the third one worked. When Rubin returned to the car, he tossed his boots into the back.

"Is there anything else?" David asked.

Rubin, slightly out of breath, shook his head.

"Are you sure?"

Rubin nodded. "Positive. Let's go. Just make sure to erase the camera footage. The button on the right side of the intercom controls the gate."

David opened the gate, closed the front door, and locked it. He tossed the house keys into the car along with his gloves and shut the boot.

As the gate opened, David put on his sunglasses, and they both ducked behind the sun visors as best as they could. When there was enough clearance, they casually pulled away and began heading back in the direction they had come from.

"So, what now?" Rubin asked, his voice heavy with adrenaline.

"Now, we are going fishing," David replied as he pressed the accelerator.

++++

Darius read the message, exhaled loudly, and gently placed his phone on the desk. "It's done, my friend."

William nodded and took a seat across from Darius. They both sat in silence, deep in thought, reflecting on their roles in the recent passing of their former board member. William leaned back in his chair and tilted his head, staring at the ceiling of Darius's office. "This was a difficult decision you've made, but I understand it needed to be done, and your asset worked quickly. Are you sure nothing will come back to us, Darius?"

"My contact and his colleague are professionals. There's always some risk in these matters, but I'm confident they will do everything they can to manage it."

"How are you going to explain this to Hugh, Ronald, and the rest of the board?" William asked.

"I'll have our IT professional send me an email from our former board member's account, stating that due to media pressure, he has decided to take an extended leave, effective immediately and is stepping down from the board. I'll instruct him to write it just like that."

"And it will appear to come from his account?"

"Of course. We use a secure network. He can make it look like it's come from any source of our choosing."

"And what about Lisa? She worries me," William said, leaning forward.

"Yes, that's a little tricky, my friend. For now, we'll keep an eye on her. As I mentioned, I suspect her resignation is imminent, especially when she finds out that her colleague has taken an extended leave. That's all I'll say about the matter in this office. Just remember, my friend, walls have ears."

William nodded as Darius turned on the television. "Let's see what our friend Alix is up to."

"Have you heard anything?" William asked.

"No, I wasn't expecting to."

On the news channel, a banner at the bottom of the screen read: "Breaking news—the Prime Minister will deliver a speech outside Downing Street at 7 p.m."

"Looks like someone else is facing a career change as well," William mused.

"It's inevitable, given the circumstances." Darius glanced at his watch. "I think I'll call Ronald and Hugh into the office for a drink; they should arrive in time to see Alix fall on his sword."

"You want them here?"

"To witness this? Yes. And as I understand it, you're returning to the States soon. Just a few measures need to be put into place."

"With Alix leaving, it may complicate things; he was a useful line of protection for us."

"He was, my friend, but his stupidity is his own doing. Besides, it doesn't matter. There is someone else."

++++

"How far are we from our destination?" Rubin asked, his breathing steadying as he reached into the back to grab his boots.

"Not much longer. That reminds me," David said, pulling the doctor's phone from his pocket. "Can you check how to unlock it? Does it use facial or fingerprint recognition?"

Rubin pressed the button on the side of the phone. "Looks like it uses facial recognition to unlock."

"Crap. Okay, I'll need to pull over. I can't have you climbing over the back while I'm driving. I know this area well. Let's take one of the side lanes and keep an eye out for cameras." David turned away from the main road. "There's a lane up ahead. I'll keep the car running. Can you open the boot and see if you can access his phone?"

"Sure, I just need to put my boots on," Rubin replied. He ducked below the visor to check for cameras as David pulled over and stopped next to a hedgerow.

"Is there anything further ahead?" Rubin asked.

"I don't think so, just an old cricket club. Okay, try it now, there's no one behind us." David turned to keep watch as Rubin quickly got out of the car and opened the boot. He moved the towels from over the body and abruptly tugged at the corpse in the back, causing the car to rock. "Alright, buddy, open your eyes."

David grimaced at Rubin's behaviour and turned away. The car's boot was slammed shut as Rubin returned, nodding with satisfaction. "Success!" he announced.

David quickly accelerated down the lane, made a U-turn, and returned to the main road. "Good. Look for the app for his security camera, and when you find it, delete all the footage."

"That won't erase it from the main server," Rubin replied.

"I know, but until it is, we might as well do that for now."

"Okay, I've found it. I might as well watch what it recorded."

"Is that really necessary?"

"It's good to know what we're up against. Oh yes, you're very identifiable. All of that looks highly suspicious," Rubin laughed to himself while David scowled and looked away.

"You can't see the body going into the back because you were too close to the front door. However, we are seen getting into the car, which reminds me." Rubin deleted the footage, removed his glasses, wig and moustache, and tossed them into the back of the car.

"Have you scrubbed the footage?" David asked.

"Yes, along with what was recorded from the gate camera."

"Good. Switch off the phone, remove the SIM card, and throw both in the back," David instructed.

"How far are we from where you're taking me? You didn't really say. When people find out he's missing, this phone line might be checked, and this will be the last known location," Rubin pointed out.

"I know, but we're still about ten minutes away from where we're heading," David replied.

"That sounds risky. The police might search the area."

"Trust me. None of this will ever be found. We'll do this quickly, and I want this car off the road as soon as possible."

"I think that would be wise," Rubin said as he tossed the doctor's shoes, SIM card, and phone into the back. "Oh, almost forgot," he leaned forward and pulled out a couple of bundles of cash. "Pound notes! Look, hard cash, this will probably be obsolete in the near future."

David glanced over in shock. "Where did you get those?"

"They were in the doctor's safe. He's not going to need them, is he?" Rubin replied casually.

"Jesus, Rubin!"

"Don't use the Lord's name in vain."

"For God's sake..."

"That's not an improvement..."

"You took those from his safe! What were you thinking?"

"What's the problem? I was wearing his shoes and used my elbow to re-close the safe. I got some blood on my gloves when he fell against me, but I didn't leave any traces, I assure you. Stop fretting."

"Fretting! That was a risk not worth taking." David watched as Rubin stuffed two bundles of money into his bag in the back.

"I'll share some with you; don't worry about it."

"I don't want it. What's wrong with you? Your greed knows no bounds; you're being paid well enough without taking these extra risks."

Rubin shrugged. "You seem agitated."

David smacked the steering wheel in anger. "Oh, that's right, you need all this money for your temple!"

"What's going on with you, David? You're not yourself."

"I'm not myself!"

They locked eyes, and Rubin could see the anger simmering beneath the surface. David's eyes were practically bloodshot. "Okay, calm down. It's done now." Rubin said, "Let's just get there in one piece."

David turned away, focusing on the road and wishing for the day to be over.

✢✢✢✢

"Are you sure you know your way around here? It looks like we're in the middle of nowhere."

"That's kind of the point," David replied, glancing at Rubin. "Have you ever heard of Lord Hawthorne?"

Rubin frowned. "Lord Hawthorne? No, he sounds like some upper-class twat to me."

"Well, he is. He lives at an estate not far from here, proper old money. That's where we're heading."

Rubin looked shocked. "You've never paid off a lord to dump weapons on his land, have you?"

"Hardly. He has no clue. He's typical of these old, wealthy, self-serving types to ignore their security."

"So?"

"So, he has an old estate lake, and that's our destination. A couple of years ago, I called him to ask if I could fish on his lake. His landline number was easy to find. In posh terms, he told me to go forth and multiply. He's not a pleasant man, and he said that no one fishes on his lake, and that's how it will stay. He annoyed me so much that I did some research and discovered an entry for the lake in the Domesday Book, which shows just how old it is. To my knowledge, it has never been fished. It's over twenty acres in size. I plumbed the depth once; it has varying depths of up to twenty-five feet."

"I'm still not following," Rubin said as David turned off the main road.

"Think of all the years of inactivity, no movements other than those of nature's ecosystem..."

"You sound like a tree-hugger," Rubin interrupted.

David sighed. "You're missing the point. Years of debris from the surrounding trees, silt buildup, and detritus make it a perfect burial ground."

"I thought we were going to the scrapyard to dump the body?"

"That's not what I mean. You'll see."

"And this lord muck guy won't see us?"

"No. There's a side lane that's completely unadopted and has awkward terrain, which leads to the lake. There's only one padlock securing the gate to that lane, and it's ancient, it takes seconds to crack."

"But he lives there?"

"Yes, but his estate covers over ninety acres, and trees surround the lake. You can drive right up to the water without being seen. Whenever I arrive, I have to make sure that no one is sitting there or using the lake in any way, but that has never happened. Other than that, it's simple enough."

"And after that, we can leave? I need to sort out this money before I head back."

David frowned as he looked at Rubin before returning his focus to the road.

++++

"Mr Neith, Ronald Ward is on the phone," Darius's personal assistant announced.

"Thank you, Claire. Please put him through," Darius replied, nodding at William.

A light began flashing on Darius's phone system. He pressed the flashing button to answer the call. "Ronald, I trust you received my message. Are you coming by later?"

"Yes, I wanted to let you know that I can make it. I assume you've seen the news about Alix giving a statement later?"

"Yes, I've seen it. William is here with me."

"Good. I wanted to inform you that I've received a message from Gatesouth. He has been speaking with Lord Hawthorne; apparently, Hawthorne is at Westminster right now. The consensus is that Alix will resign, and the Chief Whip may also step down, given the footage suggests collusion. I sense a major cleanup is underway, which may complicate business in the future."

"Indeed, processes will not be as straightforward as they were before. This situation was unforeseen, but we always find a way," Darius replied.

"If you read the broadsheet news and follow serious political debate forums, everyone is calling for accountability, which could lead to significant reform."

"Reform just means change, Ronald. It's now something beyond our control. Let the journalists feast for now, and we'll deal with the aftermath later. I really wouldn't worry, my friend."

"If you say so, Darius. I know you have your finger on the pulse."

"So, we'll see you later, before seven?"

"Yes, I'll be there."

"Good. Hugh will be here as well."

"Okay, Darius. See you soon."

Darius ended the call and turned to William.

"You know Ronald is right; there will be serious fallout from this," William remarked.

Darius nodded, sinking back into his seat. "Significant change is upon us, my friend. I don't know how he and Hugh will react if they ever find out what happened to John."

"Not well, I suspect. Let's hope they don't find out."

++++

Despite the sign stating "Private Property," David drove the car into the lane, left the engine running, and began picking at the lock securing the old gate. Rubin sat patiently, curious about what was happening and why David was going to such lengths to dispose of weapons. True to his word, the padlock opened, and David separated the chain that held the gate to the post. He then pushed the gate aside. Running back to the car, David drove forward, stopped, got out, pushed the gate back into place, and wrapped the chain around the post, leaving the padlock on the ground and out of sight. Quickly getting behind the steering wheel, he closed the door and gently accelerated up the narrow, overgrown hill.

Rubin looked thoroughly unimpressed as the car rocked back and forth over the rocky terrain. "So, is this your burial ground?" he asked.

"This is where many secrets lie," David replied.

"I hope the suspension on this old piece of crap holds out," Rubin added, noticing how focused David was, his actions seeming rehearsed. He must have made this journey many times before.

The car slowed to a crawl as they reached the top of the bank. Below them was the lake that David had brought Rubin to see.

"There's an old jetty and a boathouse down there," David said. "The boathouse is falling apart, and the jetty is a bit rocky and slippery underfoot."

They waited at the top of the bank while David surveyed the area. "It looks clear, and we have the wind at our backs. Do you see how the surface of the water is wavy and moving away from us?" Rubin didn't respond as David gently pressed the accelerator, beginning their descent toward the lake. Rubin gripped the handle above him as the family car jolted, a scraping noise emanating from beneath as the exhaust dragged along the rocks.

"I'll turn around at the bottom and park next to the jetty," David said.

Rubin shrugged, seeming uninterested.

Aside from the viewpoint in front of them, the lake appeared inaccessible from any other direction. The banks were heavily overgrown, with weeds lining the edges and lily pads rooted in the shallows. David pointed past the lily pads. "Even with the wind blowing, do you see how the colours of the water change? It looks much darker the further out you go, which is perfect for my needs."

"Yeah, I guess," Rubin replied with a nod as the car reached the bottom of the hill. David reversed up to the jetty, turned off the engine, and stared at the lake through the back window, focusing on the darker, more ominous-looking water. He got out of the car and took off his sunglasses, instantly feeling the gusting wind swirling around the lake. "Well, are you coming?" he called out to Rubin as he opened the boot. Inside, the doctor's face was exposed from where Rubin had scanned him, his lifeless eyes staring back as David retrieved the fishing rod and clear bags from the side of the doctor's body.

Rubin rolled his eyes as he watched David take out the fishing rod. "Do I have to?"

David paused and lowered his head to look through the car. "I'm going to show you how I take care of things."

With a sigh of reluctant interest, Rubin climbed out of the car.

David pointed at him, "Take my Glock out of the glove box."

Rubin did as he was asked as David walked toward the jetty with the fishing rod in one hand and the bags in the other. Rubin followed him along the length of the jetty until David paused at the end.

"What are you doing?" Rubin asked, observing David as he scanned the area in all directions.

"I need to be sure we aren't being watched."

"How can you tell?"

"This is private land. If anyone were around, they would have yelled at us by now," David said, taking a few steps toward Rubin. "Take out your gun and put it on the jetty, along with the suppressor."

"Are you getting rid of your Glock? You didn't even use it," Rubin remarked.

David knelt on the jetty and put the fishing rod down. "I'm not taking any chances after everything we've been through this week. I'll acquire more weapons as needed. Just put my Glock on the jetty, will you?"

Rubin knelt beside David and placed the Glock next to them. He also set down his firearm and silencer. "So, what are we doing here?" he asked.

"How far can you throw that weapon into the lake?"

"Eh? I have no idea. Why?"

"Not far is the answer." David removed a large single hook from one of the rod rings, and Rubin noticed it was already tied to a thick line. "Right, drop the Glock into one of those bags."

"What are these?" Rubin asked as he placed the gun into a bag.

"They're extra-strong, water-soluble PVA bags. These extra-large bags are commonly used in carp fishing; you fill them with bait to ensure precise placement right next to your hook. Now, watch this." David took the PVA bag containing the Glock from Ruben, tied the end, and pierced the bag just below the knot with the large hook. "You need a strong hook hold to prevent the hook from tearing through the bag when you cast, so always place the hook next to or through the knot." David stood up and grabbed the fishing rod, reeling in the slack line until the PVA bag hung just below the tip of the rod. As he lifted the rod overhead, the Glock swung inside the bag as he held the rod behind him and straightened his body at the end of the jetty. "Stand back a little," he instructed Rubin. Taking a deep breath, David took a couple of steps back, then quickly moved forward, snatching at the rod with an overhead cast. The sound of the powerful cast and the line peeling out at speed created a whooshing noise as the PVA bag, with the Glock inside, soared past the lilies and into the depths of the lake.

"That's impressive! So, what now?"

"Yes, even with the weight in the bag, the wind blowing from behind us helped it travel farther. Now, we need to wait a minute or two for the bag to dissolve, and then we can reel the hook back in. That Glock is now in the depths, far beyond what any human could throw, and it will never be found; it's sinking into the silt as we speak. Here, reel the rod in and take a look."

Rubin stepped to the end of the jetty and took hold of the rod. "I have to give it to you, that's an innovative disposal technique. I might have to consider doing that myself."

"Just leave it in a little longer," David replied as he stepped back. He kept a close watch on Rubin, standing at the end of the jetty as David bent over to retrieve Rubin's Smith & Wesson and the suppressor. With his back to Rubin, David ensured the weapon was loaded, then began attaching the silencer. He then turned around, holding the firearm behind his back. "You can reel it in now. Keep the rod tip high in the air so the hook doesn't get caught in the lily pads as you bring it in."

Rubin enthusiastically reeled in the fishing line. "I take it back, David. Maybe fishing is for me after all."

"Yes, brother, you can dispose of many things out here."

As the hook neared the surface, David took a couple of steps forward. "Okay, reel it in a little more, swing the hook towards you to catch it, and then place the rod down on the jetty."

Rubin caught the hook and turned around with a smile on his face, but he quickly noticed the look of resentment on David's face. "What's wrong?" he asked as he put the rod down.

David took a deep breath and stared at Rubin. "I know."

Rubin shook his head, confused about what David was referring to. "You know what?"

"I know!" David insisted.

"Yes, you said that. Is there something else on your mind, David? There's been plenty since you got back from London."

"Your laptop. It's still in the car, right?"

Rubin nodded. "Yeah, so what?"

"I saw it. The G file."

Rubin closed his eyes, let out a deep sigh, lowered his head, and placed his hands on his hips.

"You know, I thought you'd be smarter than this, but clearly I was wrong. I opened the file because I thought maybe 'G' stood for 'government' or something. In this business, I couldn't help but look."

Rubin glanced across the jetty with immediate concern. "Where's my gun?"

David revealed the loaded weapon, fitted with its silencer, from behind his back.

"Oh, come on! What the fuck is this?"

David shook his head and began pacing. "I can't believe you!" He nearly spat his words, "You haven't found God! You haven't changed at all."

Rubin kept his head bowed, unable to meet David's eyes.

"It's all about the money for you…"

Rubin snapped his head up in annoyance. "It's all about the money for both of us; that's what we do in this business!" he interrupted angrily, starting to pace. "So what? What do you care? Let me guess: no women, no children, is that your rule? We live in an age of equality; everyone's a target these days," Rubin said assertively, pointing aggressively. "And while you're at it, what about the woman you tried to blow up last week? Did she have a family? Did you even think about that?"

"She was a target! That's not what you do. You travel wherever you like, causing chaos and destroying families."

"Man, you are such a hypocrite," Rubin exclaimed, waving his arms in anger. "They should build a monument for your hypocrisy. You're in the wrong business, my friend," he continued, pointing as saliva shot from his mouth. "Too much conscience, too much thinking, it will all catch up with you one day. It always does for people like you. You'll fold, and you'll suffer." Rubin stopped pacing for a moment. "Oh man, wait," he said, shaking his head and letting out a mocking laugh. "It all makes sense now." He looked David directly in the eyes. "Your client told you to kill that family, didn't he? I bet he instructed you to take them out, and in your weakness, you let them live!" He pointed at David, "And it will come back to haunt both of us! Tell me I'm wrong."

David looked away, tapping the Smith & Wesson against his right thigh, and reluctantly nodded.

"Oh, for God's sake!" Rubin exclaimed, waving his arms in the air.

"Using the Lord's name, are you?"

"Don't patronise me, David. I'm telling you, you're in the wrong line of work."

"Did you touch those children?"

"What!"

"Did you put your hands on those young girls while I was in London?"

"What? No, of course not! How can you even say that?"

"Because some of the images I saw were of girls not much older than that."

"So, so what? They get paid, and they like me! You should venture over there and see what the real world is like!"

"How fucking dare you! Out of all the countries I've served in, I never did anything like that..."

"Never?"

"No, never! You brutalised them, Rubin! I saw some of those pictures. They were children, for God's sake, man! You're disgusting, parading yourself around as a holy man." David stopped pacing and lowered his voice. "You don't live in Nepal, do you?"

Rubin looked David in the eyes but quickly looked away.

"Honestly, G for girls! Those young girls were far from legal, and they weren't even Nepalese. We've worked with enough Gurkhas to know what Nepalese look like! They looked Indonesian, Malaysian, Thai; you've been travelling. So, tell me now and tell me the truth: you don't live in Nepal, do you?"

Rubin placed his hands on his hips, looked down at the jetty, and began tapping his right foot nervously. "No. No, I don't."

"Jesus Christ!" David exclaimed, putting his hands to his head. "That's why you have a lockup in this country! You're always here. I bet it was you who started the rumours about changing. Many knew what you were up to and the chaos you leave in your wake. That's why you disappeared for a while and then came back, reinvented with those shitty tattoos and your outrageous stories. You're disgusting, and I won't let you take all that money with you and continue your destructive behaviour."

Rubin immediately looked up. "Oh, so you're going to rob me? Is that your plan? There will be nowhere I can't find you."

David briefly bowed his head and nodded. "I know. I know." Then, from his hip, he lifted the gun, the silencer aimed directly at Rubin's chest.

Rubin raised his arms in a panic. "Attends une seconde! Je suis ton frère!" *(Wait a second! I'm your brother!)*

David shook his head vehemently. "You are no brother of mine; you're a disgrace to our regiment, and someone needs to put a stop to you."

Rubin sighed, looked up at the sky, and shook his head in disbelief. "How could I have not seen it? The dinghy and breeze blocks are meant for me, aren't they?" He lowered his head and saw David nodding. "So, this is it; you're going to shoot me with my own gun."

David maintained his focus and said softly, "Tu étais mon frère" *(You were my brother)*. Rubin understood the weight of those final words. Panic washed over his face as he murmured, "No." Suddenly, he yelled and lunged towards David. Without hesitation, David fired two rounds from his hip, hitting Rubin in the heart. He quickly stepped back, raised his arms, and took another shot, this time striking Rubin in the skull. Rubin staggered forward and fell against David. David caught him with his left arm, holding him tightly while raising his right hand to press the silencer against Rubin's temple. Rubin blinked once, attempting to speak as a small red bubble formed at his mouth and a small trickle of blood ran down his chin. David felt Rubin's body start to collapse in his grip, as the weight of the former soldier became unsteady and his legs buckled beneath him. The double tap to the heart was likely fatal; the final shot to the head was a certainty. Lowering the weapon, David felt the life draining from Rubin as he collapsed onto his back on the jetty. David took a couple of steps away, stood in silence, took a deep breath, and closed his eyes. What he had just done weighed heavily on him; it was a difficult choice, but he knew it was necessary. Remembering where he was, he opened his eyes and glanced around. He needed to move quickly. He ran back to the car, placed the firearm on the roof, took the small dinghy from the back of his car, and tore open the box. As he grabbed the rope and threw it over his shoulder, the dinghy automatically inflated. He then ran towards Rubin and began pulling him into the inflatable boat. As David dragged Rubin into the dinghy, he noticed a small red cloud drifting away with the current. A pool of blood was on the wooden boards where Rubin had fallen, seeping between the slats of the jetty and into the lake. One of the bullets must have exited Rubin's body and entered the water. David dragged the dinghy to the end of the jetty, took the rope from his shoulder, and began wrapping it around Rubin's body. He closed Rubin's lifeless eyes and went back to the car, quickly returning with two breeze blocks. After rapidly searching Rubin's body, he removed his phone, a wallet, a couple of keys and a ring from his finger and placed them in his own pockets. David then positioned the blocks on Rubin's torso and legs, threading the rope through the holes in the breeze blocks to secure them in place. He finally fastened the rope to both sides of the oar supports of the dinghy. Perspiring from the effort, David knew there was one final task to complete. He returned to the car to collect the bag of gravel.

Dropping the bag beside the dinghy, he pulled out his flick knife and cut the midsection of the bag, lifting it to allow the gravel to spill throughout the dinghy. With the wind at his back, he hoped the dinghy would drift quickly into the centre of the lake. Kneeling beside the dinghy, it took considerable effort to push the inflatable boat over the edge of the jetty. Gravel spilt onto the jetty and into the water below as the dinghy began to float. Grabbing the oar supports, he pushed as hard as he could, steering the boat away from the jetty. Carefully avoiding the small pool of blood, he rushed back to the car, quickly snatching one of the towels away from the doctor's body and returned to the jetty. As he knelt to clean up, he could see the dinghy drifting away, carried by the wind-driven current. He brushed loose gravel into the lake while dabbing at the blood pool with the towel. Leaning over the edge, he soaked the towel with lake water and diligently scrubbed away the blood on the jetty and between the slats. With each rinse of the towel, the red water cloud beneath him grew more intense. Although his cleaning efforts were not perfect, rain was forecast for tomorrow, and at this neglected lake, he hoped any evidence would be washed away quickly. After kicking the last pieces of gravel into the lake, David picked up the empty gravel bag, retrieved his flick knife and took one last look around. As he ran back to the car, he glanced over his shoulder; the dinghy was moving closer to the dark water. David tossed the gravel bag and towel onto the body of the deceased doctor and put the flick knife in his pocket. Grabbing the handgun from the roof of the car, he began walking along the length of the jetty. Taking a deep breath to steady himself, he raised the weapon, aimed and fired a shot that skimmed the water beside the dinghy. Frowning with annoyance, he fired a second shot that hit the far end of the inflatable. The third round struck the side of the dinghy, causing it to lose buoyancy and begin filling with water. David lowered the weapon as his fellow Legionnaire quickly disappeared beneath the surface. Looking around quickly, he then detached the silencer from the gun, dropped both into one of the remaining PVA bags, tied it shut, attached the bag to the fishing hook and then grabbed the fishing rod. David stood up, took a deep breath, and cast the PVA bag far from where Rubin had fallen below the water. The firearm travelled a considerable distance to remain hidden in the depths. After checking his surroundings, David reeled in the fishing line until the hook reached the rod tip and quickly made his way to the car with the unused PVA bags. He glanced at the doctor's eyes as he placed the fishing rod and bags into the car and closed the boot. As he got into the car, he paused to steady his breathing and glanced at the clock. He had just over thirty minutes to reach the crusher, and it had to be done that evening. Starting the car, as he prepared to shift into gear, he hesitated when something in the rear-view mirror caught his eye. Turning around, he stared at Rubin's money bag in the back. Leaning over, he pulled the bag towards him and thumbed through the notes inside, pausing briefly in contemplation. He put the car into gear, took one last look across the lake, put on his sunglasses, and drove away.

Chapter Thirty-Seven

"Ah, Hugh, you're the last to join us," Darius remarked as senior board director Hugh Darlington entered his office. "Please, come in and take a seat."

Hugh shook hands with William and Ronald before gratefully accepting the glass of whisky that Darius offered him.

"How are we all this evening, gentlemen?" Hugh inquired as he settled into a chair. "I'm eager to hear about any developments; these last couple of days have certainly been noteworthy."

William responded with a smirk, "That's certainly a very British way of putting it!"

The four senior board members shared a light-hearted moment as Darius leaned against his desk, raising his glass toward Hugh. "In due course, my friend, in due course." He put his glass down, picked up the television remote, and turned on Channel 8 news. "Let's listen to what our former colleague, the Prime Minister, has to say first."

Ronald stood up to get a better view of the television. "He should be speaking any moment now," he added.

"Indeed," Darius replied, crossing his arms. "He should be going on around seven. It'll be the top news story, especially for Channel 8, given their connections to all this." He smiled as he spoke, earning nods and approving murmurs from the members of his senior board.

"There she is, standing outside Number 10 Downing Street," Ronald remarked, nodding towards Hugh. "That's their news presenter, Sharron Broadhurst. Could you turn it up louder, please, Darius?"

"Sorry, Ronald," Darius replied as he pressed the volume button on the remote. "I forgot about your hearing, you old bugger."

Ronald spun around and retorted, "The cheek of it! You bloody upstart!" They all laughed. "Besides, I was asking on Hugh's behalf anyway."

"Oh, of course you were," William chuckled as they fell silent to listen to what the news anchor had to say.

"Good evening, I'm Sharron Broadhurst, broadcasting live from Downing Street in London. Tonight, we may be witnessing a historical moment: Is the resignation of Prime Minister Alix Gregory imminent? Over what can only be described as a weekend of chaotic politics, a sitting Member of Parliament made controversial remarks about a pharmaceutical company, and a covert recording suggests the Prime Minister may have been involved in a cover-up. Remarkably, these allegations appear to be based on what we believe to be the Prime Minister's own words. As of now, no official statement has been released by Number 10. However, we expect Alix Gregory to make a statement shortly. Now, we turn to our political correspondent, Simone Davies. What updates do you have for us?"

"To say that today has been tumultuous would be an understatement, Sharron. I've spent the entire day at Westminster, speaking with both government and opposition members, and we are witnessing a significant collapse in the majority view. We haven't experienced anything like this in this country for a very long time, if ever. Members of Parliament have faced scrutiny from reporters and undercover investigators far too many times to count. However, this time, the only individual taking responsibility for this astonishing story is MP Helen Lord, who brought the story and footage exclusively to Channel 8 television. Ironically, she is the same MP who is expected to face disciplinary action for allegedly bringing the House of Commons into disrepute."

"But the broadcast she did on YouTube did not occur on the grounds of Westminster. Has she really brought the Commons into disrepute?"

"In the eyes of many political commentators and institutions, the situation is, to put it succinctly, unprecedented. However, certain aspects of her behaviour allegedly violate the parliamentary code.

Any potential disciplinary action remains uncertain because the covert recording she provided has understandably taken precedence. From what I gather, people are divided about the next steps regarding Helen Lord. Some believe she has crossed the line, while others view her as a hero championing free speech. Regardless, we find ourselves in this position because of her actions."

"In her exclusive interview with me last night, she claimed that she did not make the covert recording herself. Have you heard anything different?"

"No, I haven't heard anything to the contrary. She insists that she did not record it and claims that the footage was sent to her. So far, no one else has taken responsibility for it. Wait… the door to Number 10 is opening. Perhaps we'll learn more shortly."

"Thank you, Simone. The Prime Minister is now at the podium, and we are going live to hear his statement."

Alix Gregory stood calmly at the podium as he began his speech. "Good evening. I have a short statement to make, and I will not be taking questions afterwards. Much has been said and written over the last twenty-four hours regarding a recording that has been made public. I can confirm that the recording took place last Saturday night in Lord Gatesouth's office in the House of Lords, and I acknowledge that the voice on the recording sounds like mine. However, I want to make it clear: I do not recall using those words, and we are currently investigating whether the recording has been tampered with. Regardless of the recording's authenticity, the words that were broadcast are damaging, and I categorically refute them. Although the conversation with Lord Gatesouth was private and light-hearted, the context in which it was presented may lead to misunderstandings. He and I speak frequently, and the footage's contents could easily be misinterpreted. Today, I consulted with the Parliamentary Commissioner for Standards and received advice from my cabinet and other advisors. I welcome the investigation into this recording. However, my primary concern is that while the investigation is ongoing, it may overshadow the government's essential work and undermine the positive contributions my government makes to the British people. Therefore, I will step aside during the investigation. Once the investigation is completed, I will assess my future role in government and how we can shape this great country moving forward. I was elected to serve, and it has been the proudest moment of my life. During my absence, the Deputy Prime Minister will lead the country in serving you, the British people. I ask for your patience while this investigation takes place, and I hope to return to lead this country that I love very soon."

The camera focused on Sharron Broadhurst as Alix turned away from the podium and walked back towards the Number 10 door.

"Well, there you have it. He's gone, and, well," she laughed, "that certainly won't help his headlines in the morning. As you probably just saw behind me, when the Number 10 door opened to let the former Prime Minister back in, Larry the cat ran straight out…"

Darius switched off the television as he sipped his whisky. "Gentlemen, please join me on the balcony," he said, gesturing for William to open the balcony door. The four of them stepped outside.

"I assume you're still uncomfortable speaking in your office, Darius?" Ronald asked.

"I'm not one to take chances." Darius leaned on the railing and surveyed the view of London. "Right over there is a place in chaos," he pointed in the direction of Westminster, "and that suits me just fine."

"Does the departure of Alix and the extensive media coverage of Gatesouth impede our plans?" Ronald inquired.

Darius replied with a smile, "Not in the slightest. They are merely pawns, sacrifice them when necessary. We are the kings, my friend." He addressed the three men present. "Gentlemen, let's assess the situation. An MP and a television executive were planning to expose us due to a whistleblower at our facility in Brazil, but they failed. One of them, I'm told, lies scared in the hospital, while we are about to destroy the other legally. Additionally, we had dissent within our board. William is aware of this, but I must regretfully inform you, Ronald and Hugh, that Dr John Farmer has resigned from the board, effective immediately."

The two eldest board members exchanged shocked glances. "But why?" Ronald asked. "He's a good man; his father made pioneering contributions to this company."

"Indeed, Ronald," Darius responded, "but John did not share our forward-looking perspective."

Concern washed over Ronald's face. "I should call to check on him."

"No, leave him. I received an email earlier. He's taking an extended leave abroad, and he does not want to be disturbed."

"And what about the other?" Hugh inquired.

"Lisa?" Darius snorted, "She'll be stepping down any time now."

"Darius, that could open up two new positions on the board. Do you have someone in mind?" William asked.

Darius met his eyes, "I will consider that, and I encourage all of you to do the same."

Hugh interjected with a laugh, "I think Alix Gregory is looking for a job!"

Darius grinned. "You never know; stranger things have happened." He took a sip of his whisky and, feeling his phone vibrate, pulled it from his pocket and checked the message. "Well, well. Good news, gentlemen. Our consignment has landed at the private airstrip. They are now in the UK and will be heading to our bonded warehouse in the next hour."

"That's great news, Darius!" William exclaimed. "Well done!"

"Everything is proceeding according to plan," Darius replied. "You know, my friends, I'm also considering a new product, a variant that can work alongside our new filler, if it's feasible."

"We haven't even launched this one yet, Darius!" Ronald interjected.

Darius grinned, "Touché! However, I'm thinking about developing a new weight loss drug. They are incredibly popular right now. Just imagine the potential user base and sales value!"

William laughed, "That's perfect! And consider all the issues associated with those; we could easily fit right in. We should get the lab to look into it."

Darius patted William on the back and called for the other two board members to join him. "Come over and take a look, gentlemen."

The four senior board members of Knightark Pharmaceutical stood on the balcony as the sun set over the London skyline.

"Tomorrow marks the beginning of a new era for us. Our latest product is poised to transform the market. Starting tomorrow, the first batch will be released from our secure storage, and we will initiate nationwide distribution. Within a year, it could reach a global audience." Darius paused to take a sip of his whisky. "Look at all the lights in the distance; people are going about their everyday lives, constantly seeking self-improvement and never fully satisfied with who they are or what they have. Their insecurities will work to our advantage; soon, our product will be available on every street, at every beauty clinic, and with every practitioner. The so-called death of beauty is a myth, for the beauty business has only just begun." Darius finished his whisky and smiled.

Appendix

"Hello, darling. How are you feeling today?"

Alison Harwood pushed herself up from her hospital bed and yawned. "Good morning," she said, receiving a kiss from Mike, her husband. "Are the kids okay?"

Mike dragged a chair closer to the bed and sat down. "They're fine; they're with Joanne. They miss you. Do you have any updates on when you're coming home?"

Alison rubbed her eyes. "It should be anytime now. I'm just waiting for the surgical team to come in. They want to assess the latest surgery. How does my face look?" She asked, stretching her mouth and grinding her teeth together.

"Incredible!"

"Oh, stop it. I asked you a serious question."

Mike smiled. "I know you did. You've come a long way in a short time. Your scars are healing nicely."

"Mmm, I won't be as pretty as I was, will I?"

"Yes, you will be. But please stop with those comments; you've been through an incredible trauma."

"It sounds like I'm not the only one. The former Prime Minister is all over the news, as is Helen."

"Stop it right now. What they did doesn't even compare to what you've gone through. I don't want to hear any more about that awful Helen Lord."

Alison sighed.

"How are you feeling now?"

"Surprisingly well," she replied. "I felt a bit low after they stopped giving me morphine for the pain, but over the last couple of days, I've been feeling more energetic, I'm thinking clearly, and I'm eager to get back to work."

Mike closed his eyes. "Listen to me, please. I nearly lost you; the kids nearly lost you. It's going to take a long time for you to recover from this." He stopped speaking as three members of the medical team entered the room. "Oh, good, hopefully, they can talk some sense into you!"

"Hello, Mike," said Mr Christopher Dickinson, the head of plastic surgery and facial reconstruction, as he entered the room. "How is our patient today? What's this about talking sense into you, Alison?"

"She's already talking about going back to work," Mike replied with a hint of disgust in his voice.

"Oh, I see. Well, I'm sure none of us wants to get involved in that," the surgeon smiled, glancing from side to side. "Alison and Mike, I don't think you've met Dr Warner and Dr Halford. They have been keeping a close watch on you, and Dr Halford was present during your last surgery. Dr Warner is a cosmetic professional. So, standard question: Alison, how are you feeling today? I'm guessing your talk about returning to work is a positive sign."

Mike raised his eyebrows in surprise.

"To be honest, I feel great, except for how I look. That's going to take some adjustment."

"Mental scars can indeed take the longest to heal, but I must say, I'm highly impressed with your appearance. Do you mind if we take a closer look at you?"

"No, of course not. Please, go ahead."

The chief surgeon put on gloves and glasses as he leaned over Alison. "Can you turn your head to the left, please?"

"Yes, that's good. You are healing very well and even faster than expected. Dr Warner, could you take a closer look here? Is this your work? The colouration looks good, and the facial scarring seems to have subsided in some areas."

Dr Warner joined his senior colleague and closely observed Alison's face. "Yes, it's remarkable, especially given the short time frame. The product was donated by the company specifically for Alison. They're currently making some impressive health claims about its benefits. It's encouraging to see the products working up close."

"Dr Halford, do you have anything to add?" Christopher asked.

"No, Mr Dickinson, excellent work and progress," Dr Halford replied.

"Dr Warner, when is Alison due for further filler applications?"

"Not for a few weeks yet."

Alison immediately raised her hand in alarm. "Wait, wait, what did you just say, filler? What filler?"

Doctor Warner paused his assessment of Alison's face and smiled at her. "I did give you a little procedure, just some fillers. I must say, I'm very pleased with the results."

Alison swallowed, and her hands began to shake. "Oh God," she said, looking at Mike. "Did they put fillers in me?"

Mike nodded. "Yes, as your guardian, I signed the consent forms. You have to remember that you weren't with us for a long time, and I had to sign many things on your behalf."

"But you know I'm against cosmetic treatment!"

Mike exchanged glances with the doctors, who seemed surprised by Alison's reaction after their successful work. "I know you are against it, but given what you've been through, I had to make what I believed to be the right decisions."

Alison shook her head in disbelief. "Doctor Warner, what brand of filler did you use?"

The doctor glanced at his colleagues, taken aback by her question. "It's the brand I always use. In fact, the company's CEO contacted me directly. I must say, I was thrilled to speak with him personally; he's very well known as a pioneer in the industry. He donated products specifically for you, Alison, as he is very sympathetic to what happened to you. It was really quite generous of him, actually."

Alison swallowed, "Oh God, no. Doctor, please tell me who that was?"

"Why, it was Darius Neith, the CEO of Knightark Pharmaceutical," he replied. "He's a highly respected man who is more than willing to provide you with whatever you need."

Alison gasped in shock and buried her head in her hands, her cries echoing through the corridors.

Glossary Of Terms:

If you are reading this book outside of the United Kingdom, or do not follow politics and how the government and the United Kingdom Parliament work. This book uses terms that, for many, are self-explanatory; however, they may be unfamiliar to you.

POLITICAL TERMINOLOGY:

Backbencher -	A member of parliament who sits behind the frontbench in the chamber. They hold no office within government. Some MPs remain on the backbenches, choosing to influence the front bench rather than sit on it.
Bill -	An amendment to the law or a proposal of a new law.
By-elections -	Filling a vacancy that has been created when a general election cannot be called.
Chamber (The) -	There are 650 elected MPs in the House of Commons, which is the legislative chamber of the United Kingdom Parliament.
Chief Whip -	Someone who disciplines their party members within parliament.
Constituency -	An area that the member of parliament represents (an electoral area).

Commissioner For Parliamentary Standards -	The regulator of MPs' conduct and their suitability for office.
Crossing The Floor -	When an MP changes political party from the one for which they were elected.
Cross Bench -	In the British House of Lords, someone who is cross bench or a crossbencher has no affiliation to a political party.
Despatch Box -	Situated within the chamber, they are made of wood and from which frontbench MPs deliver speeches to the chamber.
Government -	Responsible for running the country.
Hansard -	A transcript of a parliamentary debate.
Independent MP -	Not affiliated with any political party.
Minister -	The head of a ministry, for example, "Minister for Transport." A minister is part of the Government and implements policy.
MP -	Member of Parliament.
Opposition – (Shadow Cabinet) -	Official opposition to the government. Usually on the front benches.
Palace Of Westminster -	The meeting place of the UK Parliament – The Houses of Parliament are situated in London, the capital city.
Parliamentary Privilege -	Legal immunity where MPs are protected from comments they make during parliamentary proceedings within the confines of parliament.
Peer -	A person of nobility who has the right to vote in the House of Lords.

PMQs (Prime Minister's Questions) –	Officially known as Questions to the Minister - is a British convention that takes place every Wednesday for thirty minutes while the House of Commons is sitting.
Prime Minister -	A Prime Minister is the head of Government, not the Head of State. Democratically elected as the head of the cabinet and the leader of ministers.
Red And Green Seats/Benches -	Green signifies the House of Commons, and red represents the House of Lords.
Serjeant At Arms -	An official of the House of Commons dating back to 1415. The Serjeant and their department are responsible for keeping order within the Commons and parts of the parliamentary estate.
Select Committee -	A Parliamentary Select Committee investigates issues of the Government of the United Kingdom. Members of a committee from different political parties scrutinise Government business.
Surgery -	A meeting that takes place between an MP and a constituent. These generally take place on Fridays.
Upper House And Lower House -	The UK Parliament consists of two houses. The House of Commons is often referred to as the 'Lower House', and the House of Lords is often referred to as the 'Upper House'. Sitting MPs in the Commons often refer to the House of Lords as "The other place."

Withdrawal Of The Whip - To defy the party. Unless the whip is restored, the member can be expelled from the party, but not as an MP. Unless the MP stands down, they usually remain in parliament as an independent MP.

OTHER TERMS OR REFERENCES MENTIONED IN THIS BOOK:

ANPR (Police) - Automatic Numberplate Recognition System.

Cairngorm Mountains - A mountain range in the eastern Highlands of Scotland. In the Cairngorm National Park, there are over fifty Munros. A Munro is a Scottish mountain with a summit over three thousand feet.

Companies House - The UK agency that registers company information for public access. It also incorporates and dissolves limited companies.

Domesday Book - A manuscript created in 1066 for William the Conqueror. A survey of most of England and part of Wales.

FDA (The) - The Food and Drug Administration. An American administration responsible for regulating public health.

GDPR - The General Data Protection Regulation (GDPR) is a legal framework that governs the processing and collection of personal information.

Hydra-Fillixir - This is the core fictional product as

developed by Knightark Pharmaceutical. It's this range of fillers that contains the addictive property 'Lipomorphilas'.

IED - Improvised Explosive Device.

Lipomorphilas - Is a fictional opioid drug created for this book. The word takes references from diacetylmorphine/diamorphine (a morphinan opioid), and "Lipo", an abbreviation for the word Lipophilicity from Greek that means fat/friendly – a chemical compound that is "fat-loving/liking."

Lord Lucan - Richard John Bingham, 7th Earl of Lucan. Disappeared on 8th November 1974 after being suspected of murdering his children's nanny and attempting to murder his wife. Declared dead on the 27th October 1999. To date, he has never been found.

Metropolitan Police (Met) - Responsible for crime prevention and law enforcement in Greater London.

MI5 - The UK's domestic security service that protects against threats to national security.

MI6 - Also known as SIS (Secret Intelligence Service). The UK's foreign intelligence service protects British security and economic interests.

Mozambique Drill - Also known as the Failure Drill, is a close-quarters shooting technique often referred to as 'Two to the body, one to the head'. The shooter fires two rounds into the central body mass (called a double-tap) and then fires one shot to the head.

OPSS - Office for Product Safety and Standards. The national regulator for consumer products in the UK.

Phone Hacking Scandal - The obtaining of confidential information by illegal means. Victims were primarily those in the public eye whose phones were hacked by British newspapers.

Spooks - A term often used to denote spies or secret agents.

VPN - Virtual private network.

MILITARY TERMINOLOGY:

Burnt - To be compromised, to stand out or to be seen. A term often used in surveillance.

Comms - Abbreviated terms for communications.

Compromised - To be caught. End of operation.

Eyeball - "To have eyeball" is to see the person or place.

Fastball - Reacting quickly to something unexpected with a minimal amount of time.

Foxtrot - "Going foxtrot," to follow on foot, to take a walk.

Fubar - Look it up.

Foreign Legion (French) - "The Legion", a corps of the French Army that allows foreign nationals into French service.

Ghillie Suit -	A type of camouflage clothing designed to resemble a background environment, such as foliage.
Gurkhas -	Soldiers residing in Nepal and some parts of Northern India.
Recce -	Abbreviated term for the word reconnaissance.
Sitrep -	Abbreviated term for 'Situation Report.'
SP -	Subject person.
TSCM -	Tactical Surveillance Counter Measures.

Author Footnote:

The author acknowledges that scientific testing of products, in this case, tainted beauty fillers, can take days or longer to conclude. For dramatic effects and ease of story flow, this process is accelerated within the story.

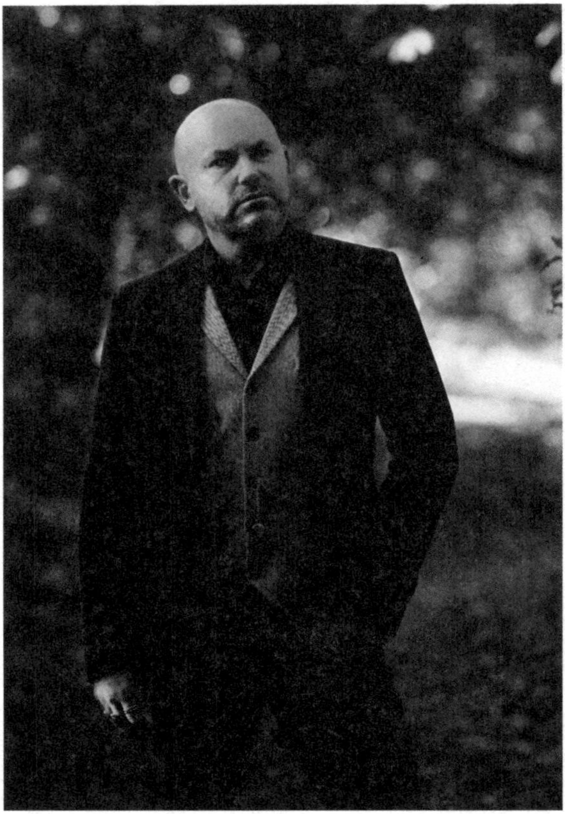

Find Kevin at:

Website: Kevinhorak.com

Facebook:

Instagram: kevinhorakofficial

About the Author:

Kevin Horak is a former Close and Executive Protection specialist with over thirty years of experience in the security industry. He has worked with royalty, business executives, parliamentarians, and prominent public figures. Although he 'retired' from the business a few years ago, he continues to consult for specialist security companies.

As an accomplished author, he has written numerous books covering a range of topics, from those related to the Close Protection sector to adult comedy. Writing under the name K.S. Horak, he is also known for the "Mildred The Crazy Cat Lady" book series.

With a passion for hard rock music and DJing, he successfully operated his own record label for eleven years before selling it to a larger independent label. He currently resides in Shropshire, UK, with his dogs and enjoys escaping to mountainous areas in his spare time. He is an enthusiastic hillwalker and weightlifter.

When asked if he is "anti-cosmetic surgery" in the lead-up to this book, he replied, "No, not in the slightest. But I wouldn't consider anything from Knightark Pharmaceutical!"

Horak regularly tours the United Kingdom, attending book signings and conventions, and is a well-known public speaker.

For further information regarding his books and updates on tour schedules, please visit kevinhorak.com or follow him on various social media channels.